Lecture Notes in Social Networks

Lecture Notes in Social Networks (LNSN) comprises volumes covering the theory, foundations and applications of the new emerging multidisciplinary field of social networks analysis and mining. LNSN publishes peer- reviewed works (including monographs, edited works) in the analytical, technical as well as the organizational side of social computing, social networks, network sciences, graph theory, sociology, semantic web, web applications and analytics, information networks, theoretical physics, modeling, security, crisis and risk management, and other related disciplines. The volumes are guest-edited by experts in a specific domain. This series is indexed by DBLP. Springer and the Series Editors welcome book ideas from authors. Potential authors who wish to submit a book proposal should contact Annelies Kersbergen, Publishing Editor, Springer

e-mail: annelies.kersbergen@springer.com

Mehmet Kaya • Sleiman Alhajj • Kashfia Sailunaz •
Min-Yuh Day
Editors

Social Network Analysis and Mining Applications in Healthcare and Anomaly Detection

Springer

Editors

Mehmet Kaya
Computer Engineering
Fırat University
Elazığ, Türkiye

Sleiman Alhajj
School of Medicine
Istanbul Medipol University
Istanbul, Türkiye

Kashfia Sailunaz
Department of Computer Science
University of Calgary
Calgary, AB, Canada

Min-Yuh Day
Graduate Inst. of Information Management
National Taipei University
New Taipei City, Taiwan

ISSN 2190-5428 ISSN 2190-5436 (electronic)
Lecture Notes in Social Networks
ISBN 978-3-031-75203-2 ISBN 978-3-031-75204-9 (eBook)
https://doi.org/10.1007/978-3-031-75204-9

This Springer imprint is published by the registered company Springer Nature Switzerland AG
The registered company address is: Gewerbestrasse 11, 6330 Cham, Switzerland

Contents

Sensitivity to Noise in Features in Graph Neural Network Learning

Guillaume Lachaud, Patricia Conde-Cespedes, and Maria Trocan

Abstract Graph Neural Networks learn with two types of information: the structure of the graph and the features of the nodes and edges. These features can be noisy or incomplete. For instance, some social network users are more active than others, and thus produce more information. In this paper, we explore the performance of Graph Neural Networks when the graph contains noisy features. We train three architectures that represent the basis of many of today's state-of-the-art methods. We use an academic citation network in which we manually add noise to the features. We investigate three types of noise: random noise, noise that targets the influential nodes, and noise that targets the most isolated nodes. We train each model in both transductive and inductive settings, i.e., when the model has access to test data at training time, or when the test data is hidden. We find that the models are most vulnerable to noise targeting the isolated nodes. Additionally, we empirically validate that some models present implicit denoising abilities. We also find that the lack of regularizing mechanisms, such as weighting schemes, negatively impact the performance of the models.

Keywords Noisy features · Graph neural networks · Deep learning · Citation network

1 Introduction

Most types of data contain some degree of noise. It can take many forms, such as blur in images, spelling or grammar mistakes in text; in audio or video recordings, some parts can be missing or distorted. The impact of noise on machine learning models varies with the severity of the noise [9]. For instance, noise in the

G. Lachaud (✉) · P. Conde-Cespedes · M. Trocan
LISITE, ISEP - Institut Supérieur d'Électronique de Paris, Issy-les-Moulineaux, Île-de-France, France
e-mail: guillaume.lachaud@polytechnique.edu; pconde@isep.fr; maria.trocan@isep.fr

M. Kaya et al. (eds.), *Social Network Analysis and Mining Applications in Healthcare and Anomaly Detection*, Lecture Notes in Social Networks,
https://doi.org/10.1007/978-3-031-75204-9_1

background of an image is less important than the background noise of an audio recording in a crowded train station. Additionally, noise can occur naturally or can be artificially injected to produce errors.

In graph structured data, the noise takes two forms: noise in the structure of the graph, and noise in the features and labels. Noise in the structure alters how nodes are connected together via the edges. Edges can be added or deleted. For example, in a social network where the nodes represent people and the edges indicate friendship, removing edges will hide the friendship between two people. In this way, a group of people forming a community might appear as disjoint groups of individuals.

Noise in the features covers the noise in the features of the nodes and the edges. As an illustration, in a products network, edges between two products indicate how many times they were bought together [3]. Because the company selling the products may have different selling points, the information can take time to be aggregated. During this time, the weight of the edges does not represent the correct number of items sold together. In a different vein, social networks such as Facebook and Twitter each record different information about their users, so the same underlying graph will not have the same features. Classification using one or the other social network will produce different outcomes.

The importance of noise in graph structured data is twofold: noise in the structure impacts how the information propagates through the graph; and noise in the features changes the messages that are passed. Firstly, many of the machine learning approaches used in graph representation learning involve a flow of information through the neighborhood of the nodes. Indeed, in Graph Neural Networks (GNNs), most models follow a Message Passing Neural Network (MPNN) framework [13]. In this framework, a message is computed between a node and each of its neighbours, and these messages are aggregated to form the new node's representation.

Secondly, while the structure determines the nodes used to update the graph's representation, it is the features which create the representation. For instance, in a social network, wrong hobbies may be attributed to a user. When machine learning models try to predict what the hobbies of their friends are, they will use the wrong hobbies which will lead to classification errors. These errors will spread to the friends of the friends, and might spread through the whole graph.

The impact of noise on the learning of GNNs can be amplified by the manner in which the learning is performed. There are two possible settings: transductive and inductive learning. In transductive learning, the GNN model has access to the validation and test features at training time; only the labels are hidden. In contrast, in inductive learning, the model is trained exclusively on the training nodes. These settings reflect different real life scenarios [35]. Transductive learning can be applied to the classification of products in an online retail store; the labelled nodes represent the bestselling items, and the goal is to predict the category of the rest of the items. In this case, the aim is to predict the category of known nodes. With respect to inductive learning, an example is the prediction of the behaviour of new users in a social network. The model must generalize to unseen nodes.

In this paper, we analyze the effects of noise in the features of the nodes on an academic citation network. We compare three architectures: Graph Convolutional

Networks, Graph Attention Networks and GraphSAGE. These models form the basis of many of today's state-of-the-art methods. We perform our experiments both in a transductive and in an inductive setting. We extend our work done in [18] where we compared the performance of several state-of-the-art models on transductive and learning tasks on an academic citation network. Our work [19] also highlighted some of the difficulties in performing multiclass classification on the same academic network. We evaluate the noise in the following settings:

- we randomly add noise to the features of the noise;
- we add noise to the most affluential nodes, i.e. the nodes with the highest degree;
- we add noise to the satellite nodes, i.e. the nodes with the smallest degree;

The paper is divided as follows: Sect. 2 presents the related works. Section 3 provides background information about graphs and the graph neural networks that are used in the paper. Section 5 presents the experiments. The section is divided as follows: Sect. 5.1 presents the dataset. Section 5.2 investigates the behaviour of the GNNs under a random noise assumption; Sect. 5.3 explores the impact of adding noise by targeting the high degree nodes first, while Sect. 5.4 focuses on targeting the small degree nodes first. Section 5.5 presents the behaviour of other types of GNNs under the presence of noise. Section 6 concludes this work.

2 Related Works

The problem of noise in graph data has been mostly studied from the point of view of noise or attacks in the structure of the graph, or in the labels.

With respect to the structure, a powerful way of disturbing the graph is to use a gradient-based attack, called *projected gradient descent* (PGD) [32], which tries to find the smallest perturbations that produce the greatest decrease in performance. To protect the GNN against such attacks, more sophisticated aggregation schemes than the mean operator, such as the Soft Medoid [11] or the Soft Median aggregators [12], must be devised.

The noise is often considered from the point of view of the downstream task, e.g. what matters is not how noisy the features are, it is how noisy labels are and how the metrics of the model are impacted by the noise. Li et al. [21] explore in great depth how neural networks react to noisy labels. Dai et al. [5] propose an architecture that is robust against noisy labels in graphs.

Instead of relying on robust architectures against noise, a different approach consist in denoising the data. This can be achieved using the graph filtering properties of GNNs [25]. Another example is the use of graph convolutions to denoise mesh data [27].

Apart from additive noise, missing data can contribute to the noise. In this case, the features can be reconstructed using graph neural networks. One approach is to create a bipartite graph consisting of observations and features; the edges between the nodes representing the value of the feature for a given observation. A GNN is then trained to perform edge weight prediction [36]. Alternatively, the features of the nodes can be propagated to the neighbours to fill in the missing values [26].

Recent studies have also shown that certain architectures of GNNs possess an internal *implicit denoising* mechanism [23]. This mechanism is studied in more depth in [22].

Parallel to the effort of denoising data, there are works which focus on creating better features that leverage the topological information available in graphs [4].

3 Background

3.1 Graphs

A graph $\mathcal{G} = (\mathcal{V}, \mathcal{E})$ is defined as a pair that comprises a set of nodes $\mathcal{V}$ and a set of edges $\mathcal{E}$. $A \in \{0, 1\}^{|\mathcal{V}|\times|\mathcal{V}|}$ is the adjacency matrix, i.e. $A_{uv} = 1$ if $e_{uv} \in \mathcal{E}$, and $A_{uv} = 0$ otherwise. If the edges are weighted, we have $\mathcal{E} = \{(u, v, \mathbf{e}_{uv}) \mid A_{uv} = 1\}$ where $\mathbf{e}_{uv}$ is the weight of the edge between u and v. $\mathcal{N}_u$ is the neighbourhood of u. X is the feature matrix of the nodes in $\mathcal{V}$.

3.2 GNNs and MPNNs

GNNs are neural networks that operate on graph structured data. They are composed of several layers and can be represented by Eq. (1). The symbol $\circ$ represents the composition operator. φ_l represents the l-th layer of the GNN. It usually consists of a graph filter and an activation function.

$$\Phi = \varphi_L \circ \varphi_{L-1} \circ \cdots \circ \varphi_1 \tag{1}$$

The hidden representation of a node at layer l is written h_v^l. Similarly, H^l is the hidden representation of all the nodes at layer l. By convention, $H^0 = X$.

GNNs that follow the MPNN framework [13] contain layers that follow Eqs. (2) and (3). m_v^{l+1} represents the intermediate message that is used to compute the new representation of node v. M_l represents the message function of layer l, while U_l denotes the function used to update the representation of the nodes.

$$m_v^{l+1} = \sum_{w \in N_v} M_l(h_v^l, h_w^l, e_{vw}) \tag{2}$$

$$h_v^{l+1} = U_l(h_v^l, m_v^{l+1}) \tag{3}$$

3.3 Graph Convolutional Networks

Graph Convolutional Networks (GCNs) were introduced in [17]. They are one of the earliest forms of MPNNs. They extend the concept of spectral convolutions on graphs by approximating the convolution with Chebyshev polynomials [7]. A GCN layer follows Eq. (4). σ represents an activation function, such as the ReLU function. $\tilde{D}$ is the normalized degree matrix, $\tilde{A}$ the normalized adjacency matrix. W^l represents the parameters of the layer.

$$H^{l+1} = \sigma\left(\tilde{D}^{-\frac{1}{2}}\tilde{A}\tilde{D}^{-\frac{1}{2}}H^l W^l\right) \tag{4}$$

3.4 GraphSAGE

GraphSAGE (Graph SAmple and aggreGatE) is a type of GNN and MPNN introduced in [15]. It is designed with the goal of performing inductive learning, i.e. to generate node embeddings for unseen data. It follows Eqs. (5)–(7). N_v represents a sampling of $\mathcal{N}_v$. Usually, N_v produces a fixed-size set. CONCATENATE is the concatenation operator. Equation (5) can be generalized by using a different operator from the sum operator, provided that the operator is still permutation invariant, i.e. produces the same result regardless of the order of the nodes.

$$h_{N_v}^{l+1} = \sigma\left(W^l\left(\frac{1}{\mid N_v \mid +1}\left(h_v^l + \sum_{v \in N_v} h_u^l\right)\right)\right) \tag{5}$$

$$h_v^{l+1} = \sigma\left(W^l \cdot \text{CONCATENATE}\left(h_v^l, h_{N_v}^l\right)\right) \tag{6}$$

$$h_v^{l+1} = \frac{h_v^{l+1}}{\|h_v^{l+1}\|} \tag{7}$$

3.5 Graph Attention Networks

Following the success of attention mechanisms in natural language processing [1], the Graph Attention Networks (GAT) extend the concept to GNNs [29]. The update rules are represented in Eqs. (8)–(10). a is an attention mechanism that takes two vectors or tensors as inputs. For example, a can be a multilayer perceptron.

$$e_{uv}^l = a\left(W^l h_u^l, W^l, h_v^l\right) \tag{8}$$

$$\alpha_{uv}^{l} = \frac{\exp\left(e_{uv}^{l}\right)}{\sum_{w \in N_v} \exp\left(e_{wv}^{l}\right)} \tag{9}$$

$$h_v^{l+1} = \sigma\left(\sum_{v \in N_u} \alpha_{uv}^{l} W^l h_u^l\right) \tag{10}$$

4 Problem Definition

Most Graph Neural Networks (GNNs) work by propagating information through the graph. They adhere to the *message passing neural network* (MPNNs) framework. What separates each MPNN architecture is the mechanism by which information is transferred. For instance, GCNs [17] use an explicit weighting scheme based on the degree of the nodes, while GATs [29] employ an implicit weighting scheme by assigning a different importance to each node via the attention mechanism.

Noise in features can take several forms, the most common of which is *additive noise*, e.g. the input can be expressed as the sum of a "clean" input and some noise. For example, the noise can be Gaussian noise. The noise can be entirely random, or follow an underlying pattern. For example, missing data in clinical studies is not always random, but may have a latent cause, such as the patient refusing to disclose personal information [14]. Similarly, if the categories contain the values "wolf" and "dog", the noise may not entirely be random.

More formally, given X the feature matrix of a graph $\mathcal{G}$, we define X_{noisy} to be the feature matrix with additive noise. Random noise is added by sampling $|\mathcal{V}| \times d \times p$ entries (u, v) in the feature matrix where d is the dimension of the features and p the probability that an entry is selected, and by adding random noise drawn from a standard normal distribution, as shown in Eq. (11). Here X_{uv} designates the feature v of node u. The features are then renormalized.

$$(X_{\text{noisy}})_{uv} = \begin{cases} X_{uv} + \epsilon, \epsilon \sim \mathcal{N}(0, 1) & \text{with probability } p \\ X_{uv} & \text{otherwise} \end{cases} . \tag{11}$$

By definition of a graph, the nodes are interconnected and are therefore not independently identically distributed. This means that the noise in one node can influence the other nodes. This raises the question: where is a GNN most vulnerable to noisy data? Is it when the noise is random, or when the noise targets a specific set of nodes, e.g. the most influential or the most isolated nodes. If the noise targets the nodes with the highest degree, the noise will reach more nodes faster than if it targets the nodes with the smallest degree. However, GNNs will often assign less importance to the features of the most influential nodes, because the more some information is used, the less it has discriminating power.

To model the targeting of nodes according to the degree, we can select nodes whose degree is below or above a threshold t, and add additive noise drawn from a standard normal distribution to $d \times p$ of the features, where d is the dimension of the features and p the probability that a feature is selected. The features are then renormalized. The noise targeting the high degree nodes can be expressed by Eq. (12), where t represents the minimum value of the degree of the target nodes.

$$(X_{\text{noisy}})_{uv} = \begin{cases} X_{uv} + \epsilon, \epsilon \sim \mathcal{N}(0, 1) & \text{with probability } p \text{ if } u.degree \geq t \\ X_{uv} & \text{otherwise} \end{cases} \tag{12}$$

Conversely, targeting the small degree nodes can be done using Eq. (13), where t is the maximal value of the degrees of the target nodes.

$$(X_{\text{noisy}})_{uv} = \begin{cases} X_{uv} + \epsilon, \epsilon \sim \mathcal{N}(0, 1) & \text{with probability } p \text{ if } u.degree \leq t \\ X_{uv} & \text{otherwise} \end{cases} \tag{13}$$

While Eqs. (12) and (13) look similar, they only overlap when there is no noise, or when all the nodes are noisy.

5 Experiments

In this section, we first present the dataset on which our experiments are made. The architectures we chose, GCN, GAT, and GraphSAGE, each represent fundamental ideas of GNNs:

- GCN belongs to the family of spectral GNNs which exploit properties of the Laplacian matrix of the graph [30];
- GAT leverages the attention mechanism, which has achieved state-of-the-art results in many fields, e.g. with Transformers in NLP [8];
- GraphSAGE uses a sampling mechanism which becomes essential when we scale GNNs to larger graphs [3].

We train the models on different versions of the dataset which we modified by adding noise to the features. We investigate three types of noise:

- we add random noise to the graph, according to Eq. (11);
- we add noise to nodes, according to Eq. (12), starting with the nodes with the highest degree and proceeding to the nodes with the smallest degree;
- we add noise to nodes, according to Eq. (13), starting with the nodes with the smallest degree and proceeding to the nodes with the highest degree.

The experiments are performed in two settings:

- *transductive learning*, where the model has access to the full graph at training time; only the validation and test labels are hidden.
- *inductive learning*, where the model is trained on the subgraph of the whole graph that contains only nodes in the training data. In this setting, edges between train and test nodes do not appear at training time.

Each model is trained for 1000 epochs. The validation accuracy is used to select the best model. We perform 5 runs to account for the randomness of the parameter initialization and the noise addition.

5.1 Dataset

We perform our experiments on the *ogbn-arxiv* dataset from the Open Graph Benchmark [16]. It is an academic citation network that contains all the papers in the arXiV Computer Science repository. It contains 169,343 nodes and 1,166,243 edges. Each node has a 128 feature vector. These features represent the average embeddings of the words in the title and the abstract. These embeddings are obtained using a word2vec model [24]. The features are normalized. The splitting of the dataset between train, validation and test is done using the year in which the articles were published: the papers up to 2017 are in the train set. Those published in 2018 are in the validation set. Papers from 2019 and 2020 constitute the test set. Motivation behind this temporal split is twofold, as advocated in [16]: this split coincides with real-world application where existing papers are used to predict the label of newly-published papers; empirical evidence further suggests that using the temporal split is more challenging than using a random split.

The labels in the dataset represent the category of the paper, e.g. machine learning, computer vision, etc. In total, there are 40 categories. They represent all the different subjects available on the ArXiV Computer Science repository.

5.2 Random Noise Perturbation

In this section, we assume that the noise is distributed randomly, i.e. follows Eq. (11).

5.2.1 Transductive Setting

The results of training a GCN, a GAT and GraphSAGE in the transductive setting with a randomly added noise are shown in Fig. 1.

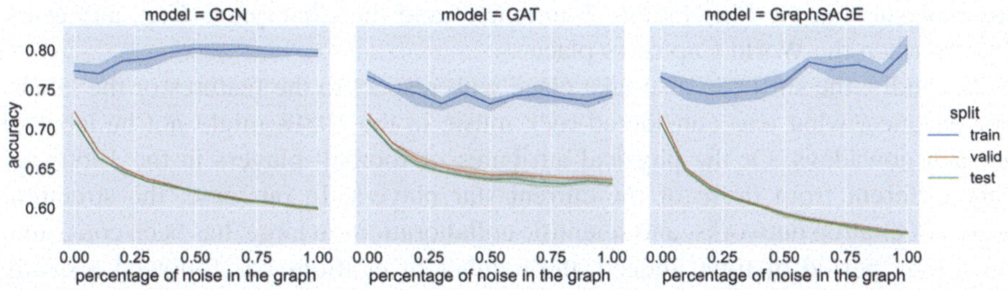

Fig. 1 Training, validation and test accuracy of three models of GNNs in the transductive learning setting. The horizontal axis corresponds to the percentage of features to which noise has been added, i.e., p in Eq. (11)

The sharpest decrease in accuracy occurs when $p \in [0, 0.2]$. When $p \geq 0.2$, the decrease follows a gentler slope. Because citation networks tend to be *scale-free* networks [2], there are nodes in the networks, called *hubs*, from which we can reach almost all the nodes in the graph in a few hops. Formally speaking, the diameter of the graph, which is the greatest distance between two nodes, is small compared to the number of nodes. Thus, when $p = 0.2$, the noise has already spread throughout the graph.

In GCN and GraphSAGE, the generalization error between train and validation is increasing as p increases. This is due to the fact that these models do not possess any graph specific regularizing mechanism. Indeed, the weighting of the neighbours for the GCN in Eq. (4) is proportional only to the degrees of the nodes. Similarly, in Eq. (5), the regularizing mechanism of GraphSAGE is its sampling of neighbourhoods. In transductive learning, the effects of regularization by sampling are lessened by the fact that the model samples from the whole graph.

Concerning the generalization error between validation and test, its existence in the first place is a result of a *distribution shift* that occurs between the different splits. This shift can manifest itself when the splitting of the dataset is not random. For instance, a good split for the Amazon dataset of products [3] is to split according to the number of sold items, because it is easier and more useful to label the bestselling items first and put them in the training set, and try to expand the labelling to the less popular items. Likewise, in citation or social networks, a challenging and natural split is to use the date information: the older nodes represent the training set while the test set comprises the most recent nodes [16].

The distribution shift can have two causes: the structure of the graph can change, or the features can evolve. Firstly, the pattern in the edges between the nodes can change over time. For example, between 2006 and 2012, the Facebook graph changed drastically as the company expanded to other states and countries. The way people used the platform between these two dates evolved as well. Additionally, the structure can change as a result of periodical events. As an illustration, the subgraph of Twitter related to rugby will see yearly spikes of interest during the championship seasons, such as the Six Nations Tournament and the Champions Cup, and every 4 years when the World Cup takes place.

Secondly, the shift can also take place with respect to the features or the labels. For instance, what was considered rock music in the 1980s might not be labelled as such nowadays. Or the physical attributes of football players in the 1960s are very different from those of the current star players. In our case, the structural aspect of citation networks, and scientific collaborations at large, has been consistent for a long period of time. Indeed, the number of citations has followed a steady exponential growth for the last 100 years [10]. This means that the shift has occurred with respect to the features and the labels.

Adding noise to the features undoes the distributional shift caused by the changing of features over time. When a certain level of noise is reached, the only remaining difference between nodes in the validation and the test set is structural. This explains the results of Fig. 1, in which by the time all the nodes have been tampered with, there is no difference between the validation and test accuracy of the GCN and GraphSAGE models.

In the case of the GAT, going back to Eqs. (8)–(10), the α^l_{uv} performs an implicit assignment of different importances to the neighbours. This mechanism allows the model to downgrade the importance of nodes once their representation contains enough noise to negatively influence the learning process, e.g. when the nodes contribute to misclassifying other nodes. In short, the GAT performs regularization via attention.

5.2.2 Inductive Setting

The results of training a GCN, a GAT and GraphSAGE in the inductive setting with a randomly added noise are shown in Fig. 2.

The first observation is that overall, the test accuracy is lower in the inductive learning setting than in the transductive learning setting. This is expected, because the inductive task is inherently a more challenging task than the transductive one

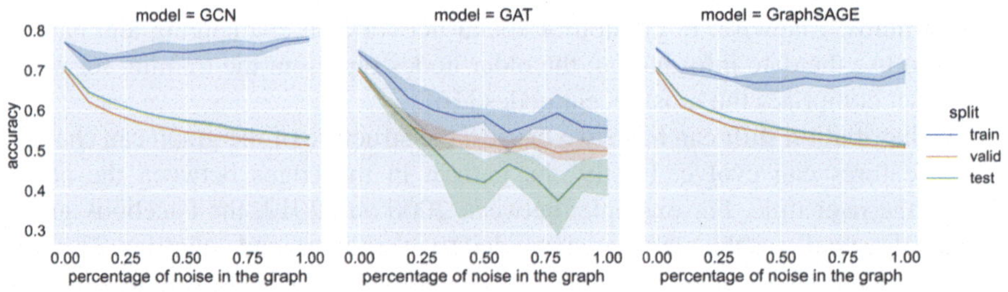

Fig. 2 Training, validation and test accuracy of three models of GNNs in the inductive learning setting. The horizontal axis corresponds to the percentage of features to which noise has been added, e.g. p in Eq. (11)

[35]. Having access to the test data at training time allows the model to fit the structure of the graph. Moreover, if there is a change in the feature distribution between training and validation, the model can adapt to this change at training time in the transductive setting.

When $p = 1$, there is still a generalization error between the validation and test accuracy in the GCN model. The lower accuracy is explained by the fact that inductive learning is inherently a more challenging task than transductive learning [35]. The gap is the result of structural differences between the training graph and the full graph. For example, since nodes become popular slowly over time, the structure may have evolved as the result of the formation of new hubs.

Conversely, the generalization error almost disappears in the case of GraphSAGE. This is the result of the sampling mechanism, which appears in Eq. (5). The sampling acts as a regularizer, which also explains why the gap between the train and validation accuracy is smaller than with the GCN. Since the sampling prevents overfitting to the structure, the gap represents the information lost via noise. When $p \geq 0.4$, most of the information in the features has been drowned in the noise.

In contrast, GAT's performance present several peculiarities. Firstly, the model performs considerably worse than in the transductive setting. It also achieves a smaller test accuracy than its GCN and GraphSAGE counterparts, with the accuracy dropping below the 50% mark. Secondly, the model presents a wider range of outcomes for the different runs. This is an indication that the model is converging to different local minima at each run. Additionally, the low training accuracy indicates that the model performs excessive regularization.

This regularization is performed via the attention mechanism presented in Eqs. (8)–(10). When we consider the backpropagation phase [20] of a single node, we see that the noise will be amplified in two ways. In the first part, neighbours who share the same class as the node, but whose features have been tampered with so that they push the model to misclassify the node, will see their α^l_{uv} coefficient reduced, e.g. the model will attribute less importance to these nodes. In the second part, neighbours with a different class but whose features push the model to correctly classify the nodes, will have an increased α^l_{uv} coefficient. In other words, information will be silenced while noise will be amplified.

5.3 *High Degree Node Perturbation*

In this section, we assume that the noise targets the high degree nodes first, according to Eq. (12).

5.3.1 Transductive Setting

The results of training a GCN, a GAT and GraphSAGE in the transductive setting with noise progressively added to the nodes, starting with the nodes with the highest

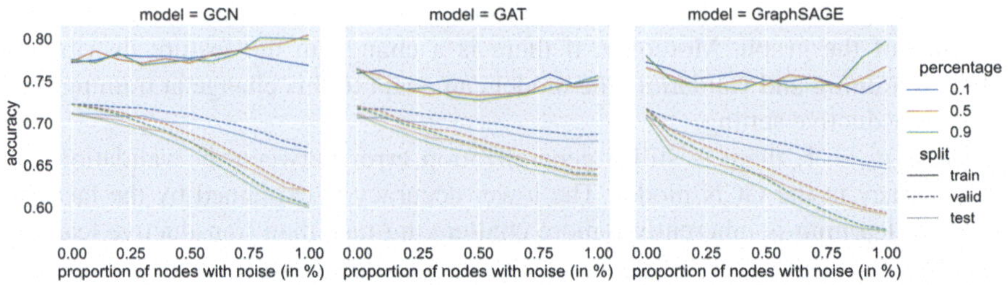

Fig. 3 Training, validation and test accuracy of three models of GNNs in the transductive learning setting. The horizontal axis corresponds to the percentage of nodes to which noise has been added. The noise targets the nodes with the highest degree first then proceeds in a decreasing manner. The percentage indicates how many of the features of each node are tampered with, e.g. 0.1 means 10% of the features contain added noise

degree, are shown in Fig. 3. The horizontal axis represents the proportion of nodes that contain noise, e.g. the normalized t in Eq. (12). Each color represents a different amount of noisy features per nodes, e.g. the p in Eq. (12). We investigate three settings: minimal noise, with $p = 10\%$; medium noise, with $p = 50\%$; and high noise, with $p = 90\%$.

For a given $t < 1$ and any p, the test accuracy of each model is higher than in the random noise setting.

Noise that spreads from an influential node will go through many nodes to reach the most isolated ones, by which time the effects of the noise will have been dampened. This phenomenon can be visualized with the following experiment, similar to the *small world* experiment [6]: the goal is to reach the best coverage of the U.S. population with the smallest group of people, in the sense that we want to select a group that minimizes the distance between any individual in the whole population and the group, e.g. each person is at least 5 hops away from the group.

If you select the members of the groups by taking the people with the highest degree, you will target people from the big cities. But you will miss the people from isolated areas. Moreover, while some people will not be within reach of a member of the group, others will be within reach of several members. When, instead of selecting the people by their degree, you pick them randomly, you reduce the overlapping of the coverage and you increase the chance of selecting members that can reach the isolated nodes. Regarding our experiment, this means what when the noise is added to the high degree nodes, some nodes will not encounter any noise because they will be beyond reach of the L neighbourhood of the high degree nodes, where L is the number of layers of the GNN. Note that this also applies to GNNs with skip connections [34], although the depth the GNN then exceeds L.

Looking at GCN and GAT, we see a only a relatively small drop in performance until at least $t \geq 0.4$. This can be explained by going back to the equations of each model. In the GCN case, the node-wise update rule can be expressed by Eq. (14). T is the transpose operator.

$$h_u^{l+1} = (W^l)^T \sum_{v \in N_u \cup \{u\}} \frac{1}{\sqrt{\hat{d}_v \hat{d}_u}} h_u^l \tag{14}$$

The weighting of the nodes in the update rule depends doubly on the degree of the nodes: the degree of the target node, i.e. the node that is updated, and the degree of the source node, that is, the neighbour from which the edge starts. At a local level, considering only a single node update, which can be done by fixing the u, the nodes with the highest degree will always have lower importance than the other nodes. More formally, given a node u, two neighbours v_1 and v_2 such that $d_{v_1} > d_{v_2}$, we have $(1/d_{v_1})^{-1/2} < (1/d_{v_2})^{-1/2}$. Likewise, given two nodes u_1 and u_2 who share a common neighbour v, by the same reasoning we find that if $d_{u_1} > d_{u_2}$, u_2 will have a greater weight than u_1. This means that the GCN's explicit weighting scheme devalues the contributions from high degree nodes. This also means that targeting the high degree nodes is the least efficient way of propagating noise in a GCN model.

Regarding the GAT model, the unnormalized attention coefficient between two nodes u and v, given by Eq. (8), is $a(W^l h_u^l, W^l h_v^l)$ where a is the attention mechanism. a can be any learnable function. For example, in the original paper [29], it is given by Eq. (15). Θ is the weight vector of the mechanism and $\|$ is the concatenation operator.

$$e_u^l v = \text{LeakyRELU}(\Theta^T [W^l h_u^l \| W^l h_v^l]) \tag{15}$$

The loss used in the training is the *cross-entropy* loss, given by Eq. (16). K is the number of classes, e.g. 40 in our case. x is the features of the node, y its label, represented as a *one-hot encoding*; and $\hat{y}$ the prediction of the GNN. $\hat{y}$ is usually taken to be a probability distribution, i.e. $\sum_{i=0}^{K} \hat{y}_i = 1$. The predicted category is the one with the highest score.

$$l(x, y) = \sum_{i=0}^{K} -y_i \log(\hat{y}_i) \tag{16}$$

When the noise targets the high degree nodes, enough noise will push the model to misclassify nodes. In terms of loss, this means that the noise will increase the loss of the model. During the backpropagation stage, the weights will be modified using gradient descent to decrease the loss. Let u be a node and v_1 one its neighbours. If v_1 contains noise that results in decreasing the score of the prediction of the correct class of u, the loss increases. To reduce the loss, the model will change its weights, and will reduce the importance of v_1 in updating u, by lowering α_{uv_1}. Because the high degree nodes will be involved in many computations, the same reasoning shows that the overall importance of these nodes will decrease. In short, the attention mechanism will silence the noise.

In terms of the percentage of features altered, we observe two phenomena: when only a few features are modified, e.g. $p = 0.1$, the performance deteriorates only slightly; and whether we set $p = 0.5$ or $p = 0.9$, the performance is similar. The second point was already observed in Sect. 5.2 regarding random noise: beyond a certain amount of noise, the performance plateaus as the noise has spread through the whole graph and there is nothing else remaining to tamper with.

A very likely explanation for the first phenomenon is the fact that many types of GNN perform some form of *implicit denoising* during their training phase [23]. In particular, the authors of [23] show that GCN and GAT can be seen as solving a specific form of denoising problem. This idea of denoising is further investigated in [22], in which the authors explore how denoising is impacted by the connectivity and the size of the graph, as well as by the architecture.

5.3.2 Inductive Setting

The results of training a GCN, a GAT and GraphSAGE in the inductive setting with noise progressively added to the nodes, starting with the nodes with the highest degree, are shown in Fig. 4.

While GraphSAGE's performance in the transductive setting was the poorest of the three models, in the inductive setting it is on par with the other models. The reason for the early drop in accuracy in the transductive and inductive settings, e.g. when $p \in [0, 0.2]$, is likely the over-representation of high degree nodes in the sampling of the neighbours. When looking at the neighbourhood sampling of all the nodes, the nodes with high degree will appear multiple times. Thus, the sampling allows the noise to spread faster. As the noise fills the whole graph, the inductive mechanism of GraphSAGE starts to be more influencial in reducing the overall noise of the messages.

In contrast with the previous experiments, we see that the validation and test gap reaches a minimum around $p = 0.6$, and starts increasing again when $p > 0.6$. In all likelihood, this is due to the fact that apart from the papers who cite and are

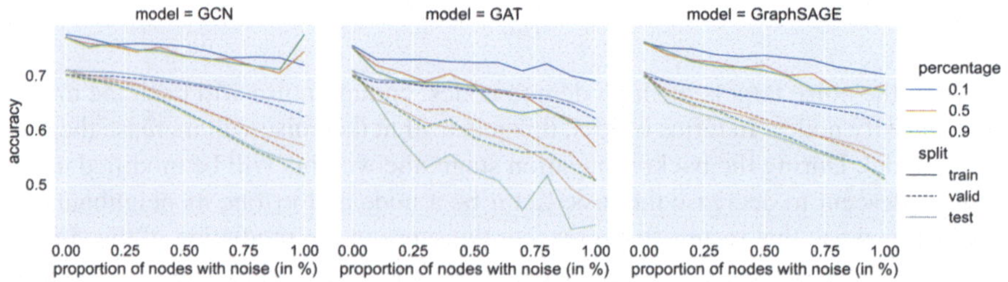

Fig. 4 Training, validation and test accuracy of three models of GNNs in the inductive learning setting. The horizontal axis corresponds to the percentage of nodes to which noise has been added. The noise targets the nodes with the highest degree first then proceeds in a decreasing manner

cited by few others, the newer papers tend to have less citations on average than the older ones, because there needs to be a certain period of time before the paper starts getting cited. By targeting the nodes with the higher degree first, we are creating a distributional shift. Indeed, the models are trained on nodes with noise while the nodes in the validation and test set contain less noise in average. This leads to the models's generalizing capabilities to decrease.

5.4 Small Degree Node Perturbation

In this section, we assume that the noise targets the small degree nodes first, according to Eq. (13).

5.4.1 Transductive Setting

The results of training a GCN, a GAT and GraphSAGE in the transductive setting with noise progressively added to the nodes, starting with the nodes with the smallest degree, are shown in Fig. 5.

The model performance drops sharply when $t \in [0, 0.3]$, then it levels off. A similar reasoning from Sect. 5.3 about the degrees of the nodes shows that the GCN model will amplify the noise: the values of the nodes with the smallest degree are weighted with the largest coefficients. Likewise, the GAT will start by penalizing heavily the small degree nodes. Only when enough noise is present in the graph will the attention mechanism be able to rescale the importance of the noisy nodes.

Because GraphSAGE proceeds with a fixed neighbourhood sampling size, there is no neighbourhood sampling for the nodes with small degree: all their neighbours are considered. Therefore, GraphSAGE has no regularizing mechanism for small degree nodes. The lack of weighting, whether implicit or explicit, does not allow GraphSAGE to penalize the noisy nodes in any other way than by modifying the

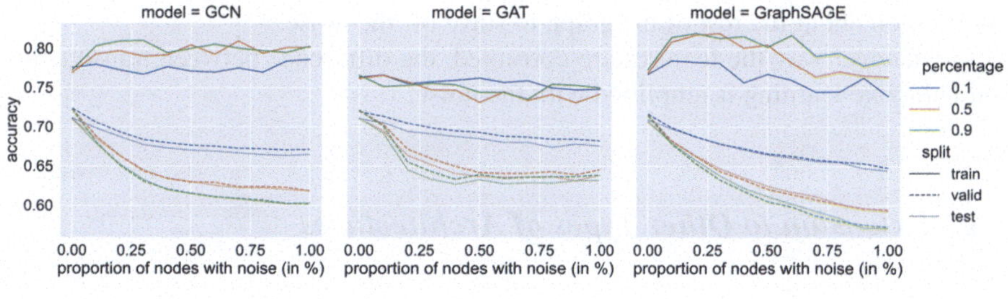

Fig. 5 Training, validation and test accuracy of three models of GNNs in the transductive learning setting. The horizontal axis corresponds to the percentage of nodes to which noise has been added. The noise targets the nodes with the smallest degree first then proceeds in an ascending manner

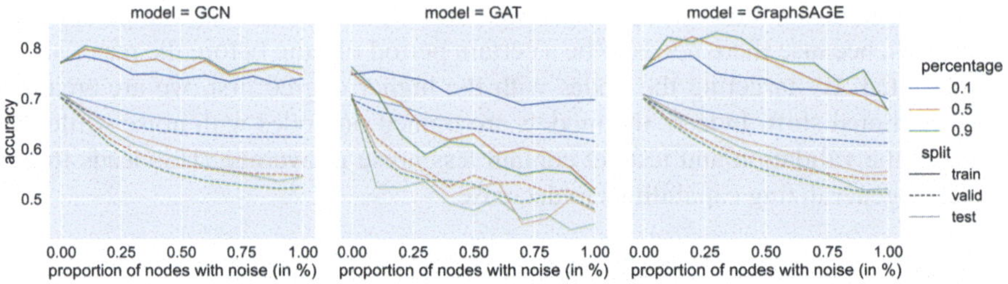

Fig. 6 Training, validation and test accuracy of three models of GNNs in the inductive learning setting. The horizontal axis corresponds to the percentage of nodes to which noise has been added. The noise targets the nodes with the smallest degree first then proceeds in an ascending manner

model's parameters, which results in low generalizing capabilities as the model is trying to fit against the noise.

We observe that, whether the noise is randomly distributed across the nodes or whether it targets high degree or small degree nodes, the presence of noise in the nodes's features is more important than the quantity of features modified. In other words, t is more important than p. Increasing t will decrease the accuracy more than if we increase p.

5.4.2 Inductive Setting

The results of training a GCN, a GAT and GraphSAGE in the inductive setting with noise progressively added to the nodes, starting with the nodes with the smallest degree, are shown in Fig. 6.

Except for the GAT, the validation accuracy is actually higher than the test accuracy. This indicates that the model is not learning properly. It is just fitting the noisy training data. The gap is consistent regardless of the amount of noise. This result hearkens back to the spread of fake news which can start more easily as a rumour then spread to infect the whole population [28]. The graph can be more easily subverted by targeting the more isolated nodes who do not possess enough information about the rest of the graph to stave off the noise.

In whatever way the features are corrupted, the difference between transductive and inductive learning is amplified with the noise.

5.5 Extension to Other Types of Architectures

In this section, we go beyond the GCN, GAT and GraphSAGE models to look at two other models: the Graph Isomorphism Network (GIN) [33], which is an MPNN model provably more powerful at discerning certain graph structures than GCN and

GraphSAGE; and Simple Graph Convolution (SGC) [31], a GNN which simplifies the computations performed in the GCN and contains only a single layer.

5.5.1 Graph Isomorphism Network

A single layer of the GIN model follows Eq. (17). MLP^l is a multi-layer perceptron. $\epsilon^{(l)}$ is either a learnable parameter, or a fixed scalar value.

$$h_v^l = \text{MLP}^l\left(\left(1+\epsilon^{(l)}\right)\cdot h_v^{l-1} + \sum_{u\in N_v} h_u^{l-1}\right) \tag{17}$$

Compared with the GCN equation, the multi-layer perceptron adds more expressivity: it allows the model to adjust on a feature per feature basis, which results in more degrees of freedom. It can capture more patterns than the explicit weighting on the degrees of the nodes. The results of the training of the GIN with random noise in transductive and inductive learning are shown in Fig. 7.

We see that the overall performance of the model, both in transductive and inductive learning, is far below that of the architectures studied above. This is due to the multilayer perceptron, or fully connected layer, that allows the model to weight each feature individually. This makes the model more sensitive to variations in the features. We also see a decrease followed by an increase in the accuracy when we increase p. This variation reflects the complexity of the task: when half the features are noisy, the model can learn to assume that half the inputs are noisy. When the ratio between clean and noisy features is different, the model might constantly oscillate to find a suitable value. This can be seen by the divergence in outcome which is less pronounced in the transductive case when $p = 0.6$.

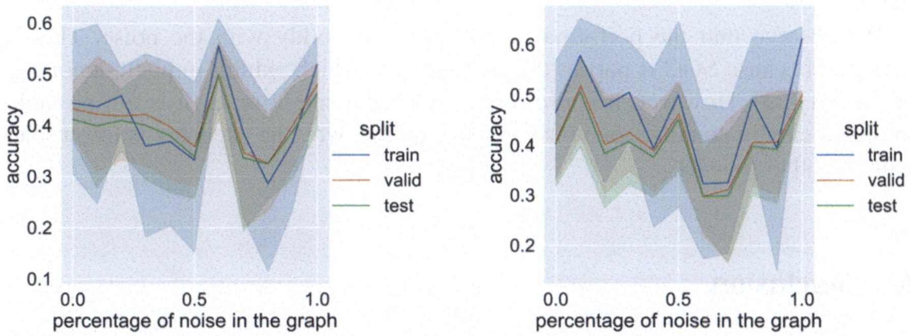

Fig. 7 Training, validation and test accuracy of the GIN model in the transductive (left) and inductive (right) learning settings. The horizontal axis corresponds to p in Eq. (11)

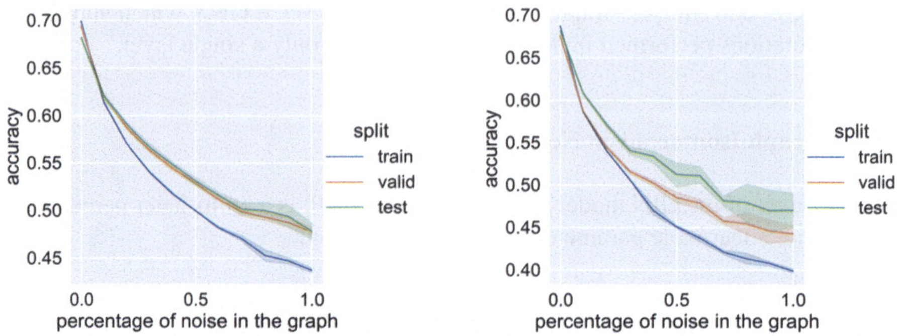

Fig. 8 Training, validation and test accuracy of the SGC model in the transductive and inductive learning settings. The horizontal axis corresponds to the percentage of nodes to which noise has been added. The noise targets the nodes with the smallest degree first then proceeds in an ascending manner

5.5.2 Simple Graph Convolution

The SGC model was conceptualized as a simplification of the GCN. By writing $S = \tilde{D}^{-1/2}\tilde{A}\tilde{D}^{-1/2}$, the SGC model follows Eq. (18). σ denotes an activation function, like the Softmax operator. K is a hyperparameter of the model. Θ represents the parameters of the model.

$$\hat{y} = \sigma(S^K X\Theta) \tag{18}$$

In comparison with the GCN model, the SGC first performs the matrix multiplication S^K, which gives the depth of neighbourhood that can be achieved, then combines the resulting power matrix with the parameters. The results of the training of the SGC with random noise in transductive and inductive learning are shown in Fig. 8.

We observe that the performance decreases smoothly with the noise. This is expected because SGC is part of the architectures which exhibit implicit denoising behaviour [23]. However, because the model has a single layer, it is not possible to incrementally penalize the noise, which explains why the accuracy is lower than with the other models.

6 Conclusion

In this paper we investigate the sensitivity of different types of graph neural networks, especially message passing neural networks, to the noise in the features of the nodes. We explored different types of noise: random noise, where noise is added randomly to the features; noise which is targeted at the high degree nodes; and noise which targets the small degree nodes. GNNs are trained both in the transductive setting and in the inductive learning, i.e. with and without access to the test data at training time. We find that weighting mechanisms, whether they are explicit, as in the GCN, or implicit, such as the attention mechanism in the GAT, help reduce the influence and the propagation of the noise.

We also found that certain architectures present an implicit denoising mechanism that allows the model to maintain a certain level of accuracy under the presence of noise. Furthermore, architectures which lack this mechanism exhibit a more chaotic pattern of learning.

Out of the three types of noise, the noise targeting the small degree nodes first is the most challenging for the models. This reflects the fact that these nodes are more isolated; thus noise will have a relatively higher impact than it would for nodes with more neighbours.

We find that random noise in transductive learning leads to overfitting of the data. In inductive learning, the gap between training and validation accuracy is large, as well as the gap between validation and test accuracy.

Perspectives for future works include analyzing similar types of perturbations for categorical features, and in temporal graphs.

References

1. Bahdanau D, Cho K, Bengio Y (2015) Neural machine translation by jointly learning to align and translate. In: Bengio Y, LeCun Y (eds) 3rd International Conference on Learning Representations, ICLR 2015, San Diego, CA, USA, May 7–9, 2015, Conference Track Proceedings
2. Barabási AL, Albert R (1999) Emergence of Scaling in Random Networks. Science (New York, NY) 286(5439):509–512. https://doi.org/10.1126/science.286.5439.509
3. Chiang WL, Liu X, Si S, et al (2019) Cluster-GCN: An Efficient Algorithm for Training Deep and Large Graph Convolutional Networks. In: Proceedings of the 25th ACM SIGKDD International Conference on Knowledge Discovery & Data Mining, pp 257–266, https://doi.org/10.1145/3292500.3330925, https://doi.org/1905.079531905.07953
4. Chien E, Chang WC, Hsieh CJ, et al (2022) Node feature extraction by self-supervised multi-scale neighborhood prediction. In: The Tenth International Conference on Learning Representations, ICLR 2022, Virtual Event, April 25–29, 2022. OpenReview.net
5. Dai E, Aggarwal C, Wang S (2021) NRGNN: Learning a label noise resistant graph neural network on sparsely and noisily labeled graphs. In: Zhu F, Ooi BC, Miao C (eds) KDD '21: The 27th ACM SIGKDD Conference on Knowledge Discovery and Data Mining, Virtual Event, Singapore, August 14–18, 2021. ACM, pp 227–236, https://doi.org/10.1145/3447548.3467364
6. de Sola Pool I, Kochen M (1978) Contacts and influence. Social Networks 1(1):5–51. https://doi.org/10.1016/0378-8733(78)90011-4
7. Defferrard M, Bresson X, Vandergheynst P (2016) Convolutional neural networks on graphs with fast localized spectral filtering. In: Proceedings of the 30th International Conference on Neural Information Processing Systems. Curran Associates Inc., Red Hook, NY, USA, NIPS'16, pp 3844–3852

8. Devlin J, Chang MW, Lee K, et al (2019) BERT: Pre-Training of deep bidirectional transformers for language understanding. In: Burstein J, Doran C, Solorio T (eds) Proceedings of the 2019 Conference of the North American Chapter of the Association for Computational Linguistics: Human Language Technologies, NAACL-HLT 2019, Minneapolis, MN, USA, June 2–7, 2019, Volume 1 (Long and Short Papers). Association for Computational Linguistics, pp 4171–4186, https://doi.org/10.18653/v1/n19-1423
9. Dodge SF, Karam LJ (2016) Understanding how image quality affects deep neural networks. In: Eighth International Conference on Quality of Multimedia Experience, QoMEX 2016, Lisbon, Portugal, June 6–8, 2016. IEEE, pp 1–6, https://doi.org/10.1109/QoMEX.2016.7498955
10. Dong Y, Ma H, Shen Z, et al (2017) A century of science: Globalization of scientific collaborations, citations, and innovations. In: Proceedings of the 23rd ACM SIGKDD International Conference on Knowledge Discovery and Data Mining, Halifax, NS, Canada, August 13–17, 2017. ACM, pp 1437–1446, https://doi.org/10.1145/3097983.3098016
11. Geisler S, Zügner D, Günnemann S (2020) Reliable graph neural networks via robust aggregation. In: Larochelle H, Ranzato M, Hadsell R, et al (eds) Advances in Neural Information Processing Systems 33: Annual Conference on Neural Information Processing Systems 2020, NeurIPS 2020, December 6–12, 2020, Virtual
12. Geisler S, Schmidt T, Sirin H, et al (2021) Robustness of graph neural networks at scale. In: Ranzato M, Beygelzimer A, Dauphin YN, et al (eds) Advances in Neural Information Processing Systems 34: Annual Conference on Neural Information Processing Systems 2021, NeurIPS 2021, December 6–14, 2021, Virtual, pp 7637–7649
13. Gilmer J, Schoenholz SS, Riley PF, et al (2017) Neural message passing for quantum chemistry. In: Precup D, Teh YW (eds) Proceedings of the 34th International Conference on Machine Learning, ICML 2017, Sydney, NSW, Australia, 6–11 August 2017, Proceedings of Machine Learning Research, vol 70. PMLR, pp 1263–1272
14. Graham JW (2009) Missing data analysis: Making it work in the real world. Annual review of psychology 60:549–576
15. Hamilton WL, Ying R, Leskovec J (2017) Inductive representation learning on large graphs. In: Proceedings of the 31st International Conference on Neural Information Processing Systems. Curran Associates Inc., Red Hook, NY, USA, NIPS'17, pp 1025–1035
16. Hu W, Fey M, Zitnik M, et al (2020) Open graph benchmark: Datasets for machine learning on graphs. In: Larochelle H, Ranzato M, Hadsell R, et al (eds) Advances in Neural Information Processing Systems 33: Annual Conference on Neural Information Processing Systems 2020, NeurIPS 2020, December 6–12, 2020, Virtual
17. Kipf TN, Welling M (2017) Semi-supervised classification with graph convolutional networks. In: 5th International Conference on Learning Representations, ICLR 2017, Toulon, France, April 24–26, 2017, Conference Track Proceedings. OpenReview.net
18. Lachaud G, Céspedes PC, Trocan M (2022) Comparison between inductive and transductive learning in a real citation network using graph neural networks. In: IEEE/ACM International Conference on Advances in Social Networks Analysis and Mining, ASONAM 2022, Istanbul, Turkey, November 10–13, 2022. IEEE, pp 534–540, https://doi.org/10.1109/ASONAM55673.2022.10068589
19. Lachaud G, Céspedes PC, Trocan M (2022) Graph neural networks-based multilabel classification of citation network. In: Nguyen NT, Tran TK, Tukeyev U, et al (eds) Intelligent Information and Database Systems - 14th Asian Conference, ACIIDS 2022, Ho Chi Minh City, Vietnam, November 28–30, 2022, Proceedings, Part II, Lecture Notes in Computer Science, vol 13758. Springer, pp 128–140, https://doi.org/10.1007/978-3-031-21967-2_11
20. Lecun Y, Bottou L, Bengio Y, et al (1998) Gradient-based learning applied to document recognition. Proceedings of the IEEE 86(11):2278–2324. https://doi.org/10.1109/5.726791
21. Li J, Zhang M, Xu K, et al (2021) How does a neural network's architecture impact its robustness to noisy labels? In: Ranzato M, Beygelzimer A, Dauphin YN, et al (eds) Advances in Neural Information Processing Systems 34: Annual Conference on Neural Information Processing Systems 2021, NeurIPS 2021, December 6–14, 2021, Virtual, pp 9788–9803

22. Liu S, Ying Z, Dong H, et al (2022) How Powerful is Implicit Denoising in Graph Neural Networks. In: NeurIPS 2022 Workshop: New Frontiers in Graph Learning
23. Ma Y, Liu X, Zhao T, et al (2021) A unified view on graph neural networks as graph signal denoising. In: Demartini G, Zuccon G, Culpepper JS, et al (eds) CIKM '21: The 30th ACM International Conference on Information and Knowledge Management, Virtual Event, Queensland, Australia, November 1–5, 2021. ACM, pp 1202–1211, https://doi.org/10.1145/3459637.3482225
24. Mikolov T, Chen K, Corrado G, et al (2013) Efficient estimation of word representations in vector space. In: Bengio Y, LeCun Y (eds) 1st International Conference on Learning Representations, ICLR 2013, Scottsdale, Arizona, USA, May 2–4, 2013, Workshop Track Proceedings
25. Rey S, Segarra S, Heckel R, et al (2022) Untrained graph neural networks for denoising. IEEE Trans Signal Process 70:5708–5723. https://doi.org/10.1109/TSP.2022.3223552
26. Rossi E, Kenlay H, Gorinova MI, et al (2022) On the unreasonable effectiveness of feature propagation in learning on graphs with missing node features. In: Rieck B, Pascanu R (eds) Learning on Graphs Conference, LoG 2022, 9–12 December 2022, Virtual Event, Proceedings of Machine Learning Research, vol 198. PMLR, p 11
27. Shen Y, Fu H, Du Z, et al (2022) GCN-Denoiser: Mesh denoising with graph convolutional networks. ACM Trans Graph 41(1):8:1–8:14. https://doi.org/10.1145/3480168
28. Shu K, Sliva A, Wang S, et al (2017) Fake news detection on social media: A data mining perspective. SIGKDD Explor 19(1):22–36. https://doi.org/10.1145/3137597.3137600
29. Velickovic P, Cucurull G, Casanova A, et al (2018) Graph attention networks. In: 6th International Conference on Learning Representations, ICLR 2018, Vancouver, BC, Canada, April 30 - May 3, 2018, Conference Track Proceedings. OpenReview.net
30. Wang X, Zhang M (2022) How powerful are spectral graph neural networks. In: Chaudhuri K, Jegelka S, Song L, et al (eds) International Conference on Machine Learning, ICML 2022, 17–23 July 2022, Baltimore, Maryland, USA, Proceedings of Machine Learning Research, vol 162. PMLR, pp 23,341–23,362
31. Wu F, Jr. AHS, Zhang T, et al (2019) Simplifying graph convolutional networks. In: Chaudhuri K, Salakhutdinov R (eds) Proceedings of the 36th International Conference on Machine Learning, ICML 2019, 9–15 June 2019, Long Beach, California, USA, Proceedings of Machine Learning Research, vol 97. PMLR, pp 6861–6871
32. Xu K, Chen H, Liu S, et al (2019) Topology attack and defense for graph neural networks: An optimization perspective. In: Kraus S (ed) Proceedings of the Twenty-Eighth International Joint Conference on Artificial Intelligence, IJCAI 2019, Macao, China, August 10–16, 2019. ijcai.org, pp 3961–3967, https://doi.org/10.24963/ijcai.2019/550
33. Xu K, Hu W, Leskovec J, et al (2019) How powerful are graph neural networks? In: 7th International Conference on Learning Representations, ICLR 2019, New Orleans, LA, USA, May 6–9, 2019. OpenReview.net
34. Xu K, Zhang M, Jegelka S, et al (2021) Optimization of graph neural networks: Implicit acceleration by skip connections and more depth. In: Meila M, Zhang T (eds) Proceedings of the 38th International Conference on Machine Learning, ICML 2021, 18–24 July 2021, Virtual Event, Proceedings of Machine Learning Research, vol 139. PMLR, pp 11,592–11,602
35. Yang Z, Cohen WW, Salakhutdinov R (2016) Revisiting semi-supervised learning with graph embeddings. In: Balcan MF, Weinberger KQ (eds) Proceedings of the 33nd International Conference on Machine Learning, ICML 2016, New York City, NY, USA, June 19–24, 2016, JMLR Workshop and Conference Proceedings, vol 48. JMLR.org, pp 40–48
36. You J, Ma X, Ding DY, et al (2020) Handling missing data with graph representation learning. In: Larochelle H, Ranzato M, Hadsell R, et al (eds) Advances in Neural Information Processing Systems 33: Annual Conference on Neural Information Processing Systems 2020, NeurIPS 2020, December 6–12, 2020, Virtual

Interpretable Ensemble Model For Associative Classification

Md Rayhan Kabir, Seeratpal Jaura, and Osmar R. Zaiane

Abstract Associative classifiers have shown competitive performance with state-of-the-art classification methods for predicting class labels. In addition to their accuracy performance, associative classifiers produce human-readable rules for classification, providing an easier way to understand their decision-making process. However, the presence of high-dimensional feature vectors in the training data impacts these models' performances. In this study, we propose an ensemble model, Dynamic Ensemble Associative Learning (DEAL), where we use associative classifiers as base learners on feature sub-spaces. We also propose a dynamic feature sampling procedure that automatically defines the number of base learners and ensures diversity and completeness among the selected features. As each of the base learners of our ensemble model is interpretable, we can collect the rules from the base learners and examine them to understand the decision process. Although, understanding this decision process can be complicated if there is a large number of base learners. To that end, we introduce another ensemble model, Classification by Frequent Association Rules (CFAR), where we make the decision process of the model easier to understand. In CFAR, instead of using a voting method for the final decision of the ensemble, we rank the generated rules based on their prevalence and select a subset of the predominant rules for predicting class labels. We use ten datasets from the UCI repository to evaluate the performance of our proposed models. Both our ensemble approaches, DEAL and CFAR, eliminate the high memory and runtime requirements of recent associative classifiers, especially for training datasets with high-dimensional feature vectors, all without jeopardizing classification accuracy. CFAR enhances the model's interpretability by removing noisy rules while achieving increased classification accuracy in most cases in our experiments. While the decision process of DEAL is human interpretable, CFAR enhances this further by collecting and ranking the rules generated by its base learners to predict the final class label.

M. R. Kabir (✉) · S. Jaura · O. R. Zaiane
Department of Computing Science, University of Alberta, Edmonton, AB, Canada
e-mail: rayhan.kabir@ualberta.ca; seeratpa@ualberta.ca; zaiane@ualberta.ca

M. Kaya et al. (eds.), *Social Network Analysis and Mining Applications in Healthcare and Anomaly Detection*, Lecture Notes in Social Networks,
https://doi.org/10.1007/978-3-031-75204-9_2

Keywords Ensemble model · Interpretable model · Associative classification

1 Introduction

With the steady increase in the use of machine learning in real-life scenarios, the importance of classification is de facto increasing. Classification is a supervised machine learning technique that labels the data in different distinct class labels. In the present context, this process is being used in various tasks like the classification of images, text, tabular data, etc. To solve classification problems, some of the popular algorithms are Logistic Regression, Decision Trees [33], Random Forest [10], Support Vector Machines [15] and Artificial Neural Networks [20]. Even though these models have good performance in classification tasks, most of the classification models work in a black-box fashion. After training the model, the model remains opaque without revealing what has actually been learned [4]. For instance, even though amazingly accurate, neural networks, after convergence of the edge weights and node biases, are not interpretable. In addition, during inference, they do not provide the necessary explanation for the prediction, which is troublesome in some application fields like medical diagnosis, financial decision-making, etc. Furthermore, while the spotlight for supervised learning is on deep learning, it was demonstrated that Tree ensemble models (such as XGBoost) outperform these deep models across multiple real-life datasets [34]. Since machine learning is becoming popular and ubiquitous, an explanation is now even legislated in many jurisdictions. This has led to many efforts attempting to explain salient features in deep learning, but also a return to rule-based classifiers. Associative classifiers are among them.

Associative classifiers use an association rule mining approach [1] to discover frequent patterns, and lately statistically significant patterns, from which to derive classification rules. The test data is then classified using the rules that are generated during the training phase. A rule is in the form of $X \rightarrow Y$ where X, the antecedent, is a conjunction of co-occurring features, and Y, the consequent, is a class label. Several associative classifiers have been proposed namely CBA [29], ARC [2], CMAR [28], CPAR [37]. Rules generated by the associative classifiers are simple and human-readable thus their predictions can be interpreted. Though the associative classifiers are competitive with the state-of-the-art classifiers and have a huge advantage of built-in explainability, they suffer from the limitation imposed by the required threshold tuning, namely support and confidence. Choosing optimal support and confidence values for a dataset requires prior knowledge about the dataset and it differs from dataset to dataset. Another disadvantage of the mentioned algorithms is that sometimes they produce noisy rules during the rule generation phase. Some of the noisy rules prevail even after the rule pruning. If any rule does not add any valid information to the class label then the rule is considered a noisy rule. Noisy rules affect the performance of the model as they hinder the classification process to classify the instance to its appropriate class label.

To solve the issue of requiring prior confidence and support values, Li and Zaiane [27] proposed SigDirect where they used the Kingfisher algorithm [21] to find statistically significant classification rules. This model removes the necessity of requiring threshold values that are different for different datasets. Sood and Zaiane [35] showed though SigDirect removes the necessity of hyperparameters, it still produces many noisy rules. Thus they proposed SigD2, a classifier based on SigDirect with a two-stage rule pruning strategy which further removes the noisy rules from SigDirect. The improvement is promising as it reduces the number of rules without compromising accuracy. In fact, it was shown that SigD2 outperforms other rule-based classifiers, as well as classical classifiers such as SVM, Bayesian, C4.5, and even simple neural networks [35]. SigD2 increases the efficiency of associative classifiers as it uses a minimum number of rules for the classification process. As we discussed earlier, one major advantage of an associative classifier is the fact that the rules produced for the classification process are human-readable. However, a large number of rules and noisy rules make it hard to understand the decision process. Using fewer rules, SigD2 makes the understanding of the decision process of the classifier easier.

Though the performance of SigD2 is very competitive, its performance is limited in terms of required memory and run-time if the feature vector of the feature space is large. This limitation persists in Sigdirect too making both the models non-scalable when the feature vector of the dataset is large. An Ensemble of classifiers, each trained on a subset of the feature space, could address this issue. However, one has to fix the size of the ensemble. To make SigDirect and SigD2 scalable, we propose an ensemble model named Dynamic Ensemble Associative Learner (DEAL) to improve the efficiency of SigD2 in terms of memory requirement and runtime without hampering the accuracy. As a base learner, we considered SigD2 as SigD2 outperforms other associative classifiers [35]. In our model, we add a dynamic feature sampling technique inspired by the work of Cao et al. [12] which eliminates the necessity of defining the number of base learners for the ensemble model and ensures diversity and coverage of the feature space among the base learners. We first sample the features randomly to form a subset of the feature vector. After sampling, we calculate the overlap of the new subset with the previously generated subsets. If the overlap of the new subset is high, we discard the subset and start another sampling. We stop the sampling procedure either if after subsequent sampling, we do not find any more subset which has low overlap with the previous subsets or if all the features are covered by the generated subsamples. We train one SigD2 model with each of the subsamples and perform max-vote among the class label predictions. The class label with the highest vote is assigned to the new test instance. Our proposed method reduces the memory requirements and makes the model faster in terms of runtime without affecting the accuracy. On top of that, even after the ensemble, the model remains interpretable as we can gather the rules from the base learners.

Classical ensemble approaches make the final class prediction by training the base learners and taking their votes. In DEAL, it is quite difficult to interpret the decision process as at first the base models who voted for the final class are to be selected and the decision process of each of the base models is to be determined which can be a tedious process. In the case of a random forest where the base learners are decision trees, the decision process of each of the trees should be considered individually to understand the decision process. We focus on this part of the ensemble to keep the ensemble model simple so that the decision process can be inferred easily. Though DEAL solves the limitation of SigD2 in the case of a dataset with high dimensional feature vector space, to understand the decision process of DEAL we have to go through the rules produced by each of the base learners. Thus we propose Classification by Frequent Associative Rules (CFAR). In this approach, we train the base learners with a subset of the feature vectors. After training, we collect all the rules generated by the base learners. We speculate some base learners can produce noisy rules which do not add any information to the decision process but rather affect the performance of the model. Thus, we rank the rules based on their frequency in the base learners. Our assumption is if a rule is produced by many base learners, that rule has more importance in the classification process. We gradually select rules from the pools of rules based on their frequency. We deploy only the selected rules for the classification of the test dataset. This approach makes the model simpler as we get a very small number of rules after the selection based on their ranking. In this process, we also have the ranking of the rules based on their frequency, thus we can understand the importance of a rule and features in the decision process. Following this strategy, the decision process becomes easy to interpret. CFAR also shows competitive performance in terms of accuracy compared to SigD2. CFAR requires less memory and is faster than base classifiers. One advantage of CFAR is that the final rules which are selected for the classification process are even less than those generated by SigD2. Thus the interpretation of the decision process of CFAR is more suitable than SigD2. The main contributions of this study are:

- Our proposed model DEAL significantly decreases memory requirement and the runtime in comparison with SigD2 without affecting the accuracy for a dataset with a large feature vector,
- We proposed a feature sampling technique that automatically determines the number of the base learner in an associative classifier bagging approach ensuring diversity and feature space coverage.
- Our second proposed model CFAR also significantly lessens the limitation of SigD2 of high memory requirement for datasets with large feature vector space.
- CFAR uses frequent rules from the base learners which helps to remove noisy and less important rules. Thus with fewer rules, the ensemble becomes more interpretable.

The following sections are organized as follows: Sect. 2 provides the necessary background and related works, Sect. 3 describes the methodology and performance of our proposed model DEAL, Sect. 4 describes the methodology and performance of our proposed model CFAR, and finally, Sect. 5 is the conclusion with some future research direction of the work.

2 Related Works

In this section, we discuss on related work on classification, associative classification, and ensemble learning models for classification.

2.1 Classification

Classification is a process of labeling a given instance to a class label. In this process, a model is trained on labeled training data. In the training phase, the model finds patterns among the data and establishes a relationship between the pattern and the class label. When a new data instance is provided for labeling, the model uses pre-discovered patterns to label the new data instance. Till now several state-of-the-art machine learning models have been designed for the classification task. Among them support vector machine(SVM), decision tree, naive Bayes classifier, and logistic regressions are noteworthy. In this section, we will discuss them briefly.

Cortes et al. [15] proposed a support vector machine. This model is widely used in a classification tasks. Support vector machine finds a separating hyperplane between the data points of two different classes. After plotting the input vector in a data plane, the support vector machine tries to find a separating plane. In this process, the kernel plays an important role. Sometimes data points that are not separable in one kernel might be separable in a high-dimensional kernel. This model is efficient when the data points are linearly separable in a high-dimensional plane. But if the datasets are very large. In that case, SVM takes a huge time to find a hyperplane between the data points of two classes.

Decision trees proposed by Quinlan [33] is another widely used classification model. One important feature of a decision tree is the decision process is interpretable. In a decision tree, data instances are split based on different features of the dataset. This forms a tree-like structure. The intermediate nodes of the tree are features. The decision of class label is taken based on these features. The leaf nodes of the tree are class labels. There are several phases in tree generation. The first step is branch generation where different branches of the trees are generated based on the data instances of the training data. The second step is the pruning phase where noisy branches are pruned from the tree. In the classification phase, when a new data instance is given to the tree for classification, the data points are considered the intermediate nodes based on the features of the instance and mapped to a leaf node. The mapped leaf node is the assigned class label of the test instance. A decision has the advantage of being explainable over other classifiers. Quinlan also proposed C4.5 [32] as an extension of the decision tree algorithm which is also very efficient and competitive. Though both decision tree and C4.5 are very competitive performances and the decision process is human understandable, they are prone to overfitting and noise in the training data affects the performance significantly.

The deep learning classification model proposed by Hagan et al. [19] follows the architecture of an artificial neural network. The working procedure of this model follows layer-by-layer data processing like a human brain. The deep learning classification model showed excellent performance in comparison to other classification models. The deep learning model consists of connected layers and in each layer, there are interconnected nodes. Input data is processed in each of the nodes and they are forwarded to the next layer. Being processed in each layer and each node, the data is passed to the output nodes to predict the final class label. Though this architecture has superior results than other classifiers there are some drawbacks. A high volume of training data is required to train deep learning classifiers which can be a problem in some domains like medical data of a particular disease. Another drawback of deep learning models is the requirement for computing resources is very high. The model needs to store the processed data from each node and each layer. Thus processing this huge amount of data requires high computing resources. As the data are processed and transformed at each layer of the model, the decision process is not human understandable which can be a problem in the case of working with sensitive data like financial decision-making. Because if there is a bias or lots of noise in the data, in the case of deep learning models, there is no way to understand its effect from the model.

For any classification model, it is very important to understand the decision process. Associative classifiers are interpretable and human understandable as they generate rules and make the classification based on the generated rules. The rules generated by the associative classifiers are human-understandable. We will discuss associative classifiers in the next section.

2.2 Associative Classification

Associative rule mining finds relations among the features in the transaction data in terms of their association and correlation. For example, association rule mining finds the relation among item 'A' and item 'B' from transactions by counting the transaction where item 'A' appears. Then it counts in how many of those transaction items 'B' appears. This simple strategy becomes very important in different scenarios like retail stores to increase their sales and profits. This strategy can be helpful to build a classification model. The rules which are generated by the association rule mining are in the form of $X \rightarrow Y$ where X, the antecedent, is a conjunction of co-occurring features, and Y, the consequent, is a class label. The relation between the features to the class label can be determined by the associative rule mining approach. Further using these rules, the class label of the test data can be predicted. Inspired by this idea, researchers studied associative classifiers extensively in the last few decades.

The concept of using association rules as class association rules were first proposed by Bayardo [8]. He used an apriori rule generation approach and a few rule pruning techniques to increase efficiency by extracting rules with high confidence.

Liu et al. [29] proposed Classification Based on Association (CBA) which uses an Apriori-based rule generation approach to generate class association rules. In their approach, all constrained association rules from the database are generated and ranked based on metrics. The highest matching rule is used for the classification task. There are three steps in the associative classification process. They are rule generation, rule pruning, and rule selection. Rule generation is the first approach of the associative classification process. As we stated earlier, the class association rules are in the form of $X \rightarrow Y$ where X, the antecedent, is a conjunction of co-occurring features, and Y, the consequent, is a class label. The rules are generated in such a way that the antecedent and the consequent class label co-occurs together in transactions. Two important measures of the rules are support and confidence. Support is calculated by the proportion of the dataset where the rules appear in the dataset. Confidence is the relationship between antecedent and consequent which is in a fraction of total transactions containing the antecedent and the consequent appearing together. Class association rules are a special type of association rules where the antecedent is the features and the consequent is the class label. Apriori proposed by Agarwal et al. [1] is the most widely used rule mining strategy. Another famous rule mining strategy is fp-growth algorithm [22]. Almost all the classifiers use one of these two strategies in rule generation.

The next step is the rule-pruning strategy. In the rule generation phase, many noisy rules are generated which affect the performance of the classifier. The rule pruning phase is very important as this removes the rules which do not add any additional information to the classification process. Different rule-pruning strategies have been proposed by different researchers over the years. In CBA, [29] database coverage strategy has been used. In another study, Zaiane and Antonie [38] proposed pruning based on finding a minimal set of class association rules. They aimed at finding a minimum set of rules for classification without jeopardizing the performance of the classifier.

The final step of the classification is to select the rules for predicting the class label of a test instance. After the rule generation and rule pruning steps, the number of rules still might be large and all of them might not be applicable to the test instance. Thus the applicable rules are to be selected from the pool of rules. After selecting the applicable rules, in most cases, the number of applicable rules is more than one. Among the applicable rules, the best rules are to be selected following heuristics. Several heuristics are there to select rules to apply to the test instance. Some of the heuristics are the sum of confidence values, the sum of support values, the average of confidence values, etc which are used to find the most effective rules. For each of the test instances, the rules are selected based on the heuristics. In the study of Sood and Zaiane [35], they used three different heuristics namely the sum of ln(p-value), the sum of confidence value and the sum of ln(p-value)*confidence for the rules of each of the class labels. From their experiment, they found in most of the cases the rules with the highest sum of the confidence values provide better results.

These three major steps are followed in all the associative classifiers. We will describe the associative classifiers in the next section.

2.3 Associative Classifier

Liu et al. [29] showed it is possible to use association rule mining to build a classifier. Their proposed Classification Based on Association (CBA) uses an Apriori-based approach to generate class association rules. In their approach, all constrained association rules from the database are generated and ranked based on metrics. The highest matching rule is used for the classification task. Their subsequent work [30] attempts to decrease noisy rules. They improved the performance of the classifier by choosing the most accurate class association rules for the classification task. Inspired by this work, many researchers came forward with different approaches to improve the performance of associative classifiers, mainly differentiating themselves by proposing different strategies to select the applicable rules during inference. Yin and Han [37] proposed a Classification based on Predictive Association Rules (CPAR). They generate association rules directly from the training data by a greedy approach. To evaluate each of the generated rules, they use an expected accuracy and finally select the best k rules for the classification task. Li et al. [28] proposed CMAR which is a Classification based on Multiple Association Rules. They extended FP-growth [22] frequent pattern mining method to construct an FP-tree for class distribution association. In this approach, the class association rules are stored in a special data structure. The generated rules are pruned based on confidence, correlation and database coverage. Using multiple strong association rules with a Weighted χ^2 measure, a datapoint is labeled to the appropriate class.

Antonie and Zaiane [2] propose another Association rule-based classifier that they apply for text categorization. They put forward two different approaches; ARC-AC, considering all generated rules from the whole training set, and ARC-BC, where data from each class is mined separately allowing the handling of unbalanced datasets. Indeed, being based on frequency, minority class risk is not being expressed in a predictive model when all dataset entries are mined together. Another approach, CCCS, proposed by Arunasalam and Chawla [5] introduces a measure named "Complement Class Support" (CCS). The authors claim CCS guarantees a positive correlation between the class label and the generated rules. Antonie et al. [3] also propose a two-stage associative classifier where associative classification rules are discovered in the first stage and in the second stage, another algorithm learns how to use those rules for class prediction. Instead of basing the selection of rules to apply during inference on some heuristics, they use a neural network to learn how to predict the best rules to apply. This approach showed improved efficiency in terms of accuracy. One limitation of associative classifiers is the generation and the need to evaluate a huge number of rules, among them many are noisy rules. To overcome this problem Zaiane and Antonie [38] performed an extensive study with the focus of reducing the number of rules without decreasing the accuracy of the classifier. The authors propose a new pruning strategy to reduce the number of class association rules. They also propose different heuristics for selecting rules which can obtain high accuracy for a given instance. However, it remains that the proper support and confidence values have to be selected and tuned.

This is one major drawback of associative classifiers inherited from association rule mining. The performance of the model largely depends on these values. It is a tedious task to find the proper confidence and support values for each of the datasets, hampering the adoption of associative classifiers.

To solve this issue, Li and Zaiane [27] propose SigDirect to find the statistically significant rules for classification, instead of frequent ones. In their strategy, they improvised the Kingfisher algorithm [21]. To find out whether a rule is significant or not, they used Fisher's exact test to measure the significance rule. In this method, they directly mined rules from the data and pruned them by following an instance-centric pruning strategy. Their method solves the limitation of requiring support and confidence values. This method also solves some other limitations of the previous associative classifier. In the previous classifier, no statistical dependency between the antecedent and the consequent was considered. Thus many rules were generated which instead of adding further information, affected the performance of the model. In addition to this, using support-confidence framework includes a large number of rules. But considering statistical significance considers only those rules which add significant information to the classification task. Their proposed method SigDirect increases the accuracy of the classifier. The main contribution of their work is eliminating the necessity of annoying support and confidence thresholds. However, SigDirect also has some limitations. Sood and Zaiane [35] showed though Sigdirect produces a very less number of rules compared to other associative classifiers, noisy rules still exist. In their study they showed, those noisy rules can be further eliminated and the elimination of noisy rules increases the efficiency of the model. Thus they proposed SigD2, a two-stage pruning technique that can reduce the number of rules without jeopardizing the accuracy of the classifier and therefore making a learned model even more practically interpretable.

Though Sigdirect and its successor SigD2 shows competitive result in terms of accuracy, with the increase of the features in the training dataset, memory requirement and runtime of the dataset increases rapidly. Using ensemble models can solve this issue which we will discuss in the next sections.

2.4 *Ensemble Classification Model*

The concept of the ensemble model was first proposed by Dasarathy and Sheela [16], where they proposed the idea of a composite model. They achieved enhanced performance by deploying two or more component classifiers each trained of a separate partition of the feature domain. The optimal domain partition criteria depend on the component classifier. The authors used the Sequential Weight Increasing Factor Technique (SWIFT) for partitioning the domain space. In their study, they showed when multiple classifiers are deployed together, they achieved better performance than each of the individual component classifiers when they are deployed separately. Following their work, several researchers worked in this field and achieved better results using an ensemble model. Bagging [9] and Boosting

[17] are the most popular ensemble models for classification problems. Several variations of bagging and boosting and different strategies to select the subset from the training data have been used in different literature. In bagging, a predefined number of subsets of the dataset are selected and one classification model is trained on each of the subsets of the dataset. These classification models which are trained on the subset of the training data are known as a base classifier of the model. At the end of the training models, each of the models makes the prediction of the test data independently. In the end, the class label with the highest vote is considered the final class label. In the case of the bagging approach, all the base learners are trained and make their predictions independently. In the bagging approach, the base learners can be trained in parallel as each of the base learners is trained independently. In contrast to bagging, in boosting algorithm, base learners are trained in series. After training one base learner, the misclassified instances are identified and the next base learner put extra weight on the misclassified instances. Weights if the instances which are correctly classified are decreased for the next base learners. The idea is to pay more attention to misclassified instances than the correctly classified instances in the next steps. This procedure continues until the number of base learners reaches a predefined number or the training error reaches to a predefined threshold. At the end of training the base learners, voting is performed. In the case of boosting algorithm, each of the base learners has a weight based on their performance. This voting strategy is called weighted voting. Though this strategy is susceptible to overfitting, it shows promising results. Later Hastie et al. [23] extended this work for multi-class classification. This boosting strategy is known as adaboosting. Another boosting strategy is gradient boosting proposed by Friedman [18]. In gradient boosting, a loss function is used and the objective is to minimize the loss function using gradient descent method. Gradient boosting also has competitive performance. In [7] the authors showed that bagging and boosting improved classification performance for demographic classification of handwriting. Prusa et al. [31] evaluated 12 different techniques that improve the classification performance on 3 datasets for Twitter sentiment classification. Based on their experimental findings, they concluded that bagging provides superior performance as compared to the rest of the techniques and significantly improved the classification performance. Another famous ensemble model is random forest [10]. Random forest follows the idea of a bagging procedure and uses a decision tree as the base learner. Unlike decision trees, a random forest uses a random selection of features to select each node for each of the trees. In this study author shows, in addition to having competitive performance, random forests are more robust to noise than boosting algorithms.

In the case of all ensemble models, the subset selection procedure plays a vital role. One of the main reasons for the superior performance of the ensemble models is the diversity among the base learners. Higher similarity among the subset results in poor performance of the model due to a lack of diversity among the base learners. Thus maximizing the diversity among the base learners is one of the main goals in the ensemble model. To create diversity, more emphasis should be given to the subset selection strategy. Brown [11] made extensive studies to define and measure the diverse error in the ensemble model. He showed diversity among the base learners can be achieved using negative correlation among the base learners. His work puts emphasis on creating diversity among the base models so that the prediction of each model becomes independent and by this maximum performance from a neural ensemble model can be achieved. Brown proved his proposition through theoretical and empirical analysis.

One drawback of the classical ensemble model is one has to fix the size of the ensemble. That is the number of the base learner in an ensemble model is predefined. But this process has a limitation. If the predefined number of the base learners is large and the number of features in the training data is small then this will result in many duplicate base learners which affect the diversity among the base learners. On the other hand, if the number of features is large and the number of a predefined base learner is small then the base learners might not cover the whole feature space thus many important features might not be considered in the decision process. In classical ensemble models, the subsample to train the base learners is selected randomly. Thus some features can be selected multiple times and some features can be omitted in the process. In the random subsampling procedure, there is no way to control the selection of the features. Thus this might create bias in the base learners. To address this issue Cao et al. [12] proposed a novel sampling procedure as a cost-sensitive adaptive random subspace ensemble. Their proposed method automatically defines the number of base learners in the ensemble process. The proposed sampling procedure considers the overlap among the subsamples and allow a maximum amount of overlap among each subsample. In this way, they ensure diversity and coverage. When the method can not produce another new subsample with the given constraints, it stops sampling and trains one base model with each of the subsamples. Thus the requirement of a predefined number of subsamples is eliminated.

In Sect. 3 we propose Dynamic Ensemble Associative learners where we propose a feature sampling technique inspired by the work of Cao et al. [12]. As we discussed in the previous subsection, associative classifiers are interpretable. After making an ensemble of associative classifiers, we can still gather the rules from the base learners and interpret the decision process. To make the interpretation process simple, in Sect. 4, we propose Classification by Frequent Association Rules (CFAR) inspired by the work of W. Pascal et al. [36]. They proposed Decision snippet Features where instead of classical max-vote strategy, they mined small frequent branches as decision snippets from the learned decision trees of the ensemble. They showed a linear model on top of the snippets provides competitive results and reduces the model size.

3 Dynamic Ensemble Associative Learning

In this section, we provide the details of our proposed model Dynamic Ensemble Associative Learning (DEAL). We further evaluate our model in comparison to other classifiers using UCI datasets.

3.1 Methodology

In this section, we describe our methodology for the bagging approach using SigD2 as a base learner. As mentioned above, SigD2 was shown to outperform other rule-based classifiers and certainly all other associative classifiers in terms of accuracy and a number of generated classification rules. In most cases of bagging, the dataset instances are randomly sampled. We instead sample the feature space and use all instances. In most known ensemble approaches, the number of classifiers in the ensemble is predetermined and fixed. Therefore, initially, we start proceeding with the same and randomly sampling the feature space for each classifier in the ensemble. This random sampling does not guarantee completeness as some features may never be picked, and does not ensure diversity among the classifiers since different classifiers in the ensemble may end up with exactly the same feature selection. For that reason, we later introduce our dynamic sampling technique that ensures completeness and diversity and automatically determines the necessary number of learners in the ensemble. The procedures are explained in detail in the next sub-sections.

Algorithm 1 Subsample generation by randomly selecting features

Input: features: all features of the feature space; **N:** Number of the features in each subsample
Output: 100 subsample of the feature space

```
all_subsample ← []
for i in range(100) do:
    new_subsample ← []
    n ← 0
    reset features
    while n < N
        f ← randomly select without replacement a feature from features
        add f to new_subsample
        n ← n + 1
    end while
    add new_subsample to all_subsamples
end for
return all_subsamples
```

3.1.1 Ensemble with Random Subsample

At first, we use 100 base learners in the ensemble model. Each of the base learners is trained on a random subsample of size N of the original feature space. We show the process of creating random subsamples in Algorithm 1. Following this method, we generate 100 subsamples and train the base learners with each of the subsamples. For the random selection of all the experiments, we use *random* python library and *time* as seed. During inference, the prediction of the class label is done with each of the base learners and a vote determines the final prediction.

Generating subsample in this way presents some limitations. A feature can be selected every time or some of the features might not be selected at all. Thus many important features which are strongly correlated with the class label can be excluded from the training process. Another limitation is the need to fix the number of base learners, in our case 100, based on common practice in the literature. If the number of features is not large enough, there is no need for 100 base learners. Indeed many base learners would be trained on the same subsample of the feature space. To solve these issues we propose a new feature sampling technique that addresses both of the limitations.

3.1.2 Ensemble with Dynamic Sampling

Our goal is to make sure all input features are used by at least one base learner, and that the set of base learners is diverse. Therefore, to subsample from the feature vector, we follow a sequential procedure until all features are selected (ensuring completeness). To ensure diversity, we make sure the feature spaces of any pair of base learners do not overlap more than some percentage threshold. Our method to generate diverse subsamples is provided in Algorithms 2 and 3. In the input of the algorithm, N is the number of features to be selected in each of the subsamples. From previous literature, we know that if the feature vector of the dataset is large, SigD2 requires a high volume of memory and run time. Therefore we limited the size of the feature vector using N. In our experiments, we have tested across different values for N but in all cases, we used a small value of N. The next parameter of the algorithm is O_v. O_v is the maximum allowed overlap between any two subsamples. The value of O_v is a percentage and ranges from 0 to 1. If we put a very small value close to 0 for O_v, all the subsamples would be almost unique, and the number of generated subsamples small, which results in a small number of base learners, defeating the purpose of the ensemble. If we use a value close to 1, the subsamples would be almost similar to subsamples generated using a random subsampling. Thus we have to find an optimum value for O_v. The last parameter is T which indicates how many times we will try to get a satisfactory new subsample with our required overlap. This is to avoid blocking infinite loops. When generating a subsample by selecting features, if there is at least one previously generated subsample with which overlap of the selected features of the new subsample is more than O_v, we discard the current subsample and generate a new one. T provides a boundary for how many times we try for a single subsample. If after trying T times we do not find any subsample with less than overlap O_v, we stop the sampling procedure. We also keep track of whether all the features are already covered by the subsamples or not. If all the features in the feature space are covered by the generated subsamples, we stop our sampling procedure.

Algorithm 2 Algorithm **GenerateSubsample**

Input: Features: all features in the feature space; **N:** Number of the features in each subsample, O_v**:** Maximum overlap between any two subsamples, **T:** maximum number of tries to generate a subsample
Output: Subsamples of the feature space

```
try=0;
all_subsamples ← []
while try < T do
    new_subsample ← subsampleGen(Features, N)
    if(Overlap(new_subsample)< O_v) then
        Add new_subsample to all_subsamples
        try ← 0
    else
        try ← try+1
    end if
    if (all_feature_covered(all_subsample) ==True) then
        break
    end if
end while
return all_subsamples
```

Algorithm 3 shows how a subsample is generated. Here we randomly select a feature from the feature space and add it to the new subsample. N indicates the number of features in each subsample.

Algorithm 3 Algorithm **SubsampleGen**

Input: Features: all features in the feature space; **N:** Number of the features in each subsample
Output: subsample of the feature space

```
subsample← []
n← 0
while n < N do
    new_feature ← randomly select a feature
    Add new_feature to subsample
    n ← n+1
end while
return subsample
```

After generating a new subsample we evaluate whether the features of the newly generated subsample have more overlap than the O_v ratio with any of the previously generated subsamples. Between two subsamples S_1 and S_2 where the features are F_{S_1} and F_{S_2} respectively and the number of features in each of the subsamples is N then the overlap between the subsamples is calculated using the following equation:

$$Current\_overlap = \frac{F_{S_1} \cap F_{S_2}}{N} \quad (1)$$

If there is at least one previously generated subsample with which the feature overlap is greater than O_v, we discard the subsample. If there is no previous subsample with which the newly generated subsample has overlap greater than O_v, we consider the current subsample satisfies the required condition and accepts the sample. After generating the subsamples, we train one SigD2 model with each of the generated subsamples. The size of the output set of subsamples determines the size of the ensemble. We use the trained base learners to predict the class label of the test dataset. The class label with the highest vote of the base learners is determined as the final predicted class label. We evaluate the model using the predicted value in terms of accuracy, memory requirement and runtime.

3.2 Result Analysis

We use 10 different UCI datasets [6] to test our model. Before using a dataset we discretize the numerical values as stated in [13]. We convert the features to a binary feature vector. We used the same vector form of discretized values for all our experiments will all contenders. Thus the results of mentioned algorithms can be slightly different from their original papers. For each of the datasets, we use 80% of the data as training data and the rest 20% as test data. We compare the result of our model DEAL with different values of N which is the number of features for each base learner, against the result of C4.5 [32], Random Forest [10], RIPPER [14], SigD2 and the ensemble using 100 random sampling of features, we denote as RS. We also experiment with an ensemble of C4.5 as a base learner using our proposed feature sampling method DEAL.

The reported result is the average of 20 runs for each of the datasets. We compare the performance of our proposed model in terms of accuracy, memory requirement and runtime. We also provide an analysis on the performance of DEAL for different values of O_v. Finally, we discuss the interpretability of the prediction by DEAL.

We compare the performance of our proposed method with SigD2 since it was demonstrated to have better performance than other associative classifiers, rule-based classifiers [27, 35]. We also include RIPPER, however, since it is a rule induction algorithm different from association rules. We also compared the performance of DEAL with C4.5 and an ensemble of C4.5. As a representative of the traditional ensemble approaches, we use Random Forest [10] to compare our results. In the case of a random sampling of the features (RS), we experiment with different values of N (i.e. number of features in each subsample) and different values of O_v (i.e. maximum overlap among the selected features of base learners). From the experiment, we find the optimum result when the value of N is between 25 and 30.

The comparison in the accuracy of C4.5, an ensemble of C4.5 using the proposed sampling method, Random Forest (RF), RIPPER, SigD2, Random feature Sampling method (RS) with DEAL using different values of N is provided in Table 1 and Fig. 1. From the table we can see, among the datasets, in comparison with

Table 1 Accuracy of C4.5, Ensemble of C4.5 using feature sampling of DEAL, Random Forest (RF), RIPPER, bagging using random sampling (RS), SigD2, and DEAL

Dataset	#cls	#rec	Feature vector size	C4.5	C4.5 with dynamic sampling	RF	RIPPER	SigD2	RS N=25	RS N=30	DEAL N=20 O_v=0.6	DEAL N=25 O_v=0.6	DEAL N=30 O_v=0.6
Zoo	7	101	35	95.24	95.24	**97.62**	85.48	94.55	85.53	85.53	91.66	92.85	**97.62**
Pima	2	768	36	76.62	73.38	67.41	76.08	76.44	77.21	79.81	75.26	**79.82**	77.61
PageBlocks	5	5473	41	93.15	92.23	**93.51**	80.37	91.67	90.04	91.23	84.16	91.84	88.53
Heart	5	303	47	50.82	52.45	52.45	**64.90**	45.90	46.86	48.51	47.54	49.18	49.18
Hepatitis	2	155	54	70.97	74.19	78.38	78.72	81.93	80.65	81.29	78.06	80.64	**82.58**
Wine	3	178	65	91.67	91.67	77.78	93.33	92.7	91.57	93.26	86.51	**94.38**	92.13
Anneal	5	898	67	97.22	86.67	**98.89**	97.5	92.22	84.41	88.86	80.51	83.85	92.2
Horse	2	368	83	78.38	75.67	75.67	80.56	78.80	70.38	81.25	80.43	**82.33**	81.79
Adult	2	48,842	95	84.06	82.31	**84.97**	83.91	84.59	79.67	81.81	80.52	84.92	81.51
Ionosphere	2	351	155	88.73	**95.78**	**95.78**	92.81	90.18	88.1	90.77	90.47	92.85	94.04
Average				82.69	81.96	82.25	82.77	82.89	79.44	83.37	79.512	83.27	**83.72**

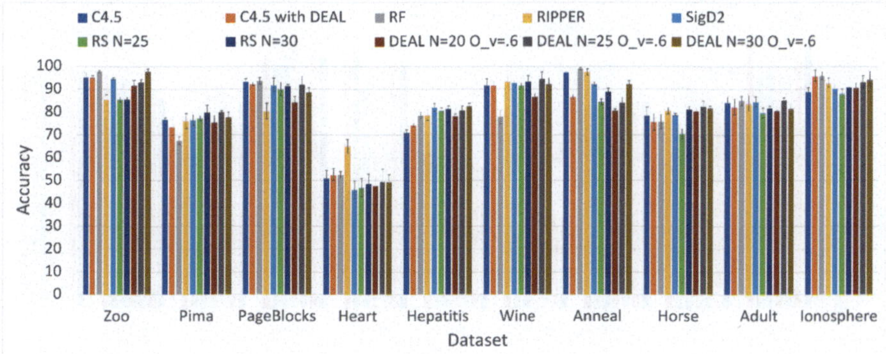

Fig. 1 Accuracy of C4.5, C4.5 using sampling of Deal, Random Forest (RF), RIPPER SigD2, and DEAL

Random Forest and C4.5, Random Forest has better performance than DEAL in 4 of the datasets while DEAL is a close runner-up, and in 4 others DEAL has better performance, with one ex aequo with the zoo dataset. In one dataset RIPPER performed better than DEAL. On average DEAL is better. In comparison with the original SigD2, we can see that apart from the Anneal dataset, DEAL presents an improvement in accuracy. The probable cause might be that some of the feature vectors in the Anneal dataset being highly correlated which plays an important role in the class prediction. DEAL selects a subset of the feature vectors thus the feature vectors that are needed to be together get separated. Further investigation is required for this dataset to find how the important features can be kept together. That might improve the performance of DEAL in those datasets where some feature vectors together play an important role in class prediction. The random sampling of the features with 100 base learners could not perform at the same level as DEAL. In comparison with SigD2 sometimes it improves the accuracy and in some cases, the accuracy is decreased. As the random sampling is completely random, many important features might not be selected for any of the base learners at all. This is the reason for the poor performance of RS. On average, DEAL with a feature vector size $N = 30$ and $O_v = 0.6$ has the best performance.

We also compare the performance of DEAL with other models in terms of precision and recall. Figures 2 and 3 show the precision and recall of the models for each dataset respectively. We can see DEAL, either with $N = 25$ or $N = 30$, has very competitive precision and recall compared to other models. We can get another interesting observation from Table 1. With the increase of N, the number of features for each of the base learners, the average accuracy increases. For a better understanding of this, we experimented with different values of N. The average accuracy for different values of N is plotted in Fig. 4. We can see a sharp increase when the value of N is increased from 15 to 25. After 25, the average accuracy continues to increase but not at the same steep rate.

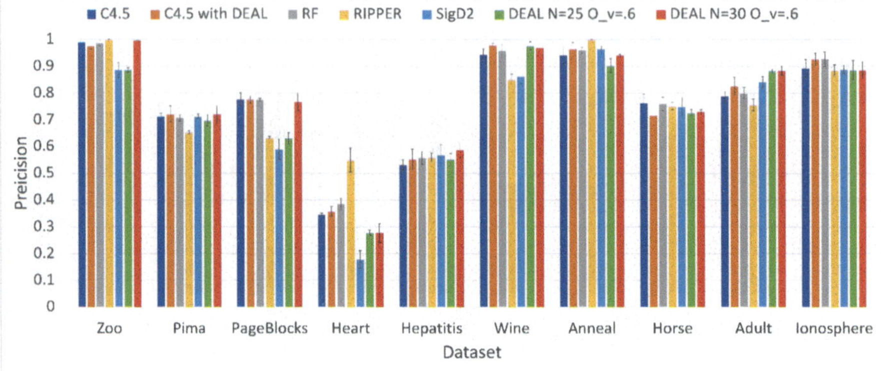

Fig. 2 Precision of C4.5, C4.5 using sampling of Deal, Random Forest (RF), RIPPER SigD2, and DEAL

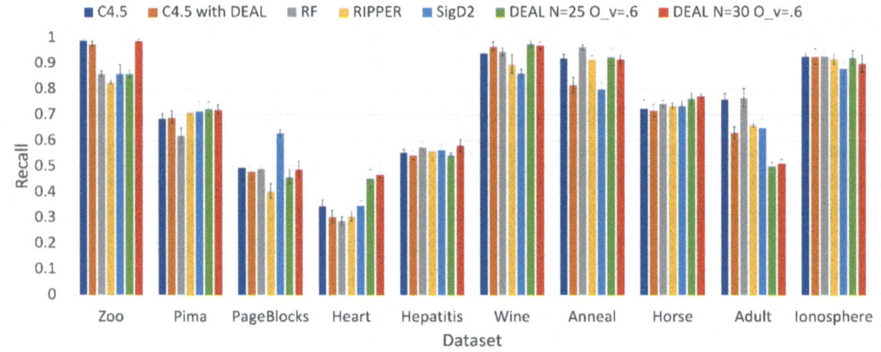

Fig. 3 Recall of C4.5, C4.5 using sampling of Deal, Random Forest (RF), RIPPER SigD2, and DEAL

There is a compromise to make with the required memory and runtime, particularly due to the aforementioned limitations of the used base learner SigD2. Therefore, we chose not to increase the number of features per base learner to more than 30. We are also interested to know the number of base learners for each of the datasets as we mentioned the number of base learners is determined automatically by DEAL. Table 2 provides the number of base learners for each of the datasets. These are significantly less than the typical 100 or even 50 used in the literature for classical ensembles.

To understand the effect of different values of O_v we also experiment with values starting from 0.1 to 0.9 increasing by 0.1 in each step. The result is provided in Fig. 5. From the figure we can see, the performance of the model is best when the value of O_v is in the middle. Because a small value results in almost unique base learners and a very small number of base learners. In the case of a large value of O_v, the results would allow repetitions of base learners like with a simple random

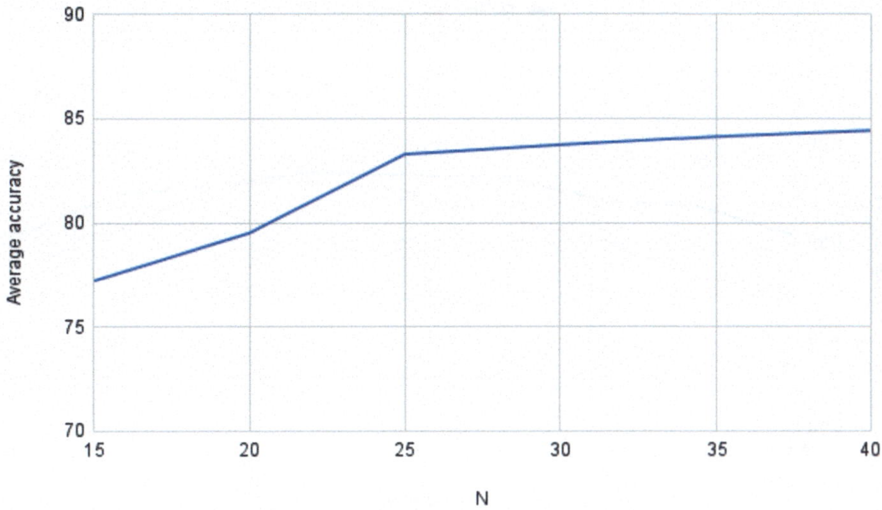

Fig. 4 Average accuracy of DEAL for different values of N(Number of selected feature for each base learner)

Table 2 Number of base learners using $N = 30$ and $O_v = 0.6$

Dataset	Feature vector size	#Base learner	Dataset	Feature vector size	#Base learner
Zoo	35	4	Wine	65	13
Pima	36	4	Anneal	67	12
PageBlocks	41	8	Horse	83	19
Heart	47	7	Adult	95	21
Hepatitis	54	10	Ionosphere	155	45

sampling procedure. Thus in both cases, the performance is affected. We can see good performance when the value of O_v is between 0.4 to 0.6 for N=30 and 0.5 to 0.7 when N=25 for the dataset we used in our experiments. Thus overlap between 0.4 to 0.7 provides an optimum result for most cases.

To understand whether the improvement in accuracy by DEAL is significant or not, we performed a statistical significance test. We carried out a student-paired t-test with the null hypothesis, that the improvement in the accuracy of DEAL is not significant. We run the whole experiment 20 times and recorded the average accuracy each time for each model. For DEAL we used $N = 30$, $O_v = 0.6$. The difference in the accuracy in each pair is calculated by Eq. (2).

$$\delta = \mathcal{M}_{DEAL}(test\_data) - \mathcal{M}_i(test\_data) \tag{2}$$

Here, $\mathcal{M}_{DEAL}$ is our proposed model, and the subscript i stands for the other models. Running the models on test data provides the accuracy of the models and δ is the difference in the accuracy.

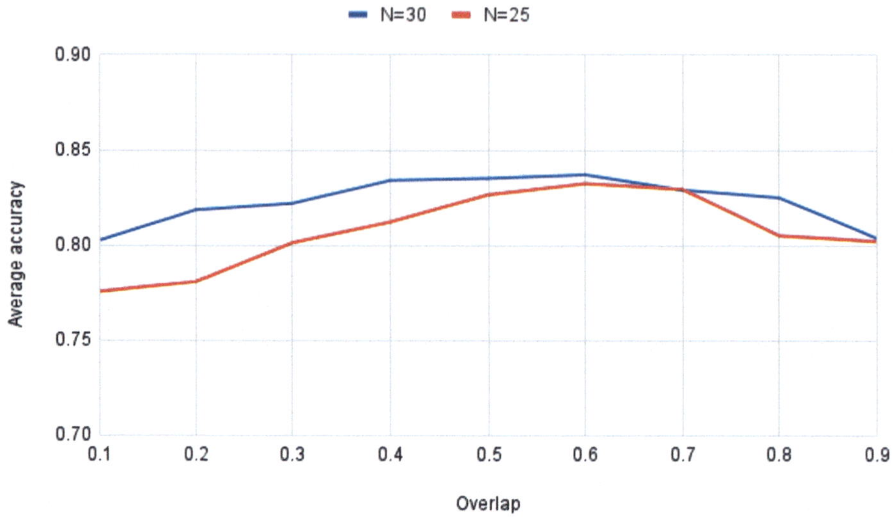

Fig. 5 Average accuracy across different values of O_v

Table 3 Statistical result

Algorithm	p-value
DEAL vs C4.5	0.0036
DEAL vs C4.5 ensemble	0.0077
DEAL vs Random forest	0.0087
DEAL vs SigD2	0.0046
DEAL vs RIPPER	0.1190

We performed the paired t-test followed by the work of Henry et al. [24] for pairwise comparison among the models and calculated the p-value. If the calculated p-value is less than the threshold alpha(0.05) then we can say the improvement by the proposed model is significant. The calculated p-values are provided in Table 3.

From Table 3 we can see the p-value for each pair is less than the threshold alpha(0.05) except for DEAL vs RIPPER. Thus, except RIPPER, for the other models we can say, the improvement in accuracy of our proposed over other models is significant.

One of the main goals of DEAL is to reduce the memory requirements for datasets having large feature vector sizes. In previous sections we showed that DEAL does not reduce the accuracy in comparison to the original SigD2 rather in almost all datasets, it increases the accuracy. Using DEAL we can reduce the memory requirements for datasets having a large number of features. The memory requirements of C4.5, an ensemble of C4.5 using the proposed feature sampling method, Random Forest, SigD2 and DEAL using N as 25 and O_v as 0.6 are shown in Table 4. Here we did not provide memory requirement using the random sampling procedure as for any given number of feature vectors in base learners, the memory requirement of SigD2 is the same. In the memory requirements, the reported result

Table 4 Memory requirement(in Megabyte) by contenders and DEAL($N = 30$ and $O_v = 0.6$)

Dataset	C4.5	C4.5 with deal	Random forest	RIPPER	SigD2	DEAL
Zoo	106	108	127	107	121	**105**
Pima	103	109	128	102	102	**101**
PageBlocks	111	117	134	111	112	**110**
Heart	105	112	129	**104**	107	**104**
Hepatitis	103	111	127	102	113	**100**
Wine	104	112	128	105	165	**100**
Anneal	107	113	129	107	150	**106**
Horse	109	112	128	109	235	**106**
Adult	195	211	252	**124**	257	252
Ionosphere	124	117	128	112	2519	**108**

Table 5 Runtime (in Seconds) by contenders and DEAL ($N = 30$, $O_v = 0.6$)

Dataset	C4.5	C4.5 with deal	Random forest	RIPPER	SigD2	DEAL
Zoo	**0.06**	0.58	0.12	0.08	3.64	6.65
Pima	1.76	3.84	**0.15**	0.41	0.47	0.89
PageBlocks	21.04	35.83	**0.24**	0.46	10.23	17.86
Heart	0.69	3.04	**0.13**	0.40	8.55	3.11
Hepatitis	0.23	2.62	**0.11**	0.26	10.41	1.25
Wine	0.17	1.27	**0.11**	0.33	0.46	1.05
Anneal	2.1	9.46	**0.14**	0.56	7.99	5.38
Horse	0.92	6.24	**0.13**	0.53	32.49	2.97
Adult	13.2	19.8	**3.19**	171.56	263.12	167.16
Ionosphere	1.86	16.13	**0.12**	0.32	1905.44	6.22

for DEAL is the highest memory used by a base learner in the process as we run the base learners sequentially. In the case of Random Forest, the trees in the forest are executed in parallel. Thus the memory requirement reported here is the memory required for running 100 decision trees in parallel.

Running base learners in parallel has a huge advantage for runtime, which we discuss in the next subsection. Further studies are required to understand whether this trade-off between memory requirement and runtime is feasible by executing the base learners of DEAL in parallel. From Table 4 we can see, DEAL decreases the memory requirements even in comparison with Random Forest. The memory requirement in SigD2 increases with the increase in features. One main reason behind this is when working with a large-size feature vector, SigD2 has to go through a huge number of class association rules (CAR). CAR increases with the increase of the feature vector size. But in our approach, with a dataset with a large feature vector size, the number of rules for each of the base learners is reduced dramatically. In the case of a dataset having a very large size of a feature vector, our proposed sampling method decreases the memory requirement to a significant extent.

We also measure the runtime of DEAL for the same datasets in comparison to Random Forest and SigD2. The runtime of the methods are provided in Table 5. In this table, we do not include random sampling (RS) as in random sampling we have to train 100 base learners in a sequential manner which would always require a longer runtime than DEAL. From Table 5, we can see Random Forest is always the fastest except for the Zoo dataset where C4.5 is faster. Despite the fact that DEAL is an ensemble and we are not running the base learners in parallel, DEAL is still faster than SigD2 in many cases. SigD2 beats DEAL when the input feature space is small because for datasets with a small feature space, DEAL still has to go through the sampling and for not having enough features, DEAL has to sample many subsamples and compare with the previously generated subsamples which increase the runtime. However, with larger feature vectors, DEAL outperforms SigD2.

One of the major advantages of our ensemble model is that the prediction of the model is interpretable. After creating subsamples of the feature space and training the base learners with each of the subsamples, base learners uncover classification rules expressed in their respective feature subspace. When predicting the class label of an instance, base learners use their own rules. There are applicable rules, applicable to the instance case, and there are applied rules, effectively used for the decision by each base learner. The applied rules that agree with the majority vote are kept. Using DEAL, we can easily gather all the applied rules selected by base learners. Those would be part of the decision explanation. In addition, the set of applied rules and the applicable rules can be used to rank features by importance vis-à-vis the final prediction. Rules gathered from the base learners can be grouped according to the class label and ranked based on their frequency among the base learners. Features are ranked by importance for a particular class label prediction. The more a feature appears in an applied rule, the more important it is. Features appearing in applicable rules get an additional boost of importance. Table 6 gives a glimpse of the individual interpretable models learned by the different base learners. In the case of the Zoo dataset, there are 4 base learners. The learned models are sets of human readable classification rules with their strength measures, typically sorted by these measures). In Table 6 we provide a subset of these rules and the feature subspace for each base learner. At inference time, each base learner finds the applicable rules for that instance and selects the rules to apply to the decision.

Table 7 shows the applicable rules per base learner for a given test instance as well as the decision for each learner before the vote. We can see that the consensus is for class 5 in this case and that there is an agreement on the importance of features 16 and 28. What constitutes the decision explanation is the list of important features but also the list of applied rules as well as applicable rules with the final class label decision as their consequent.

Table 6 Rules from the learned model in the form of "Antecedent -> Class label;(support, confidence, -ln(p-value))" where Antecedent is a conjunction of tokenised features. For interpretability, tokens are mapped back to features (attribute-value pairs)

Base learner 1		Base learner 2	
Selected features	[0, 2, 4, 6, 9, 10, 11, 12, 14, 14, 15, 15, 16, 19, 19, 19, 19, 21, 21, 23, 24, 25, 26, 29, 30, 31, 33, 33, 34, 34]	Selected features	[0, 1, 1, 3, 3, 3, 4, 4, 6, 6, 15, 15, 15, 18, 20, 20, 21, 23, 25, 25, 27, 27, 28, 29, 29, 31, 32, 32, 33, 34]
Rules	6, 23 → 3;(0.1375,1.000,−29.980) 0, 25→ 1;(0.1625,1.000,−33.384) .... 2, 34, 19 → 0;(0.3500,0.966,−28.991) 31, 2, 33, 14 → 6;(0.1125,0.750,−20.776)	Rules	27 → 6;(0.0250,1.000,−4.475)) 18, 29 → 6;(0.0750,1.000,−15.090) .... 33, 15, 21 → 2;(0.0250,0.667,−5.185) 0, 29 → 6;(0.1000,0.615,−14.797)
Base learner 3		Base learner 4	
Selected features	[1, 3, 6, 7, 7, 8, 10, 13, 14, 15, 16, 17, 19, 20, 21, 22, 24, 24, 24, 25, 27, 28, 29, 30, 30, 30, 31, 31, 32, 33]	Selected features	[0, 0, 1, 1, 1, 2, 3, 4, 5, 7, 8, 9, 9, 10, 11, 12, 12, 14, 16, 17, 17, 18, 20, 21, 22, 23, 28, 28, 30, 34]
Rules	27 → 6;(0.0250,1.000,−4.475)) 3 → 1;(0.1625,1.000,−33.384) .... 15, 6, 19 → 4;(0.0375,0.600,−9.014) 10, 6, 17, 8 → 2;(0.0375,0.600,−7.647)	Rules	7 → 0;(0.4500,1.000,−52.636) 3 → 1;(0.1625,1.000,−33.384) .... 0, 14, 17 → 1;(0.1625,0.929,−30.745) 0, 16 → 6;(0.1125,0.750,−20.776)

Table 7 Applicable rules from the generated rules by the base learners(**BL**) and decision process of DEAL

Test instance: [1, 2, 5, 6, 9, 10, 12, 14, 16, 19, 20, 22, 28, 29, 31, 33]	
Vectorized test instance: [0,1,1,0,0,1,1,0,0,1,1,0,1,0,1,0,1,0,0,1,1,0,1,0,0,0,0,0,1,1,0,1,0,1,0]	
Applicable rules by BL 1	Applicable rules by BL 2
9, 29 → 5;(0.0250,1.000,−6.267) **16**, 12 → 5;(0.0500,0.667,−11.566) 31, **16** → 6;(0.1125,0.750,−20.776)	**28** → 5;(0.0500,0.667,−11.566) 1, 20 → 0;(0.4250,1.000,−45.694)
Predicted class label: 6	Predicted class label: 5
Applicable rules by BL 3	Applicable rules by BL 4
19, **28** → 5;(0.0500,1.000,−14.274)	10, **28** → 5;(0.0500,1.000,−14.274)
Predicted class label: 5	Predicted class label: 5

4 Classification by Frequent Associative Rules

In Sect. 3, to understand the decision process of our proposed model DEAL, we need to identify the base learners who vote for the final class label and gather the rules from those base learners. If the number of base learners is large, this process can be cumbersome. To simplify the interpretation of the ensemble model, in this section we propose Classification by Frequent Association Rules (CFAR) where instead of using majority voting of the base classifiers for the final class label, we gather all the rules from the base learners. After gathering all the rules we rank and select the rules based on their ranking to determine the final class label. In this section, we compare the performance of CFAR to DEAL and other machine learning models in terms of accuracy, runtime and required memory.

4.1 Methodology

In CFAR we also use SigD2 as the base learner and one advantage of making an ensemble of SigD2 as well as other associative classifiers is that we can collect all the rules learned by the base learners from the training data set. These rules are used to label test data to a specified class label. However, selecting all the rules might include noisy rules which might affect the performance of the model. To solve this we select a subset of the rules which enhance the performance of the model. For this, we introduce the term Relative Frequency Ratio (RFR). After collecting all the rules generated by the base learners, we count the frequency of the rules. We find the Rule having the maximum frequency that we note as *max_frequency*. We calculate the RFR of any rule R by Eq. (3).

$$Relative\_frequency\_ratio(R) = \frac{Frequency(R)}{max\_frequency} \quad (3)$$

To predict the class label, we need to select rules from the generated rules. We consider a threshold T and select all the rules whose RFR is greater than or equal to T. The process of selecting rules is provided in Algorithm 4.

In this approach, we need to find an optimum value of T. But with our experiment we found this value to be different for different datasets. We show the accuracy result for our 10 datasets for different values of T in Figs. 6 and 7. We split the results of the 10 datasets in two figures for clarity.

Unfortunately as depicted on Figs. 6 and 7, there is no optimum value for T for all datasets. Therefore we design our model in such a way that the model itself can find the value of T for which we can get maximum accuracy. To achieve this goal, we outline a 3 step ensemble classifier. We describe each of the steps below:

Algorithm 4 Rules selection based on RFR

Input: Rules: all rules generated by base learners; **T:** Threshold value to select Rules.
Output: Selected_rules: rules with RFR $\geq$ T

```
Selected_rules ← []
for r in Rules do:
    if RFR(r) ≥ T:
        Selected_rules.append(r)
    end if
end for
return Selected_rules
```

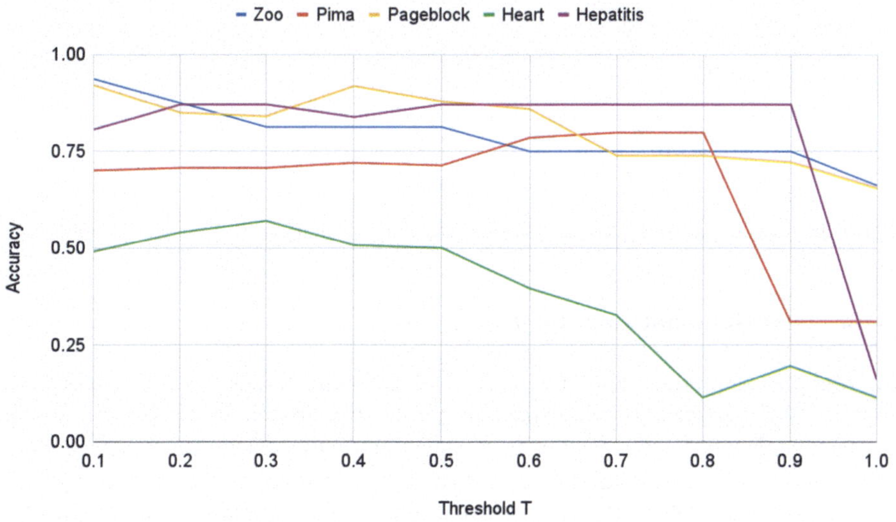

Fig. 6 Performance of the model for different values of Threshold T

4.1.1 Rule Generation

In the rule generation phase, at first, we try with the dynamic subsampling procedure of DEAL but the dynamic strategy could not perform well in this case. We will discuss this in a later section. For CFAR, we follow the random sub-sampling procedure and train 100 SigD2 base learners. We divide the dataset into train and validation data. We take 80% of the whole dataset as training data and the rest 20% as validation data. Then again we divide the training data as training and test data in the ratio of 80 and 20% respectively. To train each base learner we take a subset of the feature vector of size 30. After training 100 base learners with the training data, we gather all the rules generated by the base learners. We calculate the Relative Frequency Ratio (RFR) for each of the rules using Eq. (3).

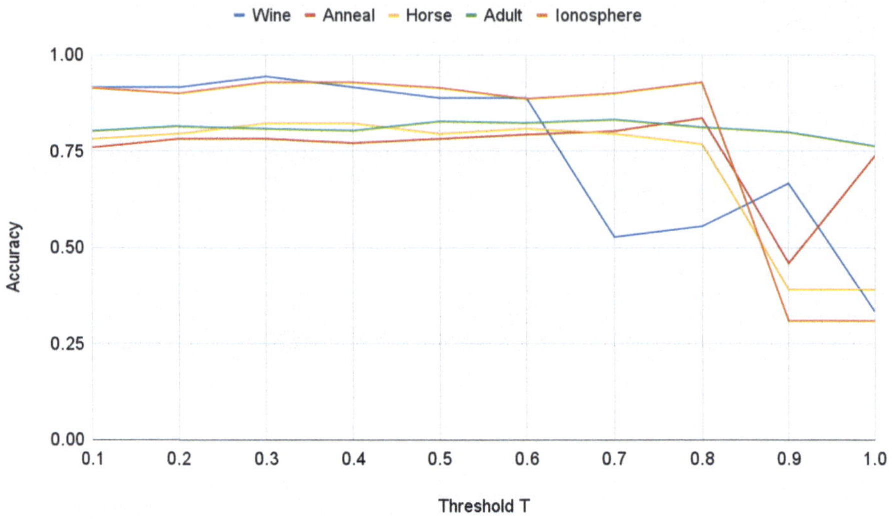

Fig. 7 Performance of the model for different values of Threshold T

4.1.2 Find Optimum Value for T

To find the optimum value for T, we try different values in a linear search fashion. We assume the importance of a rule depends on its frequency among the base learners. A rule being more frequent among base learners indicates more importance. Thus while experimenting with different values of T, at first we try with $T = 1$. We select rules from the generated rules using Algorithm 4 and predict the class label with the selected rules. In the next step, we decrease the value of T by 0.1 up to 1.0 and with that value we perform a rule selection and class prediction. In each step, we calculate the accuracy. From there we determine the optimal value of T.

4.1.3 Prediction

The last step is the prediction. From the previous step, we get the value of T which provides the best result. We select rules using that value of T and predict the class label of the validation data. With the predicted class label, we calculate the performance of the model. The whole architecture is shown in Fig. 8.

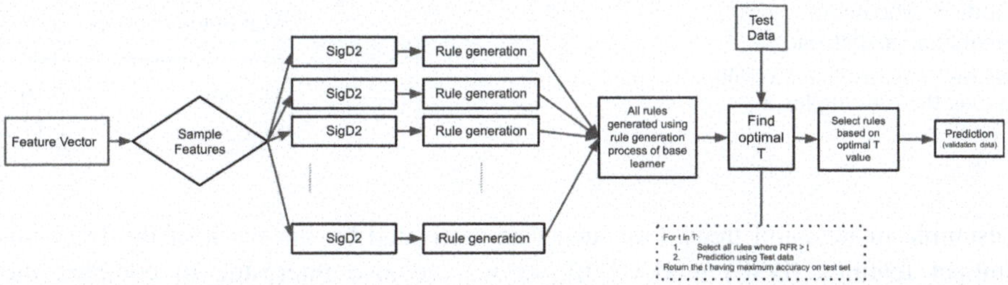

Fig. 8 Proposed model of CFAR: We generate rules by base learners using training data. We apply generated rules on test data to find the T which provides the best performance. With the help of T, we select final rules and apply them to validation data to calculate the performance of the model

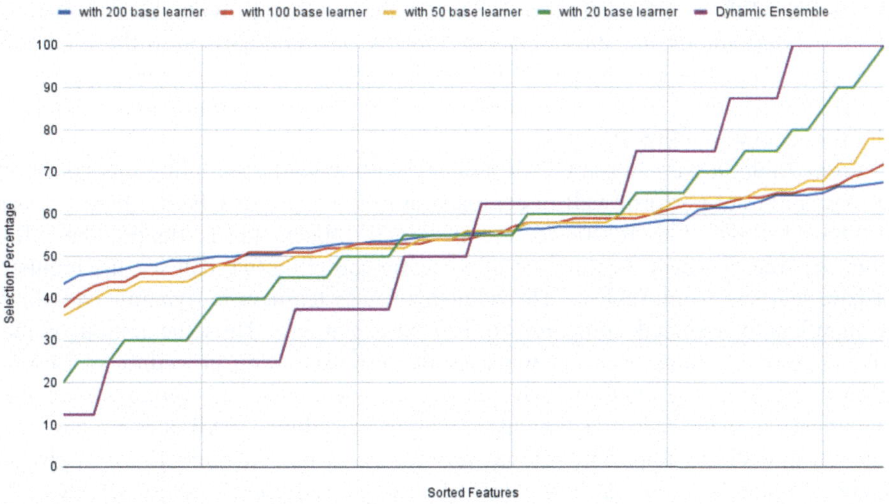

Fig. 9 Sorted frequency of appearance of the features in CFAR

4.2 Result Analysis

We use the same 10 datasets [6] with discretization [13] we mentioned in the previous section to evaluate our proposed model CFAR. As we mentioned earlier, to test our model CFAR, we use 20% of the dataset to validate our model. We further divide the rest 80% of the data into train and test data in the ratio of 80 and 20% respectively. For all other models, we use 80% of the data to train the model and rest 20% of the data is used as test data (Fig. 9).

We compare our model with SigD2 as Sood and Zaiane [35] showed SigD2 outperforms other associative classifiers, rule-based classifiers, and other state-of-the-art machine learning models. To compare the result with another interpretable model we consider C4.5 proposed by Quinlan [32]. As we are making an ensemble architecture we considered the performance of random forest [10] which is an

Table 8 Maximum, minimum, median and standard deviation of overlap among the subsamples in CFAR

Maximum overlap	0.67
Minimum overlap	0.03
Median	0.30
St. deviation	0.11

ensemble of decision trees. Our idea was motivated by the work of the Decision snippet features (DSF) model [36], so we are also interested to compare the performance of our model with it. We also considered the classical ensemble architecture where we used 100 base learners each trained with a subset of the feature vector of size 30. As we do not control the overlap of the features between the subsamples there can be different overlaps between the subsamples. We measured the overlap between the subsamples and we provide the information about overlap among the subsamples in Table 8. The comparison in the accuracy of SigD2, C4.5, Random forest, DSF model, SigD2, classical ensemble approach, DEAL, CFAR with a dynamic ensemble and CFAR is provided in Table 9. We also plot the accuracy in Fig. 10.

From Table 9, we can see CFAR strategy with dynamic sampling procedure of DEAL could not perform well in comparison to the result of CFAR where we use 100 base learners. One reason for this is, CFAR collects and learns popular rules from the base learners. In the case of dynamic sampling, we can see the number of base learners from Table 2. The number of base learners in dynamic sampling is significantly reduced compared to 100 base learners. Thus the notion of the frequency of the rules does not work for dynamic sampling procedure in CFAR. With many base classifiers, CFAR can decide which rules are important for the classification. In the case of a dynamic sampling procedure, CFAR does not have the capacity of deciding important rules as very few rules are generated. From empirical analysis, it can be seen that in the case of dynamic sampling strategy, CFAR ends up selecting all the rules every time. Thus training a large number of features is a good choice for CFAR. Another issue is when the number of base learners is small then the features are not selected uniformly. We show the frequency of appearance of the features in the base learners in Fig. 9. From the figure, we can see with the increase of base learners the uniformity of the selection of the features increases. For this reason, we go for 100 base learners with a random selection of the features.

From Table 9, we can also see in 7 among the 10 datasets CFAR has better performance than other classifiers and ensemble models. The random forest has better performance than CFAR in 3 datasets among which in Anneal dataset the margin is very large. Another interesting observation in Anneal dataset is classical ensemble approach has better performance than CFAR. That means in this dataset, the approach of CFAR where we select the rules based on the Relative Frequency Ratio (RFR) does not perform well. Further analysis is needed on this dataset to understand why CFAR is not performing well. On Average, CFAR has better performance than other models.

Table 9 Accuracy of C4.5, Random Forest(RF), Decision Snippet Features(DSF), SigD2, Classical ensemble approach(CE), DEAL, CFAR with dynamic ensemble and CFAR

Dataset	#cls	#rec	Feature vector size	C4.5	RF	DSF	SigD2	CE	DEAL	CFAR with dynamic ensemble	CFAR
Zoo	7	101	35	95.24	**97.62**	92.23	94.55	85.53	**97.62**	96.43	93.47
Pima	2	768	36	76.62	67.41	74.92	76.44	78.96	77.61	74.38	**79.22**
PageBlocks	5	5473	41	93.15	93.51	90.87	91.67	91.23	88.53	91.02	**94.42**
Heart	5	303	47	50.82	52.45	52.46	45.90	48.51	49.18	53.44	**57.38**
Hepatitis	2	155	54	70.97	78.38	74.19	81.93	76.21	82.58	81.13	**83.87**
Wine	3	178	65	91.67	77.78	92.44	92.70	81.29	92.13	90.69	**94.44**
Anneal	5	898	67	97.22	**98.89**	97.78	92.22	88.86	92.20	81.17	83.33
Horse	2	368	83	78.38	75.67	79.73	75.68	81.25	81.79	80.88	**83.78**
Adult	2	48,842	95	84.06	84.97	82.53	**84.59**	81.81	81.51	81.71	83.31
Ionosphere	2	351	155	88.73	**95.78**	88.18	90.18	90.77	94.04	91.55	92.96
Average				82.69	82.25	82.53	82.89	80.44	83.72	82.24	**84.62**

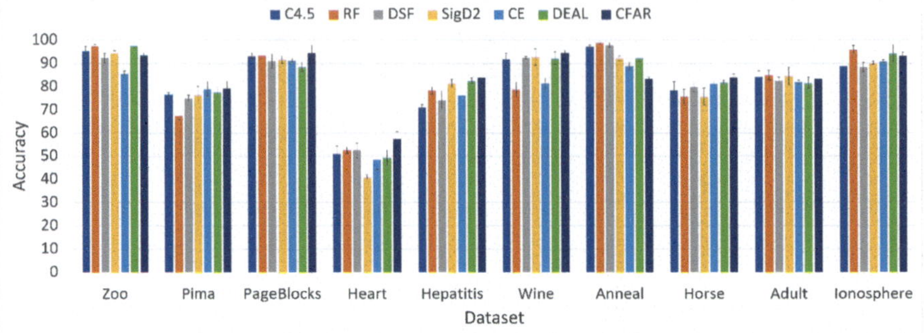

Fig. 10 Accuracy of C4.5, Random Forest(RF), Decision Snippet Features(DSF), SigD2, Classical ensemble approach(CE), DEAL and CFAR

Table 10 Statistical result

Algorithm	p-value
CFAR vs C4.5	0.0036
CFAR vs Random forest	0.0061
CFAR vs DSF	0.0007
CFAR vs SigD2	0.0001
CFAR vs Classical ensemble	5.3317e-11
CFAR vs DEAL	0.0426

We also perform a statistical test to understand whether the improvement in accuracy by CFAR is significant or not. In the test, we follow the same procedure that we mention in Sect. 3 using the null hypothesis as the improvement in accuracy by CFAR is not significant and calculate the p-value. We provide the calculated p-value in Table 10. From Table 10, we can say, in the dataset we used, except for DSF, CFAR shows significant improvement over accuracy.

From Table 10, we can see in 5 of them, the p-value is less than alpha(0.05). In the case of DSF, the p-value is large than the threshold value alpha. Thus we can say, except for DSF, in the dataset we used, CFAR shows significant improvement in accuracy.

Further, we analyze the precision and recall values of the models. Figures 11 and 12 show the precision and recall values of the models respectively. From the two figures, we can see CFAR has a very competitive performance compared to the other models in terms of precision and recall.

One of our main goals for making an ensemble of SigD2 is to eliminate the limitation of requiring very high amount of memory with the increase of the feature vector size. We measure the memory required by the models using the python library *psutil*. Table 11 shows the memory requirement for SigD2, CFAR and other contenders.

From Table 11, we can see, in the comparison of memory requirement between CFAR and SigD2 has two different scenarios. When the size of the feature vector is small, the memory requirement of SigD2 and CFAR are very close. However,

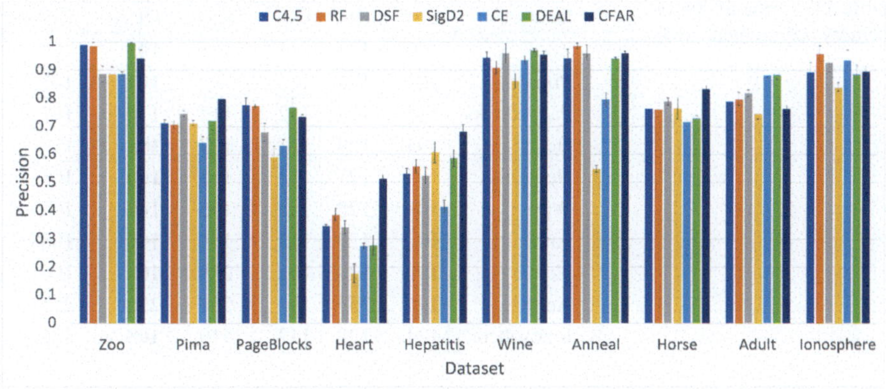

Fig. 11 Precision of C4.5, Random Forest(RF), Decision Snippet Features(DSF), SigD2, Classical ensemble approach(CE), DEAL and CFAR

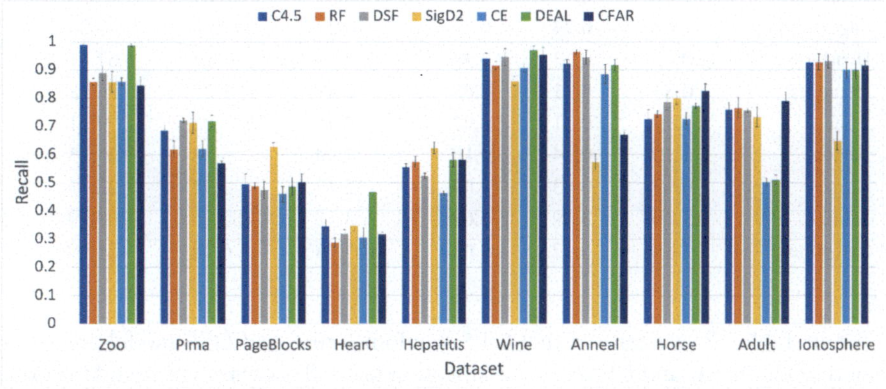

Fig. 12 Recall of C4.5, Random Forest(RF), Decision Snippet Features(DSF), SigD2, Classical ensemble approach(CE), DEAL and CFAR

with the increase in feature vector size, the memory requirement of SigD2 increases drastically while for CFAR the memory requirement remains stable. Thus we can say, CFAR eliminates the high memory requirement of SigD2 in case of a dataset with a large feature vector size. In comparison to DEAL, the memory requirement of CFAR is slightly higher than DEAL.

Another limitation of SigD2 is the runtime: it increases with the increase of feature vector space. The architecture of CFAR should solve that issue as for each of the base learners, we are taking a fixed-size subset. To understand this, we measure the runtime of CFAR, SigD2 and other contenders. The comparison is shown in Table 12. All the experiments are done on the machine with an Intel core i7 processor and 16 GB of RAM.

Table 11 Comparision of memory requirement(MB)

Dataset	C4.5	RF	DSF	SigD2	DEAL	CFAR
Zoo	106	127	112	121	**105**	106
Pima	103	128	112	102	**101**	105
PageBlocks	111	124	112	112	110	**107**
Heart	105	129	112	107	**104**	119
Hepatitis	103	127	113	113	**100**	108
Wine	104	128	112	165	**100**	107
Anneal	107	129	113	150	**106**	108
Horse	109	128	112	235	**106**	108
Adult	195	253	196	257	**252**	255
Ionosphere	124	128	113	2519	**108**	136

Table 12 Comparison of Run time(seconds)

Dataset	C4.5	RF	DSF	SigD2	DEAL	CFAR
Zoo	**0.06**	0.12	0.31	3.64	6.65	8.23
Pima	1.76	0.15	**0.10**	0.47	0.89	28.32
PageBlocks	21.04	**0.24**	0.86	10.23	17.86	21.38
Heart	0.69	0.13	**0.34**	8.55	3.11	67.51
Hepatitis	0.23	**0.11**	0.08	10.41	1.25	26.58
Wine	0.17	0.11	**0.07**	0.46	1.05	9.61
Anneal	2.10	0.14	**0.10**	7.99	5.38	23.75
Horse	0.92	0.13	**0.09**	32.49	2.97	23.33
Adult	13.20	3.19	**1.60**	263.12	167.16	200.79
Ionosphere	1.86	0.12	**0.08**	1905.44	6.22	27.09

From Table 12, we can see that C4.5, random forest, and DSF model are faster than SigD2, DEAL and CFAR in classification tasks. This was expected. However, between SigD2 and CFAR, the dataset having a small size of feature vector, SigD2 is faster than CFAR. This is also expected since CFAR has 100 base learners which are trained sequentially. No parallel processing is performed at this stage in the experiment. Thus for datasets having small feature vector size, SigD2 is faster than CFAR. When the size of the feature vector is large, CFAR wins by a significant amount despite the overhead of the ensemble running sequentially. In the comparison of the run time between DEAL and CFAR, CFAR requires more time than DEAL. While training CFAR, the model considers different values for RFR and choose the best one. Selecting rules using each RFR and evaluating them requires more time than the DEAL. We consider this as a trade-off to make the model more interpretable.

4.2.1 Performance Analysis on Different Sizes of the Subset of Feature Vector

In our whole experiments with CFAR we always selected a subset of the feature vector of size 30. This is because from experiments, we found, the performance of SigD2 to be affected if the feature vector size is greater than 30. In this section, we conduct an experiment for a different size for the subset of feature vector. We start the experiment by selecting subset of size 15 and in each step, we increase the size by 5 until a size of 40. In Figs. 13, 14, and 15 we can see the average accuracy, average memory requirement, and average runtime of the datasets for different sizes of subset of feature vector respectively.

Figure 13 shows an increase of the accuracy with the increase of the size of the subset of feature vector. In the beginning, the rate of increase in accuracy is high but with the increase in the size of the subset, the rate of increase slows down. This shows that the more features we can bundle in a feature subspace for a base learner, the more CFAR can take advantage of possible feature inter-dependence. Figures 14 and 15 show the memory requirement and runtime increase with the increase of the size of the feature subspace. Beyond 30, this increase accelerates. Therefore we conclude that 30 is a good compromise for a good accuracy while considering memory requirement and runtime.

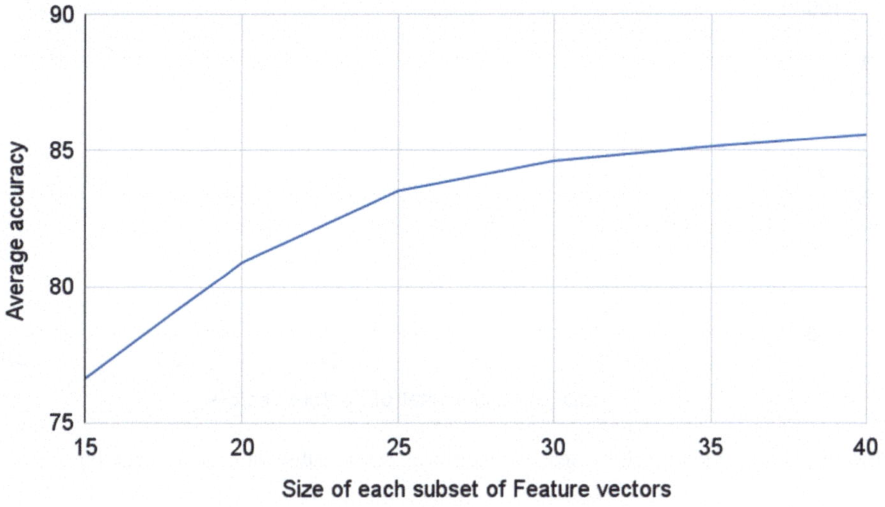

Fig. 13 Average accuracy of 10 datasets for different size of the subset of Feature vector for CFAR

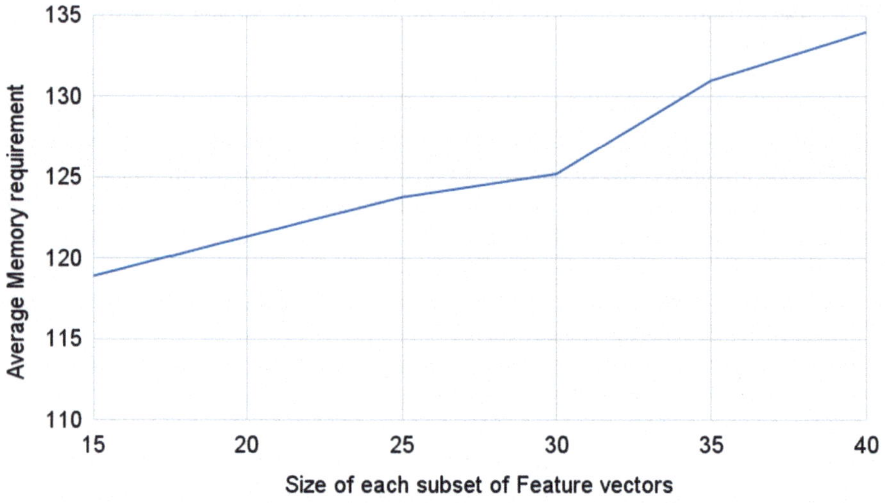

Fig. 14 Average Memory requirement of 10 datasets for different size of subset of Feature vector for CFAR

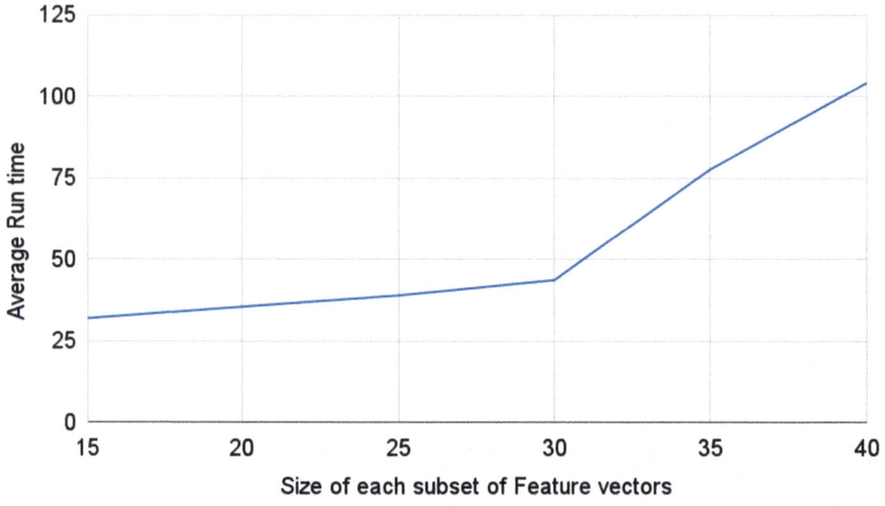

Fig. 15 Average Runtime of 10 datasets for different size of subset of Feature vector for CFAR

4.2.2 Effect of Number of Base Learners

In our model, we use 100 base learners. We are interested to know the effect of the number of base learners in CFAR. Thus we tested the model with a different number of base learners. In Fig. 16 we can see the performance of CFAR for a

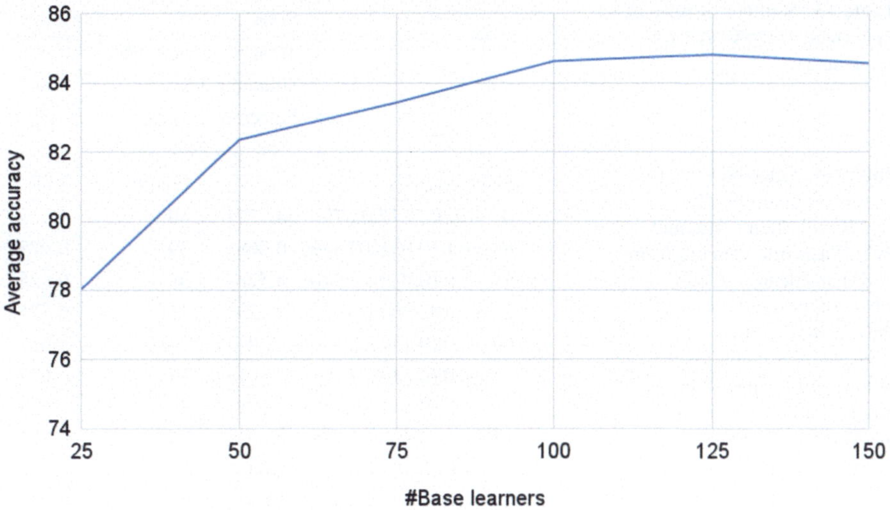

Fig. 16 Effect of number of base learners on average accuracy in CFAR

different number of base learners. In this experiment, we consider the size of the subset of the feature vector to be 30.

From Fig. 13, we can see when the number of base learners is reduced the average accuracy is low. With the increase of the base learners, accuracy increases. Beyond 100 base learners, the accuracy almost reaches a plateau then decreases. Considering the runtime there seems no advantage in having an ensemble larger than 100.

4.2.3 Interpretability and Explainability

The major advantages of the associative classifier is the production of human-readable rules and by analyzing the rules it is easier to understand the decision process of the classifier. The associative classifier is therefore in itself explainable. An ensemble, however, is not straight forwardly explainable. In the classical ensemble approach, each of the base learners predicts the class label of test instances, and the final prediction is determined by a maximum vote. In the case of the ensemble of associative classifiers, to interpret the decision process we need to keep track of the base learners who voted for the final class label and then get the rules from those base learners. In this process, the number of base learners who voted for the final class label can be quite large and we need to consider the decision process of each of the base learners. Along with this, there can be some rules which have different weights in different base learners. This way of interpreting results can be difficult and time-consuming and create huge confusion.

With the CFAR approach, instead of using the max vote strategy, we collect all the rules and select rules based on their frequency. This process reduces the number

Table 13 Number of rules at each stage of the CFAR for horse dataset

Stage	#Rules
Total generated rules	1848
Unique rules	569
Selected rules	13

Table 14 Selected rules for final class prediction by CFAR with their count and RFR. Each rule is in the form of "Antecedent → Class label;(support, confidence, -ln(p-value))" where Antecedent is a conjunction of tokenised features. For interpretability, tokens are mapped back to features (attribute-value pairs)

Selected rules	Frequency	RFR
0 → 0;(0.5277,0.873,−54.379)	40	1
63 → 1;(0.0340,0.889,−6.068)	39	0.975
49 → 0;(0.0894,0.840,−4.528)	33	0.825
1 → 1;(0.3064,0.791,−57.129)	31	0.775
64 → 0;(0.1447,0.944,−13.211)	26	0.65
55 → 0;(0.1191,0.903,−8.601)	25	0.625
60 → 0;(0.1915,0.738,−4.093)	25	0.625
15 → 0;(0.4000,0.718,−8.093)	25	0.625
48 → 0;(0.1957,0.821,−8.635)	24	0.6
54 → 0;(0.1064,0.833,−5.093)	24	0.6
78 → 0;(0.1447,0.919,−11.476)	24	0.6
62 → 1;(0.0681,0.800,−9.304)	24	0.6
12 → 1;(0.0936,0.595,−5.567)	24	0.6

of rules as well as eliminates the necessity of understanding the decision process of each of the base learners who voted for the final class label. In Table 13 we provide a comparative analysis of the number of total generated rules by the base learners, number of unique rules, and number of rules selected by CFAR for the classification process.

From Table 13 we can see, for a given datasets (Horse dataset), the total number of generated rules is very high compared to the selected rules. The total generated rules are 1848. But in the case of CFAR, only 13 rules are selected for the final prediction. Thus to understand decision process of the classifier we need to analyze only 13 rules. In Table 14, we provide the rules selected by CFAR for the final class prediction from the generated rules with their frequency and Relative Frequency Ratio (RFR). From Table 14 we can see it is very convenient to understand the decision process of CFAR.

4.3 CFAR++

In the case of CFAR, we use SigD2 as the base learner. SigD2 implements a 2-step pruning strategy to remove the rules which are not statistically significant[35]. That means in CFAR, each of the base learners goes through the two-stage pruning and outputs the rules after the pruning, before all these are combined. As CFAR selects rules from the aggregated rules, we further speculate there can be many rules in the base learner where any rule may not be statistically significant for the subset of the feature vector of that base learner but can be statistically significant considering the whole dataset. For this reason, we are interested in a different approach where we remove the rule pruning strategy from base learner SigD2 and delay it to the final stage. That is, each of the base learners only generates rules but unfiltered. We then aggregate all the rules from the base learners and select rules from the aggregated rules in the same way as CFAR. After selecting the rules, we find the statistically significant rules using the whole training dataset following the strategy of Li and Zaiane [27]. By this step, we prune rules that are not globally statistically significant. After this pruning step, the classification is done using the remaining rules. Figure 17 shows the architecture of CFAR++. This architecture is almost similar to CFAR. The only differences are in the base learners where we remove the pruning mechanism and an additional pruning step after selecting rules from the aggregated rules.

CFAR++ is our ongoing research project. We only have the preliminary result for the performance of CFAR++. We provide the comparison of CFAR and CFAR++ in Table15 in terms of accuracy and a number of selected rules for classification. From Table 15 we can see that the results of CFAR++ are very competitive to CFAR in

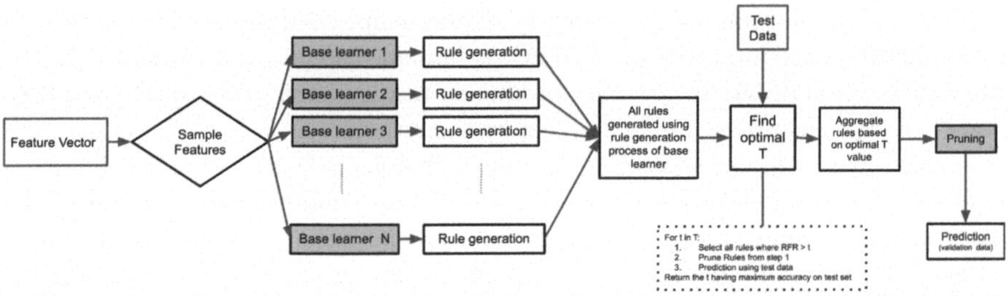

Fig. 17 Proposed model of CFAR++: We follow the same strategy as CFAR except we remove the pruning phase from the base learner and add pruning after selecting rules following the strategy of CFAR

Table 15 Comparison on accuracy and rules for classification between CFAR and CFAR++

Dataset	Accuracy		Rules for classification	
	CFAR	CFAR++	CFAR	CFAR++
Zoo	93.47	80.95	21	15
Pima	79.22	79.87	17	10
PageBlocks	94.42	91.51	38	26
Heart	57.38	54.10	141	35
Hepatitis	83.87	80.65	6	21
Wine	94.44	80.56	28	20
Anneal	83.33	96.11	26	36
Horse	83.78	75.68	13	43
Adult	83.31	82.67	57	54
Ionosphere	92.96	95.77	83	46

terms of accuracy. From the preliminary analysis, we also find, in most of the cases, in the classification process of CFAR++ there are less rules than CFAR which means there are still some noisy rules found by CFAR. Moreover, there are good rules found only by CFAR++ indicating that CFAR may not preserve all relevant rules as it does not consider the entire training dataset when pruning. In the future, we aim to evaluate the rules that are present in CFAR but not present in CFAR++ and vise-versa to get a better insight.

5 Conclusion and Future Work

In this study, we propose Dynamic Ensemble Associative Learning (DEAL) where we use SigD2 as a base learner with a feature sampling method that eliminates the need to fix the size of the ensemble while ensuring diversity and feature space coverage. Evaluating the model over different datasets reveals an increase of accuracy compared to SigD2 and other classifiers, even competing with Random Forest on average. DEAL solves the limitation of SigD2 requiring huge memory and runtime if the feature vector space is large. Memory requirement and runtime of DEAL do not increase with the increase in feature vectors like SigD2. Along with decreasing the runtime and memory requirement, we designed DEAL in such a way that the decision process of DEAL is human readable and explainable. The sampling method of DEAL provides promising results when using SigD2 as a base learner since it ensures diversity and feature space coverage.

Further, we propose another ensemble technique Classification by Frequent Association Rules (CFAR) using SigD2 as the base learner where instead of the classical max voting strategy, we aggregate all the rules generated by the base learners and select frequent rules (i.e. popular among the base learners) for the classification task. An experiment with 10 different datasets shows CFAR increases the accuracy in most cases. CFAR also eliminates the limitation of high memory requirement and runtime of SigD2 in case of a dataset having a large feature vector size. In CFAR, instead of the classical ensemble process, we design the ensemble in such a way that the decision process remains human-readable and explainable, and can be understood by analyzing a very small number remaining rules. Along with providing promising performance in terms of accuracy, memory requirement, and run time, CFAR also preserves interpretability. Understanding the decision process of CFAR is easier than any other ensemble model.

The sampling method of DEAL provides promising results when using SigD2 as a base learner since it ensures diversity and feature space coverage. Random Forest also uses a subset of the features and the subsets are chosen randomly. It would be interesting to use our sampling method in the case of Random Forest. This would eliminate the need to predetermine the number of estimators in Random Forest. DEAL is a framework where the base learner SigD2 could be replaced. A better rule based learner that is not as constrained by the dimensionality of the feature space could allow experimenting with a larger sampled feature subspace.

Our study comprises applying CFAR only to tabular data. In the future, we want to deploy CFAR on text and image data. In our model, we replace the max voting strategy with aggregating the association rules for final prediction. It would be interesting to explore the same strategy in other interpretable ensemble models. While selecting rules in CFAR we use simple criteria which we call Relative Frequency Ration (RFR) which we calculate based on the frequency of appearance of a rule. It would be worth investigating other measures to select rules.

Acknowledgments The authors gratefully acknowledge the funding from the Natural Sciences and Engineering Research Council (NSERC) of Canada and the Canada CIFAR AI Chairs Program for the Alberta Machine Intelligence Institute.

References

1. Rakesh Agrawal, Ramakrishnan Srikant, et al. "Fast algorithms for mining association rules". In: *Proc. 20th int. conf. very large data bases, VLDB*. Vol. 1215. Citeseer. 1994, pp. 487–499.
2. Maria-Luiza Antonie and Osmar R Zaiane. "Text document categorization by term association". In: *2002 IEEE International Conference on Data Mining, 2002. Proceedings*. IEEE. 2002, pp. 19–26.
3. Maria-Luiza Antonie, Osmar R Zaiane, and Robert C Holte. "Learning to use a learned model: A two-stage approach to classification". In: *Sixth International Conference on Data Mining (ICDM'06)*. IEEE. 2006, pp. 33–42.
4. Alejandro Barredo Arrieta et al. "Explainable Artificial Intelligence (XAI): Concepts, taxonomies, opportunities and challenges toward responsible AI". In: *Information fusion* 58 (2020), pp. 82–115.
5. Bavani Arunasalam and Sanjay Chawla. "CCCS: a top-down associative classifier for imbalanced class distribution". In: *Proceedings of the 12th ACM SIGKDD international conference on Knowledge discovery and data mining*. 2006, pp. 517–522.
6. Arthur Asuncion and David Newman. *UCI machine learning repository*. 2007.
7. Karthik R Bandi and Sargur N Srihari. "Writer demographic classification using bagging and boosting". In: *Proc. 12th Int. Graphonomics Society Conference*. 2005, pp. 133–137.
8. Roberto J Bayardo Jr. "Brute-Force Mining of High-Confidence Classification Rules." In: *KDD*. Vol. 97. 1997, pp. 123–126.
9. Leo Breiman. "Bagging predictors". In: *Machine learning* 24.2 (1996), pp. 123–140.
10. Leo Breiman. "Random forests". In: *Machine learning* 45.1 (2001), pp. 5–32.
11. Gavin Brown. "Diversity in neural network ensembles". PhD thesis. Citeseer, 2004.
12. Peng Cao, Dazhe Zhao, and Osmar R Zaiane. "Cost sensitive adaptive random subspace ensemble for computer-aided nodule detection". In: *Proceedings of the 26th IEEE International Symposium on Computer-Based Medical Systems*. IEEE. 2013, pp. 173–178.
13. Frans Coenen. *The LUCS–KDD software library*. 2004.
14. William W Cohen. "Fast effective rule induction". In: *Machine learning proceedings 1995*. Elsevier, 1995, pp. 115–123.
15. Corinna Cortes and Vladimir Vapnik. "Support-vector networks". In: *Machine learning* 20.3 (1995), pp. 273–297.
16. Belur V Dasarathy and Belur V Sheela. "A composite classifier system design: Concepts and methodology". In: *Proceedings of the IEEE* 67.5 (1979), pp. 708–713.
17. Yoav Freund, Robert E Schapire, et al. "Experiments with a new boosting algorithm". In: *icml*. Vol. 96. Citeseer. 1996, pp. 148–156.

18. Jerome H Friedman. "Greedy function approximation: a gradient boosting machine". In: *Annals of statistics* (2001), pp. 1189–1232.
19. Martin T Hagan, Howard B Demuth, and Maark Beale. *Neural network design*. PWS Publishing Co., 1997.
20. MT Hagan, HB Demuth, and M Beale. "Neural Network Design (PWS, Boston, MA)". In: *Google Scholar Google Scholar Digital Library Digital Library* (1996).
21. Wilhelmiina Hämäläinen and Matti Nykänen. "Efficient discovery of statistically significant association rules". In: *2008 Eighth IEEE international conference on data mining*. IEEE. 2008, pp. 203–212.
22. Jiawei Han, Jian Pei, and Yiwen Yin. "Mining frequent patterns without candidate generation". In: *ACM sigmod record* 29.2 (2000), pp. 1–12.
23. Trevor Hastie et al. "Multi-class adaboost". In: *Statistics and its Interface* 2.3 (2009), pp. 349–360.
24. Henry Hsu and Peter A Lachenbruch. "Paired t test". In: *Wiley StatsRef: statistics reference online* (2014).
25. Md Rayhan Kabir and Osmar R Zaiane. "Classification by Frequent Association Rules". In: *The 38th ACM/SIGAPP Symposium on Applied Computing (SAC '23)*. 2023.
26. Md Rayhan Kabir and Osmar R Zaiane. "Dynamic Ensemble Associative Learning". In: *2022 IEEE/ACM International Conference on Advances in Social Networks Analysis and Mining (ASONAM)*. 2022, pp. 261–268.
27. Jundong Li and Osmar R Zaiane. "Exploiting statistically significant dependent rules for associative classification". In: *Intelligent Data Analysis* 21.5 (2017), pp. 1155–1172.
28. Wenmin Li, Jiawei Han, and Jian Pei. "CMAR: Accurate and efficient classification based on multiple class-association rules". In: *Proceedings 2001 IEEE international conference on data mining*. IEEE. 2001, pp. 369–376.
29. Bing Liu, Wynne Hsu, Yiming Ma, et al. "Integrating classification and association rule mining." In: *Kdd*. Vol. 98. 1998, pp. 80–86.
30. Bing Liu, Yiming Ma, and Ching Kian Wong. "Improving an association rule based classifier". In: *European Conference on Principles of Data Mining and Knowledge Discovery*. Springer. 2000, pp. 504–509.
31. Joseph Prusa, Taghi M Khoshgoftaar, and Amri Napolitano. "Utilizing ensemble, data sampling and feature selection techniques for improving classification performance on tweet sentiment data". In: *2015 IEEE 14th International Conference on Machine Learning and Applications (ICMLA)*. IEEE. 2015, pp. 535–542.
32. J Ross Quinlan. *C4. 5: programs for machine learning*. Elsevier, 2014.
33. J Ross Quinlan. "Induction of decision trees". In: *Machine learning* 1.1 (1986), pp. 81–106.
34. Ravid Shwartz-Ziv and Amitai Armon. "Tabular data: Deep learning is not all you need". In: *Information Fusion* 81 (2022), pp. 84–90.
35. Nitakshi Sood and Osmar R Zaiane. "Building a competitive associative classifier". In: *International Conference on Big Data Analytics and Knowledge Discovery*. Springer. 2020, pp. 223–234.
36. Pascal Welke et al. "Decision Snippet Features". In: *2020 25th International Conference on Pattern Recognition (ICPR)*. IEEE. 2021, pp. 4260–4267.
37. Xiaoxin Yin and Jiawei Han. "CPAR: Classification based on predictive association rules". In: *Proceedings of the 2003 SIAM international conference on data mining*. SIAM. 2003, pp. 331–335.
38. Osmar R Zaiane and Maria-Luiza Antonie. "On pruning and tuning rules for associative classifiers". In: *International Conference on Knowledge- Based and Intelligent Information and Engineering Systems*. Springer. 2005, pp. 966–973.

Scalable Algorithms to Measure User Influence in Social Networks

Nouamane Arhachoui, Esteban Bautista, Maximilien Danisch, Anastasios Giovanidis, and Lionel Tabourier

Abstract Measuring user influence in social networks is crucial for a variety of applications. While traditional centrality metrics evaluate structural graph importance, a more recent metric known as the ψ-score takes into account users' posting and re-posting activities to provide richer information. The ψ-score is a powerful tool that generalizes PageRank for non-homogeneous node activity. However, for large datasets with N users, it becomes computationally expensive, requiring solving N linear systems of N equations. To tackle this issue, we propose three new scalable algorithms that can quickly approximate the ψ-score. The Power-ψ and Push-ψ algorithms are based on a novel equation that shows it is sufficient to solve one system of equations of size N to calculate the ψ-score. These algorithms take advantage of the fact that the solution of such a system can be recursively and distributedly approximated. Consequently, the ψ-score, which summarizes the nodes' structural and behavioral information, can be computed as quickly as PageRank. The third proposed algorithm is Push-NF. Despite aiming to solve all N systems to extract additional information on the information dynamics, it still manages to converge to the accurate user ranking faster than the current state-of-the-art alternative. To validate the effectiveness of our proposed algorithms, we release them as an open-source Python library and test them on various real-world datasets.

Keywords Social Networks · PsiScore · Ranking · Algorithms · Influence

N. Arhachoui (✉) · E. Bautista · M. Danisch · A. Giovanidis · L. Tabourier
Sorbonne Université, CNRS – LIP6, Paris, France
e-mail: nouamane.arhachoui@lip6.fr

M. Kaya et al. (eds.), *Social Network Analysis and Mining Applications in Healthcare and Anomaly Detection*, Lecture Notes in Social Networks,
https://doi.org/10.1007/978-3-031-75204-9_3

1 Introduction

1.1 Context

Measuring the importance of an individual in a network has been a focus of interest in Social Network Analysis for long. Indeed, a wealth of metrics have been developed to quantify this idea, including the well-known closeness centrality in the 1950s [1] or the betweenness centrality in the 1970s [2].

Nowadays, the ubiquitous nature of Online Social Platforms (OSPs) makes it all the more important to have relevant measurements available. For instance, it is essential for social scientists to identify the main leaders of opinion in a network in order to gain a better understanding of the dynamics that determine the roots of political polarization [3]. Also, it is crucial for companies to identify the so-called *influencers* that are believed to play a key role in the emergence of new trends [4] and thus are targeted to develop effective marketing strategies [5]. From a technical perspective, machine learning algorithms also rely on the identification of a reduced set of users with features present throughout the network, which is critical in reducing the number of parameters and avoiding the curse of dimensionality [6, 7].

In this context, many OSPs may be described using a comparable structure: users have access to a *wall* and a *news feed*, they can publish messages (*posts*) on their wall, while their news feed shows the messages posted by other specific users, known as their leaders (or followees). This archetype is well illustrated by Twitter, Facebook and Weibo among others. Users can also re-post messages from their news feed to their wall, which is the main mechanism allowing posts to spread around the network [8]. A crucial issue is to quantify the extent to which their posts and re-posts circulate throughout the network and are accessible to others, as this process can be understood as the measure of their influence.

To address the aforementioned challenge, a variety of centrality metrics have been proposed to rank network nodes according to their structural relevance [9]. But given the potentially massive size of these networks, it is crucial that these measures remain scalable. For instance, betweenness centrality measures to what extent a node falls on the shortest paths between others and thus its potential to control communication, however, the most efficient algorithms have a temporal complexity in $O(NM)$ [10] (where N is the number of nodes and M the number of edges) which makes it inappropriate for large OSPs. In addition to that, most centralities are unsuitable for assessing influence in OSPs, as they rely on a static description of the social network, while these are known to be dynamic platforms, where the activity of users is typically bursty. Nonetheless, these scores do not include user posting and sharing activity. The importance of this information is emphasized in [11], which demonstrates that people with the most followers (in-degree) may not necessarily create the most retweets or views. Therefore, influence is not solely based on the number of followers, which is mainly related to a user's popularity. In the same line of inquiry, the authors in [12] ask th question: *"Are social links valid indicators of real user interaction?"* and underline the difference between these two ideas by examining a significant user trace from Facebook. It is thus essential to get past simple structural measures.

A new metric, coined as ψ-score, has been recently introduced in [13] to overcome this limitation. The diffusion of information model presented in [13] takes into account users' behaviors by including activity features for each user. The ψ-score results from this model and provides a more accurate ranking metric of user influence in OSPs by integrating both structural information related to the graph and user activity. For instance, if users post and re-post content at different frequencies, the model incorporates this variation in the users' activity, thus yielding a more meaningful ranking metric. Furthermore, it was shown in [13, Theorem 5] that the ψ-score is equivalent to PageRank when user activity is homogeneous, *i.e.*, when all users create the same number of posts within a given time interval and share at the same rate within that interval. As a consequence, the ψ-score can be seen as a generalization of the PageRank, which is designed for situations where we have access to the nodes' activity in the network.

1.2 Goal and Contributions

A limitation of the ψ-score calculation as described in [13] is that it does not scale to large graphs. Indeed, it requires the resolution of N linear systems of N equations each, where N denotes the number of users in the network. In contrast, PageRank only requires finding the solution of a single system with N variables. This paper addresses this shortcoming by proposing new ψ-score calculation algorithms that solve this issue.

For that purpose, we reorganize these N systems into a single one whose solution can be used to easily derive the ψ-score for all users. Then, we propose two different algorithms to solve this new system:

- `Power-`ψ which is based on power-iteration rules in order to approximate the solution (see also the conference version of this work [14]). This process allows approximating the sum of a geometric series for vectors without computing any matrix inversion.
- `Push-`ψ, an algorithm inspired by the push-flow algorithm for PageRank [15, 16]. It uses an approximation vector and a residual representing the difference between the exact solution and the approximation. During each push iteration, the approximated score of a node is updated and its residual is pushed to the residual of its neighbors in order to be minimized.

In addition to this contribution, we also propose to use the push method to make a tool to analyze the influence mechanisms at a finer grain. For this purpose, we describe another push-based algorithm, named `Push-NF`, that aims to solve the original N linear systems presented in [13] instead of using the new system. While it does not allow to avoid the scalability issue aforementioned, by solving all N systems, `Push-NF` can not only extract the influence of each user on the entire network but also their influence on a specified individual. This feature provides valuable information for various applications, such as identifying opinion leaders or understanding information flow dynamics between specific users.

Finally, we provide an open-source software library[1] to facilitate the implementation of the ψ-score. This comprehensive library includes its initial baseline implementation as well as implementations of each of the improved algorithms proposed in this paper. By making this library available to the community, we aim to encourage the widespread use of the ψ-score in various fields and its adaptation to each developer's specific needs. In particular, the `psi-score` library can be used to compare the metric with PageRank, since they are equivalent when the network activity is homogeneous.

1.3 Related Works

Centrality measures have been largely used in various fields of network science, including of course social network analysis [17–19], but also transportation networks for example to improve traffic monitoring [20], communication networks to design routing protocols [21] or to improve network control [22], or even in biology, where they allow for instance to point out critical proteins in metabolic networks [23]. Another essential application of centrality measures is information retrieval: with the expansion of the web, there is an ever-increasing need for algorithms that allow one to look for precise information in a very large database. Among those, the most famous example is certainly the PageRank [24, 25]. Although these metrics are commonly used to rank nodes of a network [9], they only consider the network structure. For instance, PageRank can be described in non-technical terms as a random walk on a graph with a probability of teleporting on a random node at each step, so it does not take into account aspects such as node activity.

A standard way to compute the PageRank in a graph is to rely on a power iteration method [25, Chapter 4]. Various existing algorithms, such as Push [15] or methods using Chebyshev polynomials [26], exploit the random walk interpretation of PageRank to speed up its calculation. The Push method [15] iterates through nodes by allowing each of them to update the approximation of its own PageRank value and its neighbors' values. The method proposed in [26] uses Chebyshev polynomials to approximate the PageRank vector more efficiently than the known power-method introduced with the metric [24].

In a short version of this work [14], we have investigated the algebraic limitations of the ψ-score and proposed a novel approach to have it as scalable as the PageRank is. However, we acknowledge that other strategies to accelerate graph eigenvalue-based measures have the potential to further improve the performance of our

[1] https://github.com/NouamaneA/psi-score.

method. Moreover, they can also give us insight into the mechanisms of social influence from one individual to another. Therefore, in this study, we aim to build upon this work by considering the Push method and integrating it with our approach. Our goal is to create a novel algorithm that not only addresses the limitations of the ψ-score but also surpasses the existing methods in terms of speed.

1.4 Outline of the Paper

In Sect. 2, we describe the principles underlying the definition of the ψ-score and to what extent it measures the spread of influence on a social platform, as well as the baseline algorithm to compute it. Section 3 introduces the `Power-`ψ algorithm, which improves upon the baseline by reducing the number of equations to solve. In Sect. 4, we present the `Push-*` approach, which provides an alternative way to compute the ψ-score and also allows to compute the influence between nodes at the individual scale. Finally, in Sect. 5, we evaluate numerically the different algorithms under study in terms both of accuracy to approximate the result and in terms of time efficiency of the process.

2 Measuring the Influence of OSP Users

The authors of [13] proposed a model to describe the diffusion of posts on a generic social platform. Within this model, each user is not only a node of the social graph, but is also characterized by their own Wall and Newsfeed, as well as their own posting and re-posting activities. Using this spreading model, they compute in closed form the probabilities that a particular user's posts will appear on the Wall and Newsfeed of any other user. This allows them to derive a measure of influence in the network, that they name the ψ-score of a node.

In this section, we first give some basic elements of description of the OSP and the notations, summarized in Table 1, that will be used afterward. Then, we detail the spreading model proposed in [13] and describe how the ψ-score is defined in this context. Note however that this score is not restricted to the specifics of this model and can be defined on any network where nodes can be characterized with their activity rate.

Table 1 Notations used in the paper

Notation	Description
ψ_i	ψ-score of user i
ψ	ψ-score column-vector
$p_i^{(n)}$	Impressions of i on the Newsfeed of n
$q_i^{(n)}$	(Influence) impressions of i on the wall of n
$\mathbf{p}_i$	Vector with every $p_i^{(n)}$
$\mathbf{q}_i$	Vector with every $q_i^{(n)}$
$\mathbf{P}$	Matrix with $\mathbf{p}_i$ as column i
$\mathbf{Q}$	Matrix with $\mathbf{q}_i$ as column i
$\mathbf{b}_i$	Input vector of normalized posting activity
$\mathbf{d}_i$	Vector with the posting ratio of a user i
$\mathbf{B}$	Matrix with $\mathbf{b}_i$ as column i
$\mathbf{D}$	Diagonal matrix with $\mathbf{d}_i$ as column i
$\mathbf{1}$	Column-vector of $\mathbb{R}^N$ full of ones, i.e. $(1\ 1\ \cdots\ 1)^T$

2.1 *Network User Model and Notations*

2.1.1 Network Structure

The platform is represented as a directed and unweighted graph denoted $\mathcal{G} = (\mathcal{N}, \mathcal{E})$. Its vertices represent the users in the OSP and its edges represent the follower-leader relations: $(i, j) \in \mathcal{E}$ means that user i follows user j. The cardinalities of $\mathcal{N}$ and $\mathcal{E}$ are denoted $|\mathcal{N}| = N$ and $|\mathcal{E}| = M$. Note that a social platform where the relationships between users are reciprocal (as for instance, friendships on Facebook) can also be described by this representation, by connecting users with edges in both directions.

2.1.2 Posting Activity

As mentioned above, users are also characterized by their posting and re-posting activities. Let λ represent the vector of posting activity over the vertex set. Thus, $\lambda^{(n)}$ represents the number of wall posts per unit of time (posting frequency) created by user n. Similarly, let μ represent the vector of re-posting activity of the vertices. Then, $\mu^{(n)}$ refers to the frequency with which user n checks their Newsfeed and selects one of the current posts uniformly at random for re-posting on their Wall.

2.2 The ψ-Score: Metric of Influence

Here we present the ψ-score following the way it was introduced in [13]. It measures the nodes' influence in the OSP, not only based on the graph structure but also on the nodes' activity, as a user who shares information more frequently is bound to have more influence than users who don't. Similarly, a user whose posts are shared often by their followers is also bound to have a higher influence. The score can be computed from the graph structure and the activity vectors λ and μ only, however, it is helpful to describe the information spreading process that inspired it in order to have a better understanding of its meaning.

2.2.1 Information Spreading Model

In [13], the authors present the ψ-score as a natural way to evaluate influence within the context of a specific information spreading model on the OSP. In short, the model can be described as follows: a user in the network posts at a constant rate on their wall while messages from their leaders appear on their news feed, replacing a random older post. Regularly, this user selects randomly a post from their news feed to re-post it on the wall. This process is summarized in Fig. 1. Again, we underline that this is not necessarily a lifelike description of information spreading on an OSP, nonetheless, it is realistic enough to give a good intuition of the interpretation of the ψ-score and other intermediary quantities that are defined further.

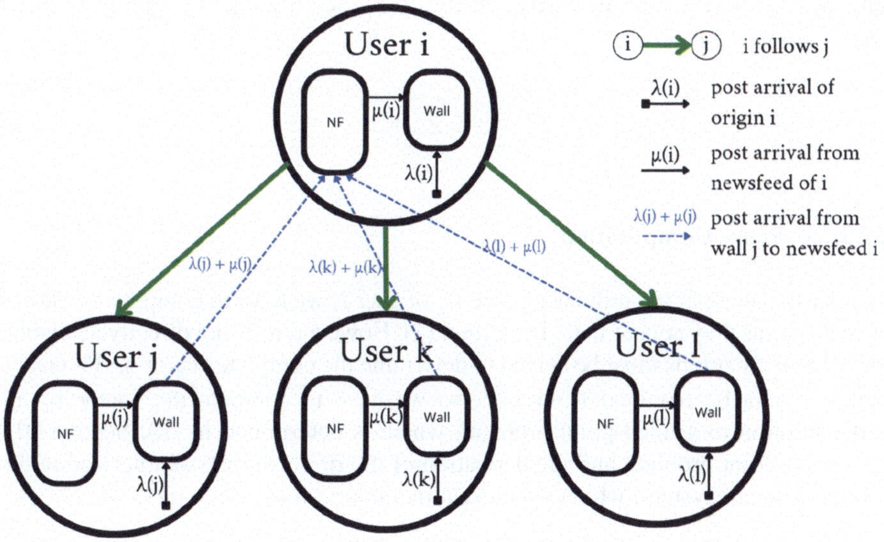

Fig. 1 A small example of the Online Social Platform from the point of view of user *i*

Precisely, this model is a continuous-time Markov chain relying on the following set of assumptions:

- *Poisson arrivals*: any user n posts on their wall according to a Poisson process with rate $\lambda^{(n)}$, and re-posts from the news feed to the wall according to a Poisson process with rate $\mu^{(n)}$.
- *Random selection policy*: we suppose that when a user checks their news feed, they randomly select one of the listed posts to re-post on their wall.
- *Random eviction policy*: a new entry on the wall or on the news feed list replaces an older entry chosen at random.

2.2.2 Influence Quantification

Now that the hypotheses of the model are set, we focus on how to quantify the influence of a user. The authors of [13] introduce two vectors related to the influence of user i in $\mathcal{N}$, which can be computed from the activity attributes of the nodes:

- $\mathbf{p}_i = (p_i^{(1)} \; p_i^{(2)} \; \cdots \; p_i^{(N)})^T$ where, for $n \in \mathcal{N}$, $p_i^{(n)}$ represents the expected proportion of posts from user i on the news feed of user n.
- $\mathbf{q}_i = (q_i^{(1)} \; q_i^{(2)} \; \cdots \; q_i^{(N)})^T$ where, for all $n \in \mathcal{N}$, $q_i^{(n)}$ represents the expected proportion of posts from user i on the wall of user n.

So, $q_i^{(n)}$ can be understood as the influence of user i on user n, which means that the more posts from i appear on the wall of n, the greater is i's influence on n. This is used to define the influence of user i throughout the whole network as the average influence of i has on all other users. This concept is formalized by the ψ-score of user i, which is defined as

$$\psi_i = \frac{1}{N} \sum_{n \in \mathcal{N}} q_i^{(n)}. \tag{1}$$

2.2.3 ψ-Score Computation

In order to calculate the influence score ψ_i of user i, we have to compute all entries of vector $\mathbf{q}_i$ as they appear in its Definition (1). However, $\mathbf{q}_i$ is not directly available: a system of equations must be solved to determine the complete vector $\mathbf{q}_i$. Precisely, each $q_i^{(n)}$ can be obtained from $p_i^{(n)}$, so we have to compute the vector $\mathbf{p}_i$. $\mathbf{p}_i$ is the solution to a fixed-point problem, which is determined in [13, Section III]. This fixed-point problem and the derivation of the $\mathbf{q}_i$ vector are summarized in the following linear system, which we present in a matrix form:

$$\mathbf{p}_i = \mathbf{A}.\mathbf{p}_i + \mathbf{b}_i \tag{2}$$

$$\mathbf{q}_i = \mathbf{C}.\mathbf{p}_i + \mathbf{d}_i \tag{3}$$

$$
\text{where} \begin{cases}
\mathbf{A} \in \mathbb{R}_+^{N\times N}, & a_{ji} = \frac{\mu^{(i)}}{\sum\limits_{\ell\in\mathcal{L}^{(j)}} (\lambda^{(\ell)}+\mu^{(\ell)})} \mathbb{1}_{\{i\in\mathcal{L}^{(j)}\}}, \\
\mathbf{b}_i \in \mathbb{R}_+^{N}, & b_{ji} = \frac{\lambda^{(i)}}{\sum\limits_{\ell\in\mathcal{L}^{(j)}} (\lambda^{(\ell)}+\mu^{(\ell)})} \mathbb{1}_{\{i\in\mathcal{L}^{(j)}\}}, \\
\mathbf{C} \in \mathbb{R}_+^{N\times N}, & c_{ji} = \frac{\mu^{(j)}}{\lambda^{(j)}+\mu^{(j)}} \mathbb{1}_{\{j=i\}}, \\
\mathbf{d}_i \in \mathbb{R}_+^{N}, & d_{ji} = \frac{\lambda^{(i)}}{\lambda^{(i)}+\mu^{(i)}} \mathbb{1}_{\{j=i\}}.
\end{cases}
$$

As shown in [13, Theorem 4], it is possible to solve (2) using a power iteration method as what is typically done to compute the PageRank. It consists in applying iteratively the following equation:

$$
\mathbf{p}_i(t) = \mathbf{A}\mathbf{p}_i(t-1) + \mathbf{b}_i \tag{4}
$$

t being the current iteration. As $t \to \infty$, the algorithm converges towards the solution $\mathbf{p}_i(t)$ independently of the initialization $\mathbf{p}_i(0)$ because $\mathbf{A}$ is a sub-stochastic matrix.[2] The Algorithm 1 given in [13] uses this equation to compute the vector $\mathbf{p}_i$.

Algorithm 1 `Power-NF`: Power method to compute the news feed probabilities $\mathbf{p}_i$ related to user i.

Input: origin user i, $N \times N$ matrix $\mathbf{A}$, vector $\mathbf{b}_i$, $\mathbf{p}$-tolerance ε
Output: vector $\mathbf{p}_i$
$\mathbf{p}_i \leftarrow \mathbf{b}_i$
$t \leftarrow 0$
$gap \leftarrow 1$
while $(gap > \varepsilon)$ **do**
  $\mathbf{p}_i^{old} \leftarrow \mathbf{p}_i$
  $\mathbf{p}_i \leftarrow \mathbf{A}\mathbf{p}_i^{old} + \mathbf{b}_i$
  $gap \leftarrow \|\mathbf{p}_i - \mathbf{p}_i^{old}\|$
  $t \leftarrow t+1$
end while
return p

Now, ranking the N users requires to compute ψ_i for each $i \in \mathcal{N}$, *i.e.*, the complete vector $\psi = (\psi_1, \psi_2, \cdots, \psi_N)^T \in \mathbb{R}_+^N$. To solve the linear system (2), the iterative approach in (4) must be used N times for each origin $i \in \mathcal{N}$. Then, mapping each vector $\mathbf{p}_i$ to $\mathbf{q}_i$ thanks to (3) and finally using (1) gives the vector ψ with all the ψ-score values.

As a side note, which will be useful for comparison purposes, the paper [13] also establishes a relationship between the ψ-score and the PageRank. Indeed,the vector ψ equals the PageRank vector π in the scenario of homogeneous activity, meaning

[2] A sub-stochastic matrix is a real square matrix having each row summing to a value strictly lower than 1.

that $\forall n \in \mathcal{N},\ \lambda^{(n)} = \lambda$ and $\mu^{(n)} = \mu$. In that specific case, the PageRank damping coefficient α is given by $\alpha = \frac{\mu}{\lambda+\mu}$ [13, Theorem 5].

2.2.4 Problem Statement

The Algorithm 1 for the ψ-score vector computation—which we are going to refer to as `Power-NF` in this paper—is highly time-consuming. By contrast with PageRank, which demands solving 1 system of N equations, we need to solve N systems of N equations separately. This is particularly challenging when attempting to calculate the ψ-score in large real-world networks in a reasonable time.

Consequently, the problem discussed in this work is the following: given a directed social graph $\mathcal{G} = (\mathcal{N}, \mathcal{E})$ and the vectors λ and μ which contain the information about the nodes posting and sharing activities, can we design an algorithm that computes the ψ-score of all nodes in the graph with a comparable speed to PageRank?

3 The Power-ψ Algorithm

In this section, we provide a first algorithm to compute the ψ-score which is faster than the baseline Algorithm 1. The principle here is to reformulate the equations as presented in Sect. 2.2 to reduce the computational cost from solving N linear systems of size N to solving a single linear system of size N that includes all users. It will allow to use the power iteration method to approximate the solution of the new linear system, which can also benefit from distributed computing. We call this process Power-ψ: an algorithm for the derivation of the ψ-score that is comparable to the PageRank in terms of computational complexity, while benefiting from the score expressiveness because of the addition of the node activity information.

3.1 Expressing the ψ-Score with a Single Linear System

We describe the ψ-score of the network in terms of the matrices **P**, **Q**, **B**, **D**, which are defined in Table 1. This matrix notation enables a vectorized expression of the ψ-score vector:

$$\psi^T = \frac{1}{N}\mathbf{1}^T\mathbf{Q} \tag{5}$$

We remind that the matrix **Q** contains the $\mathbf{q}_i = (q_i^{(1)}\ q_i^{(2)}\ \cdots\ q_i^{(N)})^T$ vectors, which components $q_i^{(n)}$ represent the influence of user i on user n. So, the task of obtaining the ψ-score is equivalent to computing a matrix $\mathbf{Q}$, the columns of which require having the vectors $\mathbf{p}_i$, according to Eq. (3).

Now, finding each $\mathbf{p}_i$ is equivalent to solving a linear system, as can be seen in Eq. (2). The Eqs. (2) and (3) call to the matrices $\mathbf{A}$ and $\mathbf{C}$, which are themselves derived from the adjacency matrix of the graph and the posting and re-posting activities of the users (λ and μ). Using [13, Lemma 2] each system solution can be written as

$$\mathbf{p}_i = (\mathbf{I} - \mathbf{A})^{-1}\mathbf{b}_i = \sum_{t=0}^{\infty} \mathbf{A}^t \mathbf{b}_i \tag{6}$$

Equation (6) is a linear equation in $\mathbf{b}_i$, which implies that the solution in matrix form for all users is

$$\mathbf{P} = (\mathbf{I} - \mathbf{A})^{-1}\mathbf{B} = \sum_{t=0}^{\infty} \mathbf{A}^t \mathbf{B} \tag{7}$$

Thus, by using Eq. (3) in its matrix form and the series in Eq. (7), we can develop Eq. (5):

$$\begin{aligned}
\psi^T &= \frac{1}{N}\mathbf{1}^T\mathbf{Q} = \frac{1}{N}\mathbf{1}^T(\mathbf{CP} + \mathbf{D}) \\
&= \frac{1}{N}\mathbf{1}^T\left[\mathbf{C}(\mathbf{I} - \mathbf{A})^{-1}\mathbf{B} + \mathbf{D}\right] \\
&= \frac{1}{N}\mathbf{1}^T\left[\mathbf{C}\left(\sum_{t=0}^{\infty}\mathbf{A}^t\right)\mathbf{B} + \mathbf{D}\right] \\
&= \frac{1}{N}\left[\left(\sum_{t=0}^{\infty}\mathbf{1}^T\mathbf{C}\mathbf{A}^t\right)\mathbf{B} + \mathbf{1}^T\mathbf{D}\right]
\end{aligned}$$

Let us define $\mathbf{c}^T := \mathbf{1}^T\mathbf{C}$ and $\mathbf{d}^T := \mathbf{1}^T\mathbf{D}$. $\mathbf{c}$ and $\mathbf{d}$ are vectors in $\mathbb{R}_+^N$ (the diagonals of the matrices $\mathbf{C}$ and $\mathbf{D}$). This allows us to formulate the following equation to compute the ψ-score:

$$\psi^T = \frac{1}{N}\left[\left(\sum_{t=0}^{\infty}\mathbf{c}^T\mathbf{A}^t\right)\mathbf{B} + \mathbf{d}^T\right] \tag{8}$$

Equation (8) demonstrates that it is not essential to solve N linear systems of size N to calculate the ψ-score. Instead, it is sufficient to solve a single N-dimensional linear system, which is written as the infinite sum of matrix-vector multiplications.

There is a drawback to this new approach, which is the fact that we do not compute explicitly the values of $\mathbf{p}_i$ and $\mathbf{q}_i$, which quantify the influence at the individual level. As (8) demonstrates, these are not required any longer to calculate the ψ-score, however, they include valuable information for practical applications, where evaluating the influence of a specific user on others is important.

3.2 Convergence and Truncation of the Sum

We state here that the infinite sum in Eq. (8) may be evaluated using a power iteration method. To show this, let us define:

$$\mathbf{s}_t^T = \sum_{\tau=0}^{t} \mathbf{c}^T \mathbf{A}^\tau, \quad \mathbf{s} = \lim_{t\to\infty} \mathbf{s}_t, \tag{9}$$

where T denotes the matrix transpose and t is the iteration index. We emphasize that Eq. (9) converges if $\mathbf{A}$'s spectral radius is strictly lower than 1 (which is a standard property of geometric series). Lemmas 1 and 2 in [13] guarantee this convergence, using the fact that $\mathbf{A}$ is a sub-stochastic matrix. Consequently, the sum in (8) may be truncated to a finite number of terms to approximate the ψ-score.

Now, let us evaluate the approximation error made when truncating the sum. The recursive expression associated with the truncated sum is

$$\mathbf{s}_t^T = \mathbf{s}_{t-1}^T \mathbf{A} + \mathbf{c}^T \tag{10}$$

where $\mathbf{s}_0 = \mathbf{c}$. This allows us to define the following gap parameter

$$\varepsilon_t = \left\| \mathbf{s}_t^T - \mathbf{s}_{t-1}^T \right\| \tag{11}$$

which is used to stop the algorithm. Any norm can be used, we opt for using the L^1-norm because it is standard when approximating series with power iterations [24]. So practically, we terminate the iterations when the following condition is met:

$$\varepsilon_t \le \varepsilon \tag{12}$$

A key question here is to evaluate how the tolerance ε impacts the approximation of the ψ-score. To answer this question, we define ψ_t to approximate ψ by substituting (10) with (8) in t terms. Then, we define the difference δ_t between two ψ-score approximations truncated at consecutive steps:

$$\delta_t = \left\| \psi_t^T - \psi_{t-1}^T \right\| \tag{13}$$

Now, we describe δ_t as a function of ε_t and identify an upper-bound relation between the two to deduce a convergence condition on the vector ψ_t from the one on $\mathbf{s}_t$. Indeed, we know from (8) that

$$\begin{aligned}\psi_t^T - \psi_{t-1}^T &= \frac{1}{N}(\mathbf{s}_t^T\mathbf{B} + \mathbf{d}^T) - \frac{1}{N}(\mathbf{s}_{t-1}^T\mathbf{B} + \mathbf{d}^T)\\ &= \frac{1}{N}(\mathbf{s}_t^T - \mathbf{s}_{t-1}^T)\mathbf{B}\end{aligned} \tag{14}$$

Equation (14) then allows to deduce that:

$$\begin{aligned}\delta_t = \frac{1}{N}\left\|(\mathbf{s}_t^T - \mathbf{s}_{t-1}^T)\mathbf{B}\right\| &\le \frac{1}{N}\left\|\mathbf{s}_t^T - \mathbf{s}_{t-1}^T\right\| \|\mathbf{B}\|\\ \Rightarrow \delta_t &\le \frac{\varepsilon_t \|\mathbf{B}\|}{N}\end{aligned} \tag{15}$$

Using this upper bound, we can choose a tolerance ε that ensures the ψ-score evolution does not deviate by more than δ. Precisely, if the algorithm is terminated by the condition $\varepsilon_t \|\mathbf{B}\| \le \varepsilon$, then δ_t is smaller than $\frac{\varepsilon}{N}$. The corresponding power iteration algorithm is designated as `Power-`ψ and described in Algorithm 2.

Algorithm 2 `Power-`ψ **:** Power method to compute the ψ-score vector.

Input: $N \times N$ matrices $\mathbf{A}$ and $\mathbf{B}$, size N vectors $\mathbf{c}$ and $\mathbf{d}$, $\mathbf{s}$-tolerance ε
Output: vector ψ with the ψ-score of all users
$\mathbf{s} \leftarrow \mathbf{c}$
$B\_norm \leftarrow \|\mathbf{B}\|$
$t \leftarrow 0$
$gap \leftarrow 1$
while $(gap > \varepsilon)$ **do**
  $\mathbf{s}_{old} \leftarrow \mathbf{s}$
  $\mathbf{s}^T \leftarrow \mathbf{s}_{old}^T\mathbf{A} + \mathbf{c}$
  $gap \leftarrow B\_norm \|\mathbf{s}_{old} - \mathbf{s}\|$
  $t \leftarrow t + 1$
end while
$\psi^T \leftarrow \frac{1}{N}(\mathbf{s}^T\mathbf{B} + \mathbf{d}^T)$
return ψ

3.3 *Relationship Between ψ-Score and PageRank*

In this section, we discuss the relationship between the ψ-score in the homogeneous activity scenario and PageRank, which highlights the contrast between our proposed method and the usual power-iteration algorithm for PageRank.

Let π denotes the PageRank vector and $\mathbf{W} = \mathbf{D}_{out}^{-1}\mathbf{L}$ is the random walk transition matrix, where $\mathbf{L}$ is the adjacency matrix of the graph that points to the leaders and $\mathbf{D}_{out}$ is the diagonal matrix whose entries (i, i) are the out-degree of node i. Theorem 5 in [13] ensures that, in the homogeneous activity scenario, where $\forall i$, $\lambda^{(i)} = \lambda$ and $\mu^{(i)} = \mu$, $\psi = \pi$ with $\alpha = \frac{\mu}{\lambda+\mu}$ as the PageRank damping factor.

In the homogeneous activity case, the vectors and matrices in the ψ-score equation of Eq. (8) are as follows:

$$\begin{cases} \mathbf{A} = \alpha\mathbf{W} \\ \mathbf{B} = (1-\alpha)\mathbf{W} \\ \mathbf{c} = \alpha\mathbf{1} \\ \mathbf{d} = (1-\alpha)\mathbf{1} \end{cases}$$

So, after replacing $\mathbf{A}$ and $\mathbf{c}$ by their expression in Eq. (10), we obtain

$$\mathbf{s}_t^T = \alpha\mathbf{s}_{t-1}^T\mathbf{W} + \alpha\mathbf{1}^T \tag{16}$$

By substituting the above expression in Eq. (8) and using the homogeneous values for $\mathbf{B}$ and $\mathbf{d}$ we get

$$\begin{aligned} \psi_t^T &= \frac{1}{N}\left(\mathbf{s}_t^T(1-\alpha)\mathbf{W} + (1-\alpha)\mathbf{1}^T\right) \\ &= \frac{1}{N}\left((\alpha\mathbf{s}_{t-1}^T\mathbf{W} + \alpha\mathbf{1}^T)(1-\alpha)\mathbf{W} + (1-\alpha)\mathbf{1}^T\right) \\ &= \alpha\left(\frac{1}{N}(\mathbf{s}_{t-1}^T(1-\alpha)\mathbf{W} + (1-\alpha)\mathbf{1}^T)\right)\mathbf{W} + \frac{(1-\alpha)}{N}\mathbf{1}^T \\ &= \alpha\psi_{t-1}^T\mathbf{W} + \frac{(1-\alpha)}{N}\mathbf{1}^T \end{aligned} \tag{17}$$

The power method for PageRank computation translates as

$$\pi_t^T = \alpha\pi_{t-1}^T\mathbf{W} + \frac{1-\alpha}{N}\mathbf{1}^T. \tag{18}$$

so, we can see that we find similar expressions, consistently with the result from [13, Theorem 5].

Now, the proposed `Power-`ψ algorithm in the general case uses a power iteration to first estimate the series $\mathbf{s}$ up to a truncation based on the desired tolerance. Following convergence, the product by $\mathbf{B}$ and addition of $\mathbf{d}$ at the end of Algorithm 2 prevent superfluous matrix-vector multiplications. This is the main implementation difference compared to PageRank power iteration. As shown above, both approaches converge to the same result in the homogeneous situation; however, the tolerance for ψ-score is defined on the $\mathbf{s}$-vector, whereas for PageRank, it is defined on π itself.

3.4 Computational Complexity

We analyze the computational complexity of the `Power-`ψ algorithm. The main computational cost of the algorithm is the power iteration, which is performed until the convergence condition is met. Let us denote $k(\varepsilon)$ the number of iterations required to reach convergence. Each iteration requires a matrix-vector multiplication, which is of complexity $O(M)$ where M is the number of non-zero entries in the matrix, i.e. the number of edges in $\mathcal{G}$. There is also a vector addition, which is of complexity $O(N)$, and a scalar-vector multiplication, which is in $O(N)$. So the total complexity of each iteration is in $O(M + N)$. The total complexity of the algorithm is then $O(k(\varepsilon)(M + N))$. This result is comparable to the complexity of the PageRank power iteration, which is also in $O(k(\varepsilon)(M + N))$.

4 Push Approach for Influence Quantification

In this section, we design a push-based algorithm approach to our problem of influence quantification on a social network. This approach can be applied to two different sets of equations with two distinct purposes. On the one hand, we can use it on Eq. (10) in a similar manner as what has been done for PageRank [15, 16]. In this case, the goal is to find more efficiently the vector $\mathbf{s}$, which in turn allows for the direct calculation of the ψ-score of each node. On the other hand, the push method can also be employed to solve Eq. (2), and the purpose here is to compute faster the ψ-score of a single user; by providing $\mathbf{p}_i$ and $\mathbf{q}_i$, it gives much more details about the mechanism of influence on the network at an individual level. Note that the application of the push approach to our problem is the main theoretical addition to the shorter version of this work [14].

4.1 Intuition Behind the Push Approach

The push method can be thought of as a message-passing algorithm. The intuitive general idea is to iteratively propagate information across the graph, in order to calculate the importance of each node based on its connections to other nodes.

Practically, it works by initializing a residual value for each node and its approximate score, where the residual represents the amount of information that still needs to be propagated from that node to its neighbors. The algorithm then iteratively updates the approximate score for each node based on the residual that it gets from its neighbors. At each iteration, a node "pushes" its residual to its neighbors, proportionally to the strength of the connection between the two nodes (encoded by the matrix $\mathbf{A}$ in the case of ψ-score and the propagation matrix for PageRank). The node then updates its own approximate score based on the residuals that it received from its neighbors. This process continues until the residuals converge towards 0, indicating that the approximate score vector has converged to the actual score.

Note that the push method can be implemented in a distributed way since each node updates its own score, making it very efficient at solving linear systems of a large number of equations.

4.2 General Formulation of the Approach Push-*

Let us first rewrite Eq. (10) as follows:

$$\mathbf{s} = \mathbf{A}^T.\mathbf{s} + \mathbf{c} \tag{19}$$

so that it has exactly the same form as Eq. (2). Now, while they contain and return different quantities, Eq. (2) on $\mathbf{p}_i$ and (19) on $\mathbf{s}$, they allow us to describe the application of the push method on both of them with some generic notations:

$$\mathbf{x} = \mathbf{M}.\mathbf{x} + \mathbf{r} \tag{20}$$

where $\mathbf{x} \in \mathbb{R}^N$ is the unknown vector, $\mathbf{r} \in \mathbb{R}^N$ and $\mathbf{M} \in \mathbb{R}^{N\times N}$. In the case of Eq. (2), $\mathbf{x} = \mathbf{p}_i$, $\mathbf{M} = \mathbf{A}$ and $\mathbf{r} = \mathbf{b}_i$ and in the case of Eq. (19), $\mathbf{x} = \mathbf{s}$, $\mathbf{M} = \mathbf{A}^T$ and $\mathbf{r} = \mathbf{c}$. Taking advantage of this formal similarity, from now on we refer to the method and algorithm that we develop as `Push-*`, then we will describe them as `Push-NF` for Eq. (2) and `Push-`ψ for Eq. (19) when necessary.

It is important here to notice that Eq. (20) does not have the same form as the one that computes the PageRank since $\mathbf{r}$ has different components while the second term of the PageRank equation is homogeneous. Consequently, we cannot use the push-based algorithm described in [15] or [16]. Thus we adapt the method to the specific case under consideration.

Let us first observe that the solution $\mathbf{x}$ is a function of the vector $\mathbf{r}$, so that we can re-write Eq. (20) as

$$\mathbf{x}(\mathbf{r}) = \mathbf{M}.\mathbf{x}(\mathbf{r}) + \mathbf{r} \tag{21}$$

Rearranging this equation, it becomes

$$\mathbf{x}(\mathbf{r}) = (\mathbf{I} - \mathbf{M})^{-1}\mathbf{r} = \sum_{n=0}^{\infty} \mathbf{M}^n \mathbf{r} \tag{22}$$

The next step is key and specific to the push method. Let χ_u be the unit vector with only the u-th entry equal to 1 and all the other components equal to 0. Also, we denote $\mathbf{r}(u)$ the u-th entry of $\mathbf{r}$. Using only Eqs. (21) and (22) (which is linear), we have the following expressions:

$$\begin{aligned}
\mathbf{x}(\mathbf{r}) &= \mathbf{x}\left(\mathbf{r} - \mathbf{r}(u)\chi_u + \mathbf{r}(u)\chi_u\right) \\
&= \mathbf{x}\left(\mathbf{r}(u)\chi_u\right) + \mathbf{x}\left(\mathbf{r} - \mathbf{r}(u)\chi_u\right) \\
&= \mathbf{M}.\mathbf{x}(\mathbf{r}(u)\chi_u) + \mathbf{r}(u)\chi_u + \mathbf{x}\left(\mathbf{r} - \mathbf{r}(u)\chi_u\right) \\
&= \mathbf{M}\sum_{n=0}^{\infty} \mathbf{M}^n \mathbf{r}(u)\chi_u + \mathbf{r}(u)\chi_u + \mathbf{x}\left(\mathbf{r} - \mathbf{r}(u)\chi_u\right) \\
&= \sum_{n=0}^{\infty} \mathbf{M}^n \mathbf{M}\mathbf{r}(u)\chi_u + \mathbf{r}(u)\chi_u + \mathbf{x}\left(\mathbf{r} - \mathbf{r}(u)\chi_u\right) \\
&= \mathbf{x}\left(\mathbf{M}\mathbf{r}(u)\chi_u\right) + \mathbf{x}\left(\mathbf{r} - \mathbf{r}(u)\chi_u\right) + \mathbf{r}(u)\chi_u \\
&= \mathbf{x}\left(\mathbf{r} - \mathbf{r}(u)\chi_u + \mathbf{M}\mathbf{r}(u)\chi_u\right) + \mathbf{r}(u)\chi_u \\
&= \mathbf{r}(u)\chi_u + \mathbf{x}(\mathbf{r}'),
\end{aligned} \tag{23}$$

where we define the vector $\mathbf{r}'$ as

$$\mathbf{r}' := \mathbf{r} - \mathbf{r}(u)\chi_u + \mathbf{M}\mathbf{r}(u)\chi_u. \tag{24}$$

So, we have derived a new expression of the solution as the sum of two components:

$$\mathbf{x}(\mathbf{r}) = \mathbf{r}(u)\chi_u + \mathbf{x}(\mathbf{r}') \tag{25}$$

where the first part is an approximation of the solution $\mathbf{x}(\mathbf{r})$ and the second, $\mathbf{x}(\mathbf{r}')$ can be interpreted as a residual and denoted $\mathbf{x}'$.

4.3 Convergence of the Residual

Following the above approach, we can put (24) and (25) in an iterative algorithm to derive the solution of (20) with a convergence criterion related to the residual. The problem is that the exact expression of the residual $\mathbf{x}(\mathbf{r}')$ is not available. However, we know its argument $\mathbf{r}'$ from (24). In addition, $\mathbf{r} \mapsto \mathbf{x}(\mathbf{r})$ is a linear map, as shown by Eq. (22), so that $\mathbf{x}(\mathbf{0}) = \mathbf{0}$, where $\mathbf{0}$ is a vector of 0. Thus, we set a convergence criterion related to the infinite norm of the residual argument of the form $\left\|\mathbf{r}'\right\|_\infty < \varepsilon$.

Now, we investigate if we can bound the volume of the residuals. As long as $\|\mathbf{M}\| < 1$, we have that

$$\begin{aligned} \|\mathbf{x}(\mathbf{r}')\| &= \left\| \sum_{n=0}^{\infty} \mathbf{M}^n \mathbf{x}' \right\| \leq \left\| \sum_{n=0}^{\infty} \mathbf{M}^n \right\| \cdot \|\mathbf{x}'\| \\ &\leq \varepsilon \cdot \sum_{n=0}^{\infty} \|\mathbf{M}\|^n = \frac{\varepsilon}{1 - \|\mathbf{M}\|}, \end{aligned} \tag{26}$$

Note that this inequality is true for the L^1 norm of a right sub-stochastic matrix, such as $\mathbf{A}$, and for the L^∞ norm of a left sub-stochastic matrix. In the case of Eq. (2) (Push-NF), $\mathbf{M} = \mathbf{A}$ and in the case of Eq. (19) $\mathbf{M} = \mathbf{A}^T$ (Push-ψ). So, we have the following cases of induced norms

- in the case of Push-NF:

$$\|\mathbf{x}(\mathbf{r}')\|_1 \leq \frac{\varepsilon}{1 - \|\mathbf{A}\|_1} = \frac{\varepsilon}{1 - \max_{1 \leq u \leq N} \sum_{v \in \mathcal{F}(u)} \mathbf{A}(v, u)}, \tag{27}$$

- in the case of Push-ψ:

$$\|\mathbf{x}(\mathbf{r}')\|_\infty \leq \frac{\varepsilon}{1 - \|\mathbf{A}^T\|_\infty} = \frac{\varepsilon}{1 - \max_{1 \leq u \leq N} \sum_{v \in \mathcal{L}(v)} \mathbf{A}^T(u, v)} \tag{28}$$

Where $\mathcal{F}(u)$ designates the set of followers of user u while $\mathcal{L}(v)$ is the set of leaders of user v.

As a consequence, we can choose the tolerance ε to be an upper bound of $\frac{\varepsilon}{1-\|\mathbf{M}\|}$ as a convergence criterion by taking the appropriate norm for $\mathbf{M}$.

4.4 The Push-* Algorithm

We propose our Push-* algorithm following this expression to derive the solution $\mathbf{x}(\mathbf{r})$ of the generic equation. Each iteration of Push-* works as follows: the u-th entry of the approximation vector is incremented by $\mathbf{r}(u) > \varepsilon$, which will be then set to 0 as indicated by the first part of (24). Next, for every v follower (respectively leader) of u for (2) (respectively for (19)), the value $\mathbf{M}(v, u).\mathbf{r}(u) > 0$ is added to $\mathbf{r}(v)$ (second part of (24)). The algorithm stops when the value of the residual is small enough according to what has been discussed in Sect. 4.3.

Algorithm 3 Push-*: the Push algorithm for **x**

Input: $N \times 1$ vector $\mathbf{r}$, $N \times N$ matrix $\mathbf{M}$, ε
Output: Calculate the $N \times 1$ vector $\mathbf{x}(\mathbf{r})$
Initialization: $x(v) = 0$, for $v = 1, \ldots, N$
FIFO $\leftarrow$ CreateFIFO()
for user u with $\mathbf{x}(u) > \varepsilon$ **do**
    FIFO.add(u)
    Mark(u)
end for
while FIFO not empty **do**
    $u \leftarrow FIFO.pop()$
    $\mathbf{x}(u) \leftarrow \mathbf{x}(u) + \mathbf{r}(u)$
    for user v in $\mathbf{M}(:, u) > 0$ **do**
        $\mathbf{r}(v) \leftarrow \mathbf{r}(v) + \mathbf{M}(v, u) \cdot \mathbf{r}(u)$
        if $\mathbf{r}(v) > \varepsilon$ and (v not marked) **then**
            FIFO.add(v)
            Mark(v)
        end if
    end for
    $\mathbf{r}(u) \leftarrow 0$
    Unmark(u)
end while

5 Numerical Evaluation

In this section, we evaluate the performances of the three algorithms presented in this work: Power-ψ, Push-ψ and Push-NF. We compare their performances to the baseline algorithm Power-NF described in [13]. In the case where the posting and re-posting activities of nodes are identical for all nodes, the ψ-score is equivalent to the PageRank, it allows us to compare the results to the ones obtained with the PageRank in this homogeneous scenario.

First, we briefly present the package which has been developed and released for this project. Second, we describe the different datasets that are investigated in the experiments. Then we precise some important elements of the experimental protocol, before reporting the results of the performance evaluation.

5.1 *The* psi-score *Python Package*

The *psi-score* project is a software library that we have developed in Python. It is open source and licensed under the terms of the MIT license, allowing free usability. It is currently available at the address https://github.com/NouamaneA/psi-score.

This package is a practical tool for the community to easily use the ψ-score metric in projects without the need to develop each algorithm individually. All methods mentioned in this work are accessible: the baseline Power-NF as well as

Table 2 Datasets used for evaluation

Dataset name	Type	#Nodes	#Edges	Sources
`DBLP`	Citation network	12,590	49,759	[31]
`Twitter-ICWSM`	Social network	465,017	834,797	[32]
`ego-Twitter`	Social network	23,370	33,101	[33]
`Russian`	Social network	181,621	515,419	[30]

the proposed algorithms `Power-`ψ, `Push-`ψ and `Push-NF`. To simplify its usage, the project has a similar Application Programming Interface (API) as the one used in *scikit-network* [27] and *scikit-learn* [28].

5.2 Datasets

For the numerical evaluation of our methods, we choose four real-world datasets which are listed in Table 2. Three of them are publicly available in *the KONECT project*[3] [29] which is a network dataset repository. These three datasets do not include any information about the nodes' activity in the network so we decided to generate λ and μ uniformly at random. The last dataset has been downloaded from *Kaggle* dataset repository[4] [30]. It is a Twitter trace that contains a million tweets and retweets from 181,621 users during the 2018 Russian elections, we can therefore derive the actual posting and re-posting activities (respectively λ and μ) of all users.

5.3 Experiments

5.3.1 Unit of Comparison

The complexity of the methods is compared using the number of messages required to reach a targeted tolerance ε, which is the number of vector entries updated at each iteration during the process. We use the term "messages" because we can interpret each update as a signal that propagates across the network from a node to one of its neighbors. By contrast with the computation time, this measure has the advantage of allowing the comparison between sequential and distributed algorithms, regardless of the technology used to implement them.

Note here that each one of the algorithms (`Power-`ψ, `Power-NF`, `Push-*` and `PageRank`) have a different notion of tolerance, depending on the criterion of convergence. Specifically, for `Push-*` we name it **r**-tolerance because the convergence

[3] http://konect.cc/.

[4] https://www.kaggle.com.

is based on the norm of the residual vector, as expressed by the equation $\|\mathbf{x}'\|_\infty < \varepsilon$. For Power-NF we name it **p**-tolerance because the convergence is based on the norm of the news-feed **p**-values. For Power-ψ we refer to **s**-tolerance because the convergence is based on the norm of the series **s**-values. For PageRank we consider π-tolerance because the convergence is based on the norm of the PageRank vector. Also, we underline that further processing is needed after convergence to eventually derive the resulting ψ-scores. So, when we set some value ε for the x-tolerance according to a specific method, we obtain some approximation of the ψ-score ψ_ε, however, we are interested in evaluating the relative error of this method compared to the exact value ψ_{true}, defined as follows:

$$error = \frac{\|\psi_{true} - \psi_\varepsilon\|_2}{\|\psi_{true}\|_2} \tag{29}$$

Note that to compute the ψ_{true} vector, we use the solver from the `sparse` module of the SciPy Python library [34] which employs matrix factorization to solve the system (10).

5.3.2 Design of the Experiments

We conducted three series of experiments to evaluate the performance of our proposed algorithms. The first series of experiments aims to validate their ability to approximate the exact ψ-score by comparing the approximation error of the algorithms to the exact ψ-score value. In the second series, we aim at validating the algorithms ability to return the actual user ranking based on the ψ-score. In the third series, we compare the algorithms' performance with that of Power-NF, in terms of messages, which is the unit of comparison previously defined. To do this, we used the Kendall τ correlation coefficient to compare the rankings returned by each algorithm to the rankings returned by the true ψ-score values.

5.3.3 Scenarios

For each series of experiments, we consider two scenarios:

(*i*) In the *heterogeneous scenario*, we set the activity parameters λ and μ to be heterogeneous. It means that in the cases of ego-Twitter, DBLP and Twitter-ICWSM, where no temporal activity data is available, we draw λ and μ uniformly at random in the interval [0, 1]. In the case of Russian, we use the actual activities measured on the dataset.

(*ii*) In the *homogeneous scenario*, we set the activity parameters λ and μ to be homogeneous, *i.e.*, we set $\lambda = 0.15$ and $\mu = 0.85$ for all nodes. According to Sect. 3.3, this corresponds to the case where the ψ-score is equivalent to the PageRank with a damping factor $\alpha = 0.85$ (which is a typical value for the damping factor). Besides, we run in this scenario the experiments on the giant connected component of the graph, as the equivalence between the ψ-score and the PageRank is ensured only within these settings, as stated in [13].

5.3.4 Series 1: Quality of the ψ-Score Approximation

In the first series of experiments, we evaluate the accuracy of our proposed algorithms in approximating the ψ-score vector by measuring the error and comparing them to `Power-NF` in both scenarios and to `PageRank` in the homogeneous scenario only.

The corresponding results for the heterogeneous and homogeneous activity scenarios are respectively presented in Figs. 2 and 3. The x-axis of the figure represents the fixed **p**-, **s**-, **r**- and π-tolerance for each algorithm, while the y-axis represents the computed error from Eq. (29). Notably, the `Power-`ψ method exhibits significantly lower approximation error than the other algorithms, which can be attributed to the fact that the measured gap at each iteration is multiplied by $\|\mathbf{B}\|$ to ensure that the gap in the ψ-score approximation is below the chosen tolerance when the algorithm converges. We also notice that the power method is systematically more accurate than the corresponding push method: the error

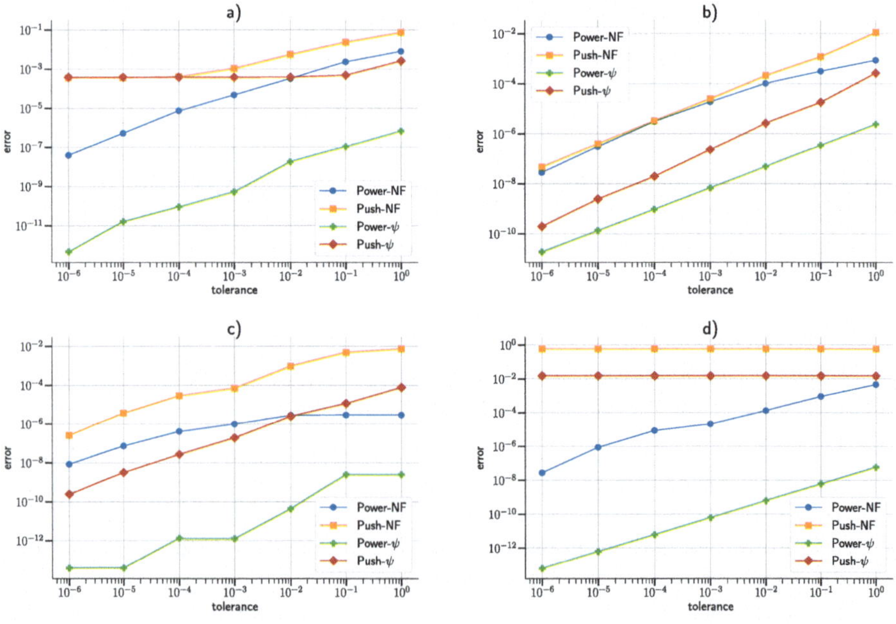

Fig. 2 (*i*) Heterogeneous scenario. Experiment 1 with (**a**) `DBLP`, (**b**) `ego-Twitter`, (**c**) `Twitter-ICWSM` and (**d**) `Russian`: Precision assessment of the proposed algorithms compared to the baseline

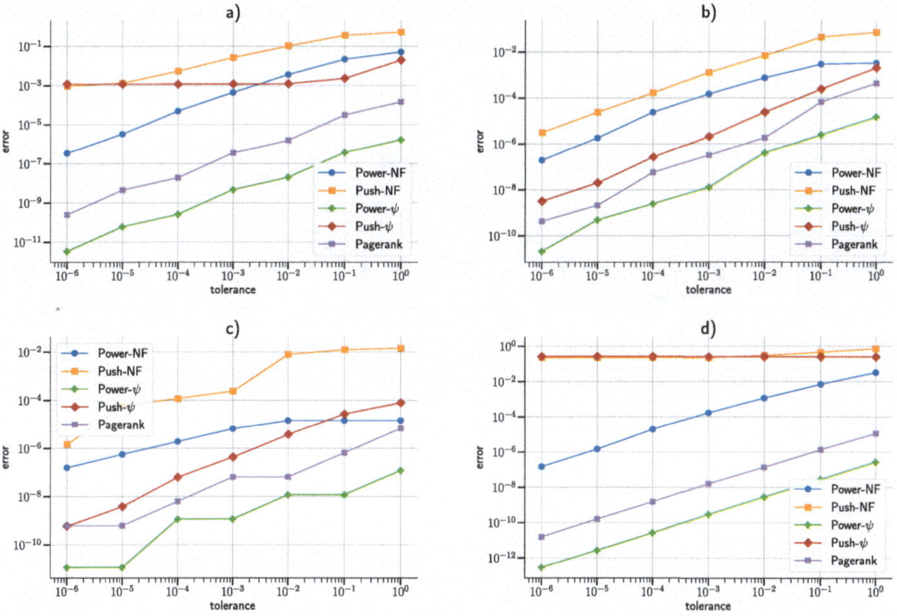

Fig. 3 (ii) Homogeneous scenario. Experiment 1 with (**a**) `DBLP`, (**b**) `ego-Twitter`, (**c**) `Twitter-ICWSM` and (**d**) `Russian`: Precision assessment of the proposed algorithms compared to the baseline

committed with `Power-`ψ is lower than the one of `Push-`ψ and similarly, the error with `Power-NF` is lower than with `Push-NF`. It is expected, as the tolerance is more directly related to the quantity targeted with a power method than it is with a push method since the latter bases its convergence on the norm of the residual. In the homogeneous scenario, Fig. 3 shows that `Power-`ψ is more accurate than `PageRank` in the sense that a similar tolerance implies a lower error.

5.3.5 Series 2: Quality of the Ranking Approximation

When using centrality measures, we are in general less concerned by the absolute value of the score than we are by the ordering of the nodes. Thus, to evaluate how the error presented in the first series of experiments translates in terms of ranking, we investigate in this series the quality of the approximations in view of the ranking that they produce.

To assess this, we compute the correlation between the rankings produced by each algorithm to the one generated by the exact ψ-score using Kendall's τ correlation coefficient. Introduced in [35], this metric is used to measure the similarity between two rankings. It involves counting the number of concordant and discordant pairs (resp. n_C and n_D) between the two rankings x and y, as well as the

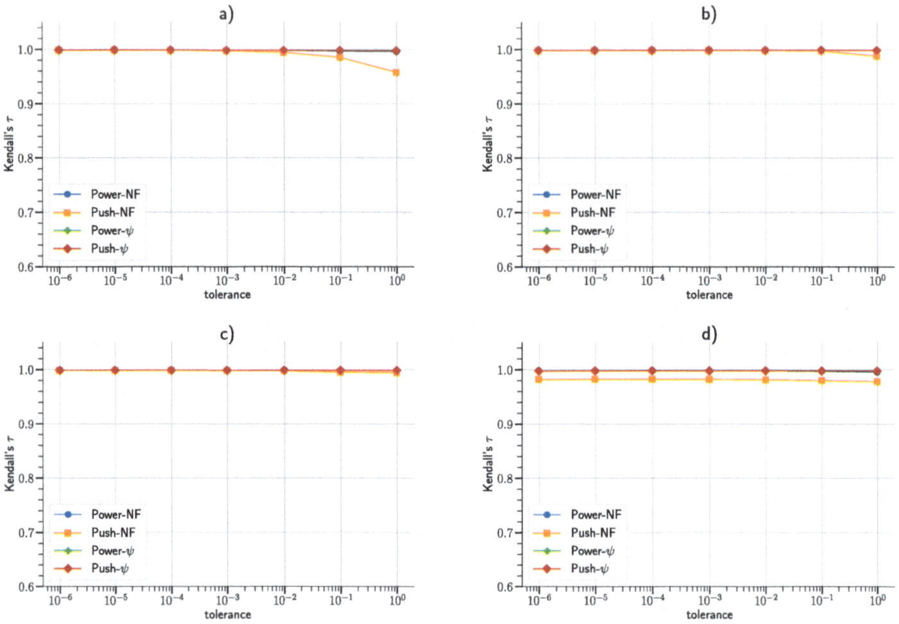

Fig. 4 (*i*) Heterogeneous scenario. Experiment 2 with (**a**) `DBLP`, (**b**) `ego-Twitter`, (**c**) `Twitter-ICWSM` and (**d**) `Russian`: Evaluation of the algorithms ability to return an accurate ranking compared to the one returned by the exact ψ-score. 1 means a perfect correlation, 0 means no correlation at all and -1 means a full anti-correlation

number of ties t_x and t_y within each ranking. Then, the coefficient is computed as follows:

$$\tau(x, y) = \frac{n_C - n_D}{\sqrt{(n_C + n_D + t_x)(n_C + n_D + t_y)}}$$

The results of this series of experiments in the heterogeneous and homogeneous scenarios are respectively displayed in Figs. 4 and 5. We represent Kendall's τ scores as a function of the tolerance on all four datasets and for each algorithm. As can be seen, all three proposed algorithms (`Push-`ψ, `Push-NF`, and `Power-`ψ) perform very well in terms of user ranking, in the sense that the Kendall τ scores are very close to 1, even with relatively high tolerance values. This means that the algorithms are able to effectively rank users in the same way as the actual ψ-score does. In the homogeneous activity scenario, we notice a decrease in the ranking quality of `Push-NF` when increasing the tolerance: a significant drop occurs around a tolerance of 10^{-2} in the cases of `DBLP`, `ego-Twitter` and `Russian` and around a tolerance of 10^{-3} concerning `Twitter-ICWSM`.

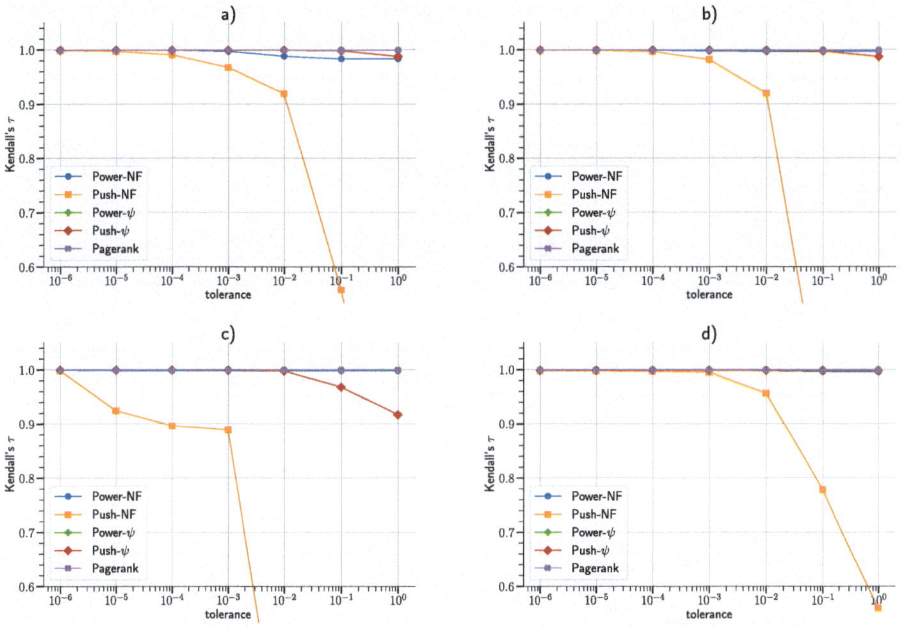

Fig. 5 (*ii*) Homogeneous scenario. Experiment 2 with (**a**) `DBLP`, (**b**) `ego-Twitter`, (**c**) `Twitter-ICWSM` and (**d**) `Russian`: Evaluation of the algorithms ability to return an accurate ranking compared to the one returned by the exact ψ-score/PageRank. 1 means a perfect correlation, 0 means no correlation at all and -1 means a full anti-correlation

5.3.6 Series 3: Message Complexity

In the third series of experiments, we focus on the scalability of these algorithms by evaluating their performance in terms of the number of messages required to achieve a given level of precision in approximating the result. It is worth noticing that achieving the same precision for all algorithms is not always possible. This is because, as discussed previously, the tolerance is not equivalent for all algorithms, so the resulting approximation error on the exact score may vary. To compare the performances of the algorithms to the baseline, we run them with various tolerance parameters (the same ones used in the first series of experiments) and measure the number of messages required to reach convergence. We then calculate the relative error using (29) to compare the algorithms performance under a specific level of precision. Note that the message-based complexity can be simply related to the number of iterations of a power method. Indeed, a complete iteration consists of sending M messages through the network, where M is the number of edges in the network. So the value $k(\varepsilon)$ mentioned in Sect. 3.4 is related to the total number of messages n_{mes} sent by the relation $k(\varepsilon) = n_{mes}/M$.

The results of this series of experiments are respectively reported in Figs. 6 and 7 for the heterogeneous and homogeneous scenarios. Consistently with the findings of

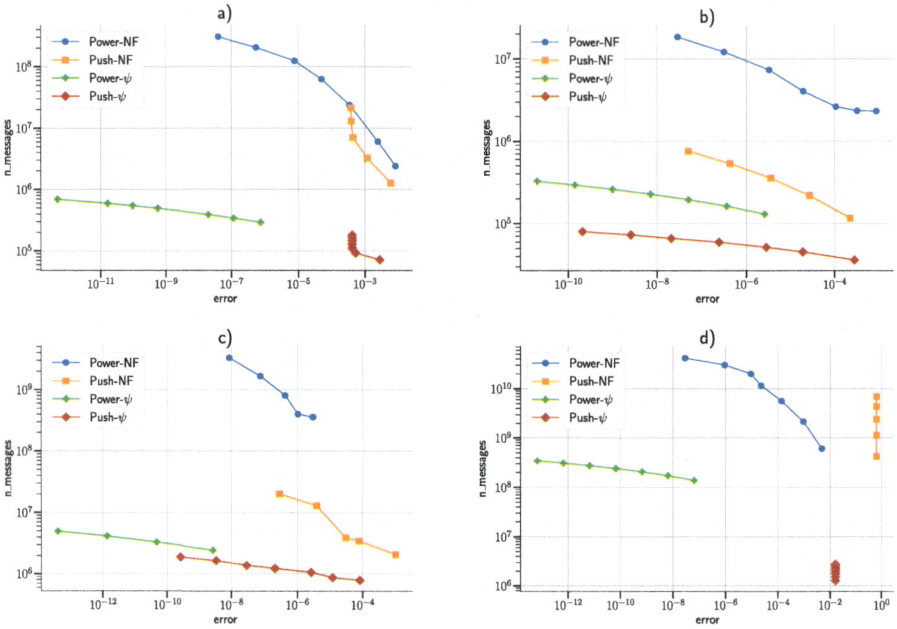

Fig. 6 (*i*) Heterogeneous scenario. Experiment 3 with (**a**) `DBLP`, (**b**) `ego-Twitter`, (**c**) `Twitter-ICWSM` and (**d**) `Russian`: Comparison of the proposed algorithms with the baseline (Power-NF) in terms of the number of messages to reach convergence

the short version of this work [14], we observe that `Power-ψ` significantly outperforms `Power-NF` due to the reduced number of equations to solve. The `Push-*` algorithms also bring some very interesting results, as `Push-NF` requires fewer messages than `Power-NF`, and `Push-ψ` requires fewer messages that `Power-ψ`. The authors of [26] reported a specificity of push methods, which is that they are not competitive to obtain very precise approximations as they require a large number of messages to decrease the error. Such a trend is confirmed by the `DBLP` and `Russian` datasets. We even notice a peculiar trend in Fig. 6d with `Russian`, for which we do not succeed in improving the approximation error even when largely increasing the number of messages of the push methods. This might be due to the fact that, unlike the other datasets, the activity parameters λ and μ are measured from the dataset (see Sect. 5.2) itself and we noticed that almost half of the nodes in this social network are inactive. However, we do not notice such a dramatic trend with datasets `ego-Twitter` and `Twitter-ICWSM`. An important observation in Fig. 7 is that `Power-ψ` and `Push-ψ` converge faster than `PageRank` in the homogeneous scenario. This makes the ψ-score a very interesting alternative to PageRank for ranking users in social networks as its complexity has been reduced to the same level as PageRank.

Finally, the overall picture that we draw from these experimental investigations is that push methods are steadily faster than power methods but allow less control over

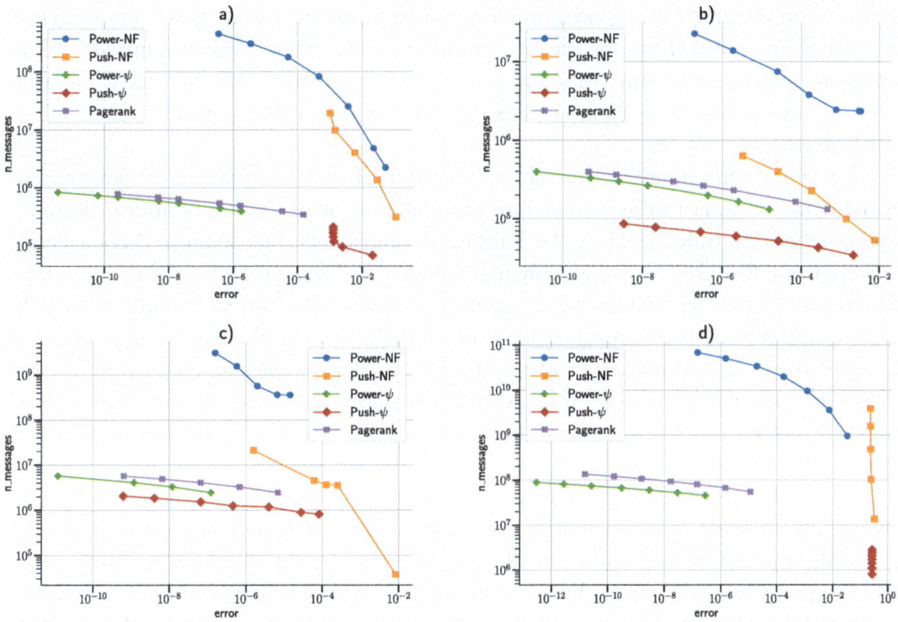

Fig. 7 (*ii*) Homogeneous scenario. Experiment 3 with (**a**) `DBLP`, (**b**) `ego-Twitter`, (**c**) `Twitter-ICWSM` and (**d**) `Russian`: Comparison of the proposed algorithms with the baselines `Power-NF` and `PageRank` in terms of the number of messages to reach convergence

the error committed on the ψ-score. Consequently, we suggest that both methods will not be used for the same applications, depending on the precision or speed required for the computation. Also, in the case of the datasets investigated, the fact that the push methods are limited to larger errors does not significantly impact the algorithms performance at ranking users, as we have seen in the previous series of experiments.

6 Conclusion and Future Work

In conclusion, the ψ-score is a powerful metric that generalizes PageRank for non-homogeneous node activities. It combines the structural information of the graph with the temporal information of the users' activities to rank their influence in the social network. In this work, we have proposed three scalable algorithms for approximating the ψ-score. The `Power-`ψ and `Push-`ψ algorithms take advantage of a novel equation that reduces the system we need to solve for the ψ-score calculation, while the `Push-NF` algorithm provides additional insights on the information dynamics at the individual level. Through our experiments, we have shown that these algorithms perform well on various real-world datasets both in terms of precision of the approximation and in terms of speed; however, someone interested in controlling the error committed will favor power methods while someone interested in time efficiency will favor push-methods. We have released them as an open-source Python package for the research community to use and improve upon.

This score suits many real-world applications. It has been specially designed to evaluate the notion of influence on online social platforms, typically micro-blogging social networks. Indeed, while the PageRank only takes into account the structural information, the ψ-score also considers nodes posting and re-posting activities, which are known to be important features on these platforms. It could thus help identify influential users on social networks. However, it could also be an interesting score to evaluate influence in other contexts, such as scientific citation networks, where an author posting corresponds to a new publication and re-posting would be a citation. Here as well, we expect the users' activity to have a significant effect on their visibility and influence in the network.

This study opens several interesting avenues for future work. A possibility is to investigate in what way the heterogeneous patterns of activities in real networks affect the spread of influence on the platform: for instance, does it allow some specific posts to reach some distant users faster? Another one could be to measure to what extent the idealized process underlying the ψ-score definition differs from the actual diffusion process and possibly identify anomalous behaviors from these differences. For instance, we can think that if a post of a user is largely re-posted while they have a relatively low ψ-score, it might convey a specific message that is worthy of analysis.

Acknowledgments This work is funded by the ANR (French National Agency of Research) through the FairEngine project (grant ANR-19-CE25-0011) and the FiT LabCom project (grant FiT-ANR-19-LCV1-0005).

References

1. A. Bavelas, The journal of the acoustical society of America **22**(6), 725 (1950)
2. L.C. Freeman, Sociometry pp. 35–41 (1977)
3. M.S. Alvim, B. Amorim, S. Knight, S. Quintero, F. Valencia, in *International Conference on Formal Techniques for Distributed Objects, Components, and Systems* (Springer, 2021), pp. 22–41
4. D. Kempe, J. Kleinberg, E. Tardos, in *Proceedings of the Ninth ACM SIGKDD International Conference on Knowledge Discovery and Data Mining* (Association for Computing Machinery, New York, NY, USA, 2003), KDD '03, p. 137–146. URL https://doi.org/10.1145/956750.956769
5. K. Bok, Y. Noh, J. Lim, J. Yoo, Electronic Commerce Research **21**(3), 671 (2021)
6. C. Musto, P. Lops, M. de Gemmis, G. Semeraro, Knowl. Based Syst. **216**, 106806 (2021). URL https://doi.org/10.1016/j.knosys.2021.106806
7. V. Cabannes, L. Pillaud-Vivien, F. Bach, A. Rudi, Advances in Neural Information Processing Systems **34** (2021)

8. S. Goel, D.J. Watts, D.G. Goldstein, in *Proceedings of the 13th ACM Conference on Electronic Commerce* (Association for Computing Machinery, New York, NY, USA, 2012), EC '12, p. 623–638. URL https://doi.org/10.1145/2229012.2229058
9. Z. Wan, Y. Mahajan, B.W. Kang, T.J. Moore, J.H. Cho, IEEE Access **9**, 104773 (2021). URL https://doi.org/10.1109/ACCESS.2021.3094196
10. U. Brandes, Journal of mathematical sociology **25**(2), 163 (2001)
11. M. Cha, H. Haddadi, F. Benevenuto, K. Gummadi, Proceedings of the International AAAI Conference on Web and Social Media **4**(1), 10 (2010). URL https://ojs.aaai.org/index.php/ICWSM/article/view/14033
12. C. Wilson, A. Sala, K.P.N. Puttaswamy, B.Y. Zhao, ACM Trans. Web **6**(4) (2012). URL https://doi.org/10.1145/2382616.2382620
13. A. Giovanidis, B. Baynat, C. Magnien, A. Vendeville, IEEE/ACM Trans. Netw. **29**(5), 2198 (2021). URL https://doi.org/10.1109/TNET.2021.3085201
14. N. Arhachoui, E. Bautista, M. Danisch, A. Giovanidis, in *2022 IEEE/ACM International Conference on Advances in Social Networks Analysis and Mining (ASONAM)* (2022), pp. 526–533. URL https://doi.org/10.1109/ASONAM55673.2022.10068673
15. J.J. Whang, A. Lenharth, I.S. Dhillon, K. Pingali, in *Euro-Par 2015: Parallel Processing*, ed. by J.L. Träff, S. Hunold, F. Versaci (Springer Berlin Heidelberg, Berlin, Heidelberg, 2015), pp. 438–450
16. R. Andersen, F. Chung, K. Lang, in *2006 47th Annual IEEE Symposium on Foundations of Computer Science (FOCS'06)* (2006), pp. 475–486. URL https://doi.org/10.1109/FOCS.2006.44
17. A. Landherr, B. Friedl, J. Heidemann, Wirtschaftsinformatik **52**, 367 (2010)
18. C. Correa, T. Crnovrsanin, K.L. Ma, IEEE Transactions on Visualization and Computer Graphics **18**(1), 106 (2012). URL https://doi.org/10.1109/TVCG.2010.260
19. P.R. Miller, P.S. Bobkowski, D. Maliniak, R.B. Rapoport, Political Research Quarterly **68**(2), 377 (2015). URL https://doi.org/10.1177/1065912915580135
20. R. Puzis, Y. Altshuler, Y. Elovici, S. Bekhor, Y. Shiftan, A. Pentland, J. Intell. Transp. Syst. **17**(1), 91 (2013). URL https://doi.org/10.1080/15472450.2012.716663
21. P. Hui, J. Crowcroft, E. Yoneki, in *Proceedings of the 9th ACM international symposium on Mobile ad hoc networking and computing* (2008), pp. 241–250
22. A. Tizghadam, A. Leon-Garcia, IEEE Network **24**(6), 10 (2010). URL https://doi.org/10.1109/MNET.2010.5634437
23. M. Ashtiani, A. Salehzadeh-Yazdi, Z. Razaghi-Moghadam, H. Hennig, O. Wolkenhauer, M. Mirzaie, M. Jafari, bioRxiv (2017). https://doi.org/10.1101/149492. URL https://www.biorxiv.org/content/early/2017/10/09/149492
24. L. Page, S. Brin, R. Motwani, T. Winograd. The pagerank citation ranking: Bringing order to the web (1998)
25. A.N. Langville, C.D. Meyer, *Google's PageRank and beyond: The science of search engine rankings* (Princeton university press, 2006)
26. E. Bautista, M. Latapy, Soc. Netw. Anal. Min. **12**(1), 31 (2022). URL https://doi.org/10.1007/s13278-022-00860-5
27. T. Bonald, N. de Lara, Q. Lutz, B. Charpentier, Journal of Machine Learning Research **21**(185), 1 (2020). URL http://jmlr.org/papers/v21/20-412.html
28. L. Buitinck, G. Louppe, M. Blondel, F. Pedregosa, A. Mueller, O. Grisel, V. Niculae, P. Prettenhofer, A. Gramfort, J. Grobler, R. Layton, J. VanderPlas, A. Joly, B. Holt, G. Varoquaux, in *ECML PKDD Workshop: Languages for Data Mining and Machine Learning* (2013), pp. 108–122
29. J. Kunegis, in *Proc. Int. Conf. on World Wide Web Companion* (2013), pp. 1343–1350. URL http://dl.acm.org/citation.cfm?id=2488173
30. B. Chumichev. Russian election 2018 — twitter user activity. https://www.kaggle.com/datasets/borisch/russian-election-2018-twitter (2018)
31. M. Ley, in *String Processing and Information Retrieval, 9th International Symposium, SPIRE 2002, Lisbon, Portugal, September 11–13, 2002, Proceedings, Lecture Notes in Computer*

Science, vol. 2476, ed. by A.H.F. Laender, A.L. Oliveira (Springer, 2002), *Lecture Notes in Computer Science*, vol. 2476, pp. 1–10. URL https://doi.org/10.1007/3-540-45735-6_1
32. M. De Choudhury, Y.R. Lin, H. Sundaram, K.S. Candan, L. Xie, A. Kelliher, in *Proceedings of the 4th International AAAI Conference on Weblogs and Social Media* (2010). URL http://www.public.asu.edu/~mdechoud/pubs/icwsm_10.pdf
33. J. McAuley, J. Leskovec, in *Proceedings of the 25th International Conference on Neural Information Processing Systems - Volume 1* (Curran Associates Inc., Red Hook, NY, USA, 2012), NIPS'12, p. 539–547
34. P. Virtanen, R. Gommers, T.E. Oliphant, M. Haberland, T. Reddy, D. Cournapeau, E. Burovski, P. Peterson, W. Weckesser, J. Bright, S.J. van der Walt, M. Brett, J. Wilson, K.J. Millman, N. Mayorov, A.R.J. Nelson, E. Jones, R. Kern, E. Larson, C.J. Carey, İ. Polat, Y. Feng, E.W. Moore, J. VanderPlas, D. Laxalde, J. Perktold, R. Cimrman, I. Henriksen, E.A. Quintero, C.R. Harris, A.M. Archibald, A.H. Ribeiro, F. Pedregosa, P. van Mulbregt, SciPy 1.0 Contributors, Nature Methods **17**, 261 (2020). URL https://doi.org/10.1038/s41592-019-0686-2
35. M.G. Kendall, Biometrika **30**(1–2), 81 (1938). URL https://doi.org/10.1093/biomet/30.1-2.81

Detecting Comorbidity Using Machine Learning

Yanessa Mari Lacsamana, Zain Sheikh, Camilla Suarez Viltres, Ahmed Al Marouf, Kashfia Sailunaz, and Reda Alhajj

Abstract Comorbidity between mental disorders is a topic of great interest as professionals in the field have been recognizing emerging patterns between a variety of disorders. This research experimented with neural networks to find if machine learning could be as accurate as professional diagnoses and concluded with two neural network models that provided the highest accuracy for diagnosing comorbidity. The training data used was retrieved from "Psychiatric Comorbidity in Patients from the Addictive Disorders Assistance Units of Galicia: The COPSIAD Study," (Pereiro et al., PLoS One 8(6):66451, 2013) as it pertains to comorbidity and doing statistical calculations on its real-world data and visualizing it for use as training data in the machine. The result concluded with the two models predicting certain relationships very well while others did not. More data will be needed to improve the accuracy of a professional diagnosis but the possibility of machine learning being used as a method of diagnosis may be possible in the future, as exhibited in this research.

Keywords Comorbidity · Machine learning · Algorithm · Mental illness

Y. M. Lacsamana · Z. Sheikh · C. S. Viltres · A. A. Marouf · K. Sailunaz
Department of Computer Science, University of Calgary, Calgary, AB, Canada
e-mail: yanessamari.lacsaman@ucalgary.ca; zain.sheikh1@ucalgary.ca; camilla.suarezviltres@ucalgary.ca; ahmedal.marouf@ucalgary.ca

R. Alhajj (✉)
Department of Computer Science, University of Calgary, Calgary, AB, Canada

Department of Computer Engineering, Istanbul Medipol University, Istanbul, Turkiye

Department of Heath Informatics, University of Southern Denmark, Odense, Denmark
e-mail: alhajj@ucalgary.ca

M. Kaya et al. (eds.), *Social Network Analysis and Mining Applications in Healthcare and Anomaly Detection*, Lecture Notes in Social Networks,
https://doi.org/10.1007/978-3-031-75204-9_4

1 Introduction

1.1 Comorbidity Definition

In contemporary society, mental health wellness is starting to become popular. Becoming more open to mental illnesses is less taboo and advocacy for mental health is everywhere these days but despite these positive developments, mental illness remains a significant source of disability for many individuals. It is also known that symptoms can be different for everyone with the same mental disorder, and many could emerge with known symptoms existing and others not. This complicated web of intricacies when dealing with mental disorders provokes the need for further study on the topic. By exploring such studies, we allow for a better understanding of these disorders amongst patients and professionals alike.

Comorbidity as defined is "co-occurring or coexisting conditions" [2, 3]. In this case, the presence of two or more mental disorders within an individual is considered comorbidity. The higher chances of two or more disorders in the same person is proven statistically for both physiological and psychological issues and the research shows that the significance cannot be dismissed as mere coincidence [4]. Mental disorder comorbidities are not always only mental disorders [5], but are often physiological issues [6], alcohol, drug, and tobacco usage [7], etc. and/or the mental disorders are caused by these physiological problems.

In the largest population-based study of 2019 with nearly 6 million people and 83.9 million person-years' worth of data, it was found that diagnosis of a first mental disorder was associated with a twofold to 48-fold increased risk of diagnosis with a subsequent mental disorder with risks being the highest in the first year of the first diagnosis but persists even 15 years later [8]. Research such as this provides very important insights into the true complexity of mental illnesses.

1.2 Purpose of the Research

The purpose of this research is to attempt to find if diagnosis of comorbidity using machine learning is just as effective as diagnosis through an actual person. One of the questions the research asks is: Given a set of certain symptoms and diagnosed disorders, is the result of a model from a machine-learned algorithm nearly as accurate as a professional diagnosis of another comorbid disorder? Professional diagnoses usually involve rigorous questions to ask the patient with. These professional diagnoses are usually done by therapists or sometimes, physicians. Although healthcare is free in Canada, many other countries do not have this case with therapist/physician diagnoses costing money that not many people can afford. This research, although not as reliable as a professional diagnosis, may help with shedding light on the possible comorbid illnesses that a person may not be aware of without the burden of the costs of a professional diagnosis.

The rest of the paper is organized as follows: Sect. 2 includes reviews of some relevant research works, Sect. 3 explains the datasets, Sect. 4 discusses the methodology with experimental results, and finally Sect. 5 concludes the paper with possible future extensions.

2 Literature Overview

2.1 Popular Traditional Methods of Research

Comorbidity analysis for mental disorders has been a well-known research topic for decades. Medical professionals and health-science researchers have been exploring various patterns for detections and predictions using classic and AI-based models. Researchers have been working on mental disorder comorbidities as well as comorbidities of mental and physical disorders with their association patterns [9, 10]. Some researchers focused on literature review to find relevant research works according to some specific conditions and timeline and included the summaries of similar existing research works [11, 12]. Hakobyan et al. [13] published a review on mental disorder comorbidities by summarizing 24 papers after filtering them from 8041 relevant publications over 20 years. Their analysis provided common patterns between disorders to assist future researchers in comorbidity detections. They also discussed the necessity of integrated approaches for managing diagnosis and treatments of different disorders more efficiently.

Another mental disorder comorbidity review was discussed in [14], but it focused specifically on children and adolescents. They analyzed 9 relevant research and showed that the possibility of 30%-50% mental disorder comorbidities existed for children and adolescents with intellectual disability. A literature review was used in [15] for comparisons of research to identify the possibility of mental disorder comorbidities in children younger than 7 years of age. The study showed that almost 20.1% children among 18,282 under 7 were affected by mental disorders and the significant percentages of ODD, ADHD, depression, etc. can be decreased with proper and early intervention.

Almost, if not all, research surrounding comorbidity usually involves time-tested methods such as interviews and questionnaires. A meta-analysis of PTSD comorbidity diseases in prison settings gathered studies involving clinical interviews, validated instruments leading to Diagnostic and Statistical Manual of Mental Disorders (DSM) or International Classification of Diseases (ICD) diagnoses, or validated self-report questionnaires such as the Post-Traumatic Stress Disorder (PTSD) checklist [16]. Another study involving ADHD comorbidity in Iranian children used structured psychiatric interviews assessing lifetime psychiatric disorders by DSM-IV criteria, using the Farsi version of the Schedule for Affective Disorders and Schizophrenia [17].

Another questionnaire based psychiatric disorder detection was discussed in [18] that used SOmatization study of the University of Leiden (SOUL) study for analyzing comorbidity with anxiety and depressive disorders using DSM-IV diagnoses as golden standard. Toussaint et al. [19] showed a similar study with DSM-5 for Patient Health Questionnaire-15 (PHQ-15), Somatic Symptom Scale - 8 (SSS-8), and Somatic Symptom Disorder - B Criteria Scale (SSD-12). A dataset collected by face-to-face interview was used in [20] for comorbid analysis of mental disorders related to adverse childhood experiences (ACE) and showed that most people with higher ACE that belonged to sexual minority groups were more perceptible to comorbid substance usage and mental disorders. McGrath et al. [21] used a survey-based approach to compare and confirm the possibility of all 548 pairs of mental health issues of 24 DSM-IV mental disorders.

Fox et al. [22] investigated the distinct possible patterns of ICD-11 PTSD comorbidities and showed that it was highly comorbid with other psychopathologies and mostly detectable later in life. A comorbidity analysis of 24,915 prisoners for mental disorders and substances uses was discussed in [23]. They discovered two major comorbidities of substances uses- major depression and non-effective psychosis. The comorbidity of mental disorders and their associations with premature mortality was explored in [24]. They showed that mental disorders affected the mortality rates and people with mental disorders had higher mortality rates and the highest mortality rate was associated with substance uses. Their study provided some new research ideas related to comorbid mental disorders in people with substance use and how they influence mortality.

And lastly, A total of 3585 (84.7% of 4231 births) children aged 6 years were assessed using the Development and Well-Being Assessment (DAWBA) from southern Brazil [25]. DAWBA is defined as "a novel package of questionnaires, interviews, and rating techniques designed to generate ICD-10 and DSM-IV psychiatric diagnoses on 5-16-year-olds" [25]. In general, for performing interviews or questionnaires, popular criteria such as the DSM are used as a reference for the questions that were made.

2.2 Discussion

Deducing from these studies, interviews and questionnaires are the most common when it comes to research involving mental comorbidity. These interviews follow very specific criteria that create the questions themselves. A major advantage when using interviews and questionnaires is that the criteria used to make it are established methods, meaning that quality information would come out from following specific and well-known criteria. The second advantage is that interviews can provide detailed information about an individual's experiences and feelings, allowing a more nuanced understanding of their mental illness. This is especially important as people do not experience mental illnesses the same. The third advantage is flexibility because interviews can be tailored to an individual. The interviewer can also follow up with responses or clarification that can provide more meaningful data. Questionnaires in turn are cost-effective and can be administered to large populations. It is also objective due to its standardized nature. There also is anonymity with participants where they may feel more comfortable disclosing private information.

Interview and questionnaire methods also have their disadvantages. Constructing interview questions or self-report questionnaires may be time-consuming to conduct and analyze, especially if the sample size is large. There may also be bias in the resulting data as participants may be reluctant to discuss sensitive topics or admit to certain behaviors. This will skew the data and may not provide any good accurate information. For questionnaires, there is also limited information compared to interviews as questionnaires are usually limited to close-ended questions which may not provide any detailed information about an individual's experiences. There may also be bias in questionnaires where participants may not answer truthfully or may not take the questions seriously. Questionnaires can also have missing or incomplete data for all questions, hence creating imbalanced datasets.

All in all, interviews and questionnaires are not perfect methods to gather data, but oftentimes most research around mental illness and comorbidity usually use these methods due to their advantages when it comes to nuance and the ability to gather the most personal experiences of an individual using simple questions.

3 Data

The concept of using criteria such as the DSM, ICD, validated self-report questionnaires, DAWBA, etc. is similar to the concept of nodes in a neural network. Each node may represent a check in a checklist or criteria in the questionnaire that would go through stages, similar to layers in a neural network. The goal is to simulate these stages and criteria such that the result of a machine-learned algorithm is as or nearly as accurate as a professional diagnosis by a therapist or physician or at least as accurate as the aforementioned criteria that physical interviews and questionnaires follow.

3.1 Database

The dataset selected for exploration is "Psychiatric Comorbidity in Patients from the Addictive Disorders Assistance Units of Galicia: The COPSIAD Study," which captures the presence of various psychiatric disorders in patients receiving treatment for addictive disorders [1]. The dataset contains information for 2300 patients, with each row representing a patient and the columns indicating, in binary form, whether the patient tested positive for a specific disorder.

The columns are classified as general disorders and specific disorders. The general disorders consist of eight categories being Cognitive Disorder (Deldermamn), Schizopsychiatric Disorder, Mood Disorder, Anxiety Disorder, Eating Disorder, Adjustment Disorder, Personality Disorder, and Impulse Control Disorder. The database also captures specific psychiatric disorders within each of these broader categories, such as specific types of mood disorders or personality disorders. For example, if a patient is identified as having a "manic disorder", the database will also indicate that the patient has a mood disorder. This level of detailed data has proven crucial in developing precise predictive machine learning models.

3.2 Dataset Statistics

A more general overview of the database was performed to get an understanding of surface-level comorbidities between the general categories of psychiatric disorders. The comorbidity between any two disorders was calculated as follows:

$$\frac{(count(disorder A)) \cap (count(disorder B))}{(count(disorder A)) \cup (count(disorder B))}. \tag{1}$$

The subsequent table and heat map depict the results of the aforementioned calculations. From this general analysis, it became apparent that the comorbidity rates among the different mental health disorders were relatively low, with the highest rate being 11% between mood and anxiety disorders. Despite the low rates, there is still a certain level of comorbidity that warrants further exploration through more advanced machine learning protocols.

Table 1 contains the comorbidity ratios calculated to gain a quick overview of the general disorder category comorbidities with Fig. 1 visualising this finding. It is evident that comorbidity between two different general classifications is not the most common but still occurs in the dataset. It is also evident that individuals with mood, anxiety, impulse control, personality, and schizophrenic disorders have somewhat enough correlation for machine learning.

The totals for individuals diagnosed with each general category of mental disorders were also computed. However, for certain categories such as cognitive disorders (6/2300 entries), eating disorders (26/2300 entries), and adjustment disorders (39/2300 entries), the available data was insufficient for machine learning purposes. Therefore, a decision was made to exclude these specific illnesses as output from predicting comorbidity diagnosis using the machine.

Table 1 Comorbidity ratios

	Cognitive disorder	Schizo psychiatric disorder	Mood disorder	Anxiety disorder	Eating disorder	Adjustment disorder	Personality disorder	Impulse disorder
Cognitive disorder	1	0.0057	0	0	0	0	0.0021	0
Schizo psychiatric disorder	0.0057	1	0.0338	0.0221	0.0256	0.0048	0.0600	0.0250
Mood disorder	0	0.0338	1	0.1120	0.0186	0.0073	0.0882	0.0466
Anxiety disorder	0	0.0221	0.1120	1	0.0254	0.0109	0.0581	0.0638
Eating disorder	0	0.0256	0.0186	0.0254	1	0	0.0141	0.0292
Adjustment disorder	0	0.0048	0.0073	0.0109	0	1	0.0159	0.0133
Personality disorder	0.0021	0.0600	0.0882	0.0581	0.0141	0.0159	1	0.0383
Impulse disorder	0	0.0250	0.0466	0.0638	0.0292	0.0133	0.0383	1

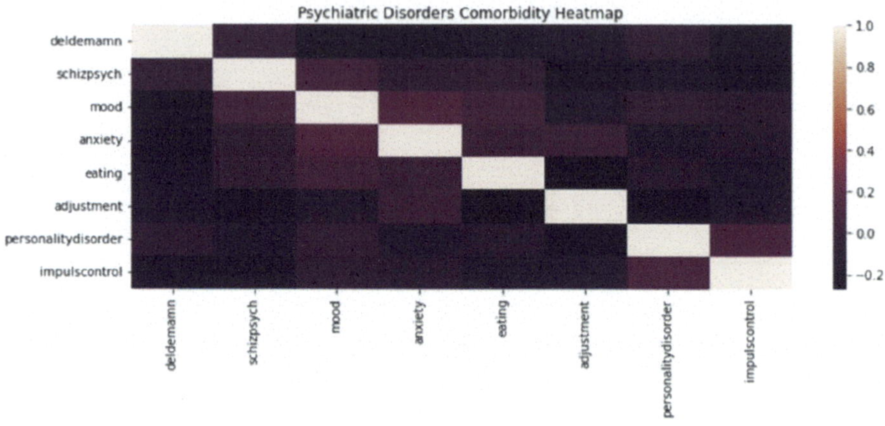

Fig. 1 Heat map

3.3 *Final Data for Machine Learning*

To get a better idea of these comorbid relationships, here is a second measure of comorbidity which will be used as data for the machine learning task:

$$\frac{(count(disorder A)) \cap (count(disorder B))}{count(disorder A)}. \tag{2}$$

The criteria for choosing which two general categories to correlate with each other is if at least 5% of people with the 'primary' disorder has the indicated second mental disorder. The highest occurrence of comorbidity in the dataset was observed between anxiety disorders and mood disorders, with 28.7% of individuals diagnosed with anxiety disorders also having a diagnosed mood disorder. The following is the comorbidity ratios of each general categories:

- Schizophrenia and other psychotic disorders: 169 in total
  - Mood disorders = 23/169 = 13.6%
  - Anxiety disorders = 11/169 = 6.5%
  - Personality disorders = 38/169 = 22.5%
- Mood disorders: 511 in total
  - Personality disorders = 86/511 = 16.8%
  - Anxiety disorders = 94/511 = 18.4%
  - Impulse control disorders = 29/511 = 5.7%
- Anxiety disorders: 328 in total
  - Personality disorders = 46/328 = 14.6%
  - Mood disorders = 94/328 = 28.7%
  - Impulse control disorder = 28/328 = 8.5%

- Personality disorders: 464 in total
  - Mood Disorders =86/464 = 18.5%
  - Anxiety Disorders = 46/464 = 9.9%
- Impulse control disorders: 111 in total
  - Personality disorders = 22/111 = 19.8%
  - Anxiety disorders = 28/111 = 25.2%
  - Mood disorders = 29/111 = 26.1%

4 Machine Learning

To further investigate the comorbidity among psychiatric disorders, a machine learning model was developed to effectively predict whether a patient would test positive for a specific disorder, given data on their other specific disorders.

4.1 Input and Output Variables

For testing comorbidity within the database, challenges arose due to the size of the table. Obtaining the list of individuals with a diagnosed disorder for their primary condition resulted in a reduction of available data. Additionally, the ratio of those with a diagnosis versus those without in the smaller primary diagnosis table presented a concern for machine learning. To address these issues, a compromise was reached to group specific disorders into their general categories of disorders, specifically for the outputs. This approach provided a higher level of granularity, allowing for the development of more accurate machine learning models.

Using the previous data, the four general categories that would be used for outputs would be the predictions of anxiety disorder, personality disorder, impulse disorder, and mood disorder. Input 'primary' diagnoses for predicting comorbid anxiety disorder are schizophrenia and other psychotic disorders, mood disorders, personality disorders, and impulse disorders. Input 'primary' diagnoses for predicting comorbid personality disorder are schizophrenia and other psychotic disorders, mood disorders, anxiety disorders, personality disorders, and impulse disorders. Input 'primary' diagnoses for predicting comorbid mood disorder are schizophrenia and other psychotic disorders, anxiety disorders, personality disorders, and impulse control disorders. Input 'primary' diagnoses for predicting comorbid impulse control disorder are mood disorders and anxiety disorders.

4.2 The Models

To predict whether a patient would test positive for a specific disorder, a binary classification approach was used. Multiple hidden layers were created to achieve an accurate model for this classification problem. The initial layers included up to 50 nodes, which were gradually reduced to 1 node for the final layer with sigmoid activation code to provide the binary classification. The priority is accuracy of the diagnosis and since for the binary output, binary cross entropy was used as a base.

The first attempt involved the use of the reLu activation function. Which resulted in generally high accuracy. The problem of this activation function is the 'dying reLu problem'. It was not preferable for the machine to completely disregard certain input variables since people experience mental illness differently. So, the research omitted this option of using reLu in general. The following Fig. 2 is one of the first attempts with using reLu layers and 10 epochs.

The accuracy achieved in the training and testing data for the models was as follows (train/test):

- Output: Personality Disorder:
  - Input: Schizo-psychiatric disorder = 91.6%/92.5%
  - Input: Mood disorder = 80.3%/86.0%
  - Input: Anxiety disorder = 90.0%/90.3%
  - Input: Impulse Control disorder = 95.4%/94.6%
- Output: Mood Disorder:
  - Input: Schizo-psychiatric disorder = 94.4%/100.0%
  - Input: Personality disorder = 81.9%/88.3%
  - Input: Anxiety disorder = 81.6%/81.6%
  - Input: Impulse Control disorder = 93.4%/98.1%
- Output: Impulse Control Disorder:
  - Input: Mood disorder = 73.9%/73.9%
  - Input: Anxiety disorder = 70.5%/91.3%

Fig. 2 First attempt involving reLu activation functions

```
tf.keras.layers.Dense(59, activation='relu'),
tf.keras.layers.Dropout(0.5),
tf.keras.layers.Dense(30, activation='relu'),
tf.keras.layers.Dropout(0.5),
tf.keras.layers.Dense(15, activation='relu'),
tf.keras.layers.Dropout(0.5),
tf.keras.layers.Dense(4, activation='relu'),
tf.keras.layers.Dropout(0.5),
tf.keras.layers.Dense(1, activation='sigmoid')
```

- Output: Anxiety Disorder
  - Input: Schizo-psychiatric disorder = 96.6%/97.0%
  - Input: Personality disorder = 87.4%/80.3%
  - Input: Mood disorder = 71.4%/71.2%
  - Input: Impulse Control disorder = 91.6%/90.9%

Furthermore, it was also found that increasing the number of epochs optimized the accuracy of the predictions greatly. As the following experiments increased epochs the results started to flatten at around 100. This, accompanied with the adam optimizer and a binary cross entropy loss function yielded the best results.

The research also started to experiment with TanH activation and seLu functions which greatly affected the accuracy as shown in Figs. 3 and 4.

The accuracy achieved in the training and testing data for the models was as follows (train/test):

- Output: Personality Disorder:
  - Input: Schizo-psychiatric disorder = 77.0%/79.4%
  - Input: Mood disorder = 81.9%/88.3%
  - Input: Anxiety disorder = 87.4%/80.3%
  - Input: Impulse control disorder = 78.4%/87.0%
- Output: Mood Disorder:
  - Input: Impulse control disorder = 73.9%/73.9%
  - Input: Schizo-psychiatric disorder = 89.6%/85.3%

Fig. 3 Attempt using TanH functions and more layers

```
tf.keras.layers.Dense(num_columns),
tf.keras.layers.Dropout(0.5),
tf.keras.layers.Dense(50, activation='tanh'),
tf.keras.layers.Dropout(0.5),
tf.keras.layers.Dense(50, activation='tanh'),
tf.keras.layers.Dropout(0.5),
tf.keras.layers.Dense(50, activation='tanh'),
tf.keras.layers.Dropout(0.5),
tf.keras.layers.Dense(50, activation='tanh'),
tf.keras.layers.Dropout(0.5),
tf.keras.layers.Dense(30, activation='tanh'),
tf.keras.layers.Dropout(0.5),
tf.keras.layers.Dense(15, activation='tanh'),
tf.keras.layers.Dropout(0.5),
tf.keras.layers.Dense(5, activation='tanh'),
tf.keras.layers.Dropout(0.5),
tf.keras.layers.Dense(1, activation='sigmoid')
```

Fig. 4 Another attempt involving tanh with the last layer's activation function being TanH

```
tf.keras.layers.Dense(num_columns),
tf.keras.layers.Dropout(0.5),
tf.keras.layers.Dense(50, activation='selu'),
tf.keras.layers.Dropout(0.5),
tf.keras.layers.Dense(50, activation='selu'),
tf.keras.layers.Dropout(0.5),
tf.keras.layers.Dense(50, activation='selu'),
tf.keras.layers.Dropout(0.5),
tf.keras.layers.Dense(50, activation='selu'),
tf.keras.layers.Dropout(0.5),
tf.keras.layers.Dense(1, activation='tanh')
```

  - Input: Anxiety disorder = 71.4%/71.2%
  - Input: Personality disorder = 80.3%/86.0%

- Output: Impulse Disorder:
  - Input: Schizo-psychiatric disorder = 95.6%/97.1%
  - Input: Anxiety disorder = 91.6%/90.9%
  - Input: Mood disorder = 93.4%/98.1%
  - Input: Personality disorder = 95.4%/94.6%

- Output: Anxiety Disorder:
  - Input: Schizo-psychiatric disorder = 92.6%/97.1%
  - Input: Mood disorder = 84.1%/81.6%
  - Input: Personality disorder = 90.6%/90.3%
  - Input: Impulse control disorder = 70.5%/91.3%

The accuracy achieved in the training and testing data for the models was as follows (train/test):

- Output: Personality Disorder:
  - Input: Schizo-psychiatric disorder = 77.0%/79.4%
  - Input: Mood disorder = 81.9%/88.3%
  - Input: Anxiety disorder = 87.4%/80.3%
  - Input: Impulse control = 78.4%/87.0%

- Output: Mood Disorder:
  - Input: Impulse control = 73.9%/73.9%
  - Input: Schizo-psychiatric disorder = 86.7%/85.3%
  - Input: Anxiety disorder = 71.4%/71.2%
  - Input: Personality disorder = 80.3%/86.0%

- Output: Impulse Disorder:
  - Input: Schizo-psychiatric disorder = 95.6%/97.1%
  - Input: Anxiety disorder = 91.6%/90.9%
  - Input: Mood disorder = 93.4%/98.1%
  - Input: Personality disorder = 95.4%/94.6%
- Output: Anxiety Disorder:
  - Input: Schizo-psychiatric disorder = 92.6%/97.1%
  - Input: Mood disorder = 81.6%/81.6%
  - Input: Personality disorder = 90.0%/90.3%
  - Input: Impulse control disorder = 70.5% /91.3%

Since the TanH activation code is just a modified version of the sigmoid activation code—both to be used for binary classification—the research attempted to use TanH as the final layer, to see if it made any significant difference. The result was that the differences were very minute and that using TanH in the final layer did not help with the accuracy of the model.

4.3 Results

The experimentations with the neural networks concluded with two models that provided the highest accuracy for predicting the outputs. The following code snippets mentioned in Figs. 5 and 6 are coded in Keras and TensorFlow both using 100 with seLu being a big factor. This, accompanied with the adam optimizer and a binary cross entropy loss function well.

Results from the experiment concluded that predictions of a comorbid personality disorder and predictions of a comorbid impulse disorder were more efficient with the first model. Predictions of a comorbid mood disorder and predictions of a comorbid anxiety disorder yielded more accuracy with the second model.

The accuracy achieved in the training and testing data for the models was as follows (train/test):

Fig. 5 First model

```
tf.keras.layers.Dense(num_columns),
tf.keras.layers.Dropout(0.5),
tf.keras.layers.Dense(50, activation='selu'),
tf.keras.layers.Dropout(0.5),
tf.keras.layers.Dense(30, activation='selu'),
tf.keras.layers.Dropout(0.5),
tf.keras.layers.Dense(15, activation='tanh'),
tf.keras.layers.Dropout(0.5),
tf.keras.layers.Dense(4, activation='tanh'),
tf.keras.layers.Dropout(0.5),
tf.keras.layers.Dense(1, activation='sigmoid')
```

Fig. 6 Second model

```
tf.keras.layers.Dense(num_columns),
tf.keras.layers.Dropout(0.5),
tf.keras.layers.Dense(50, activation='selu'),
tf.keras.layers.Dropout(0.5),
tf.keras.layers.Dense(30, activation='selu'),
tf.keras.layers.Dropout(0.5),
tf.keras.layers.Dense(15, activation='selu'),
tf.keras.layers.Dropout(0.5),
tf.keras.layers.Dense(5, activation='selu'),
tf.keras.layers.Dropout(0.5),
tf.keras.layers.Dense(1, activation='sigmoid')
```

- Output: Personality Disorder:
  - Input: Schizo-psychiatric disorder = 77.0%/79.4%
  - Input: Mood disorder = 83.3%/87.4%
  - Input: Anxiety disorder = 87.4%/80.3%
  - Input: Impulse Control disorder = 78.4%/87.0%
- Output: Mood Disorder:
  - Input: Schizo-psychiatric disorder = 73.9%/73.9%
  - Input: Personality disorder = 91.1%/85.3%
  - Input: Anxiety disorder = 91.1%/85.3%
  - Input: Impulse Control disorder = 81.7%/86.0%
- Output: Impulse Control Disorder:
  - Input: Mood disorder = 93.6%/98.1%
  - Input: Anxiety disorder = 91.6%/90.9%
- Output: Anxiety Disorder:
  - Input: Schizo-psychiatric disorder = 96.3%/100.0%
  - Input: Personality disorder = 91.4%/89.2%
  - Input: Mood disorder = 84.3%/81.6%
  - Input: Impulse Control disorder = 70.5%/91.3%

By utilizing specific, granular disorders as predictors and implementing a multi-layered neural network, the models were able to somewhat accurately predict the presence of a particular disorder based on the presence of other disorders and others somewhat do not. Good accuracy in this research's metric would be 90% above since the diagnosis of illnesses must be very accurate. From this experiment, there are some relationships that the machine has not predicted quite well such as the relationship between any of the indicated disorders predicting impulse control disorders where accuracy for using the models only yielded low results with the highest only being 81.7% training accuracy. Mood disorder predicting personality, impulse control predicting mood, and mood predicting anxiety yielded accuracies in the low eighties, and anxiety disorder predicting personality disorder resulted in train accuracy in the high eighties.

5 Conclusion

This research aimed to answer the question: Given a set of certain symptoms and diagnosed disorders, is the result of a model from a machine-learned algorithm nearly as accurate as a professional diagnosis of another comorbid disorder?

Through this careful analysis of data on psychiatric disorders, provided the right data, machine learning can be used to create decently accurate predictions of the comorbidity of psychiatric disorders amongst patients. With accuracy rates of 96% in this experiment, the models proposed in this paper suggest that not only are there very real and prominent comorbidity patterns between disorders, but that individuals can use modern technology to make predictions of existing disorders, before the conclusion of a professional physician. This allows the potential for patients to look out for possible comorbid disorders they may have without the need for paying for a diagnosis. In places where healthcare is not free, such models can help guide patients toward discovering the patterns in their health. However, detailed information about specific disorders and symptoms must be taken into account in order to begin creating accurate predictive models.

This being said, the research was not able to create a model that yielded high accuracies for every single comorbid disorder. Some disorders simply did not share enough correlation with others or there was not enough data and thus found that some disorders were much harder to predict. With this variation in accuracy, the model was able to be extremely accurate for specific disorders and not as accurate for others. Therefore, depending on the disorder, there is indeed a machine learning model that can predict comorbidity within psychiatric patients, nearly as accurately as a professional diagnosis. However, the variation in accuracy from disorder to disorder ultimately limits the use of the machine learning model as a loose prediction, rather than a substitute for a professional diagnosis.

References

1. Pereiro, C., Pino, C., Florez, G., Arrojo, M., Becona, E., Group., C.: Psychiatric comorbidity in patients from the addictive disorders assistance units of galicia: The copsiad study. PLoS One. **8**(6), 66451 (2013)
2. Balingit, A.: Comorbidity: Definition, Types, Risk Factors, Treatment & More. Healthline www.healthline.com/health/comorbidity#definition (2022)
3. Angold, A., Costello, E.J., Erkanli, A.: Comorbidity. The Journal of Child Psychology and Psychiatry and Allied Disciplines. **40**(1), 57–87 (1999)
4. Bonavita, V., De Simone, R.: Towards a definition of comorbidity in the light of clinical complexity. Neurological Sciences. **29**, 99–102 (2008)

5. Nock, M.K., Hwang, I., Sampson, N.A., Kessler, R.C.: Mental disorders, comorbidity and suicidal behavior: results from the national comorbidity survey replication. Molecular Psychiatry. **15**(8), 868–876 (2010)
6. Goodell, S., Druss, B.G., Walker, E.R., Mat, M.J.: Mental disorders and medical comorbidity. Robert Wood Johnson Foundation. (2011)
7. Jane-Llopis, E.V., Matytsina, I.: Mental health and alcohol, drugs and tobacco: a review of the comorbidity between mental disorders and the use of alcohol, tobacco and illicit drugs. Drug and Alcohol Review. **25**(6), 515–536 (2006)
8. Gamse, C.: Mental Health Comorbidity: One Thing Leads to Another. Medpagetoday www.medpagetoday.com/resource-centers/mental-health-focus/mental-health-comorbidity-one-thing-leads-another/2408 (2019)
9. Asanova, R., Sharapova, D., Turayev, B., Shernazarov, F.: Features of the treatment of patients with mental disorders and cardiovascular pathology. Science and Innovation. **2**(D12), 545–550 (2023)
10. Momen, N.C., Plana-Ripoll, O., Agerbo, E., Benros, M.E., Børglum, A.D., Christensen, M.K., Dalsgaard, S., Degenhardt, L., Jonge, P., Debost, J.C., Fenger-Grøn, M.: Association between mental disorders and subsequent medical conditions. New England Journal of Medicine. **382**(18), 1721–1731 (2020)
11. Sharma, E., Sharma, L.P., Balachander, S., Lin, B., Manohar, H., Khanna, P., Lu, C., Garg, K., Thomas, T.L., Au, A.C., Selles, R.R.: Comorbidities in obsessive-compulsive disorder across the lifespan: a systematic review and meta-analysis. Frontiers in Psychiatry. **12**, 703701 (2021)
12. Janse Van Rensburg, A., Dube, A., Curran, R., Ambaw, F., Murdoch, J., Bachmann, M., Petersen, I., Fairall, L.: Comorbidities between tuberculosis and common mental disorders: a scoping review of epidemiological patterns and person-centred care interventions from low-to-middle income and brics countries. Infectious Diseases of Poverty. **9**, 1–8 (2020)
13. Hakobyan, S., Vazirian, S., Lee-Cheong, S., Krausz, M., Honer, W.G., Schutz, C.G.: Concurrent disorder management guidelines. systematic review. Journal of Clinical Medicine. **9**(8), 2406 (2020)
14. Einfeld, S.L., Ellis, L.A., Emerson, E.: Comorbidity of intellectual disability and mental disorder in children and adolescents: A systematic review. Journal of Intellectual and Developmental Disability. **36**(2), 137–143 (2011)
15. Vasileva, M., Graf, R.K., Reinelt, T., Petermann, U., Petermann, F.: Research review: A meta-analysis of the international prevalence and comorbidity of mental disorders in children between 1 and 7 years. Journal of Child Psychology and Psychiatry. **62**(4), 372–381 (2021)
16. Ghanizadeh, A., Mohammadi, M.R., Moini, R.: Comorbidity of psychiatric disorders and parental psychiatric disorders in a sample of iranian children with adhd. Journal of Attention Disorders. **12**(2), 149–155 (2008)
17. Petresco, S., Anselmi, L., Santos, I.S., Barros, A.J., Fleitlich-Bilyk, B., Barros, F.C., Matijasevich, A.: Prevalence and comorbidity of psychiatric disorders among 6-year-old children: 2004 pelotas birth cohort. Social Psychiatry and psychiatric Epidemiology. **49**, 975–983 (2014)
18. Waal, M.W., Arnold, I.A., Spinhoven, P., Eekhof, J.A., Assendelft, W.J., Hemert, A.M.: The role of comorbidity in the detection of psychiatric disorders with checklists for mental and physical symptoms in primary care. Social Psychiatry and Psychiatric Epidemiology. **44**, 78–85 (2009)
19. Toussaint, A., Hüsing, P., Kohlmann, S., Löwe, B.: Detecting dsm-5 somatic symptom disorder: criterion validity of the patient health questionnaire-15 (phq-15) and the somatic symptom scale-8 (sss-8) in combination with the somatic symptom disorder-b criteria scale (ssd-12). Psychological Medicine. **50**(2), 324–333 (2020)
20. McCabe, S.E., Hughes, T.L., West, B.T., Evans-Polce, R.J., Veliz, P.T., Dickinson, K., McCabe, V.V., Boyd, C.J.: Sexual orientation, adverse childhood experiences, and comorbid dsm-5 substance use and mental health disorders. The Journal of Clinical Psychiatry. **81**(6), 19478 (2020)

21. McGrath, J.J., Lim, C.C., Plana-Ripoll, O., Holtz, Y., Agerbo, E., Momen, N.C., Mortensen, P.B., Pedersen, C.B., Abdulmalik, J., Aguilar-Gaxiola, S., Al-Hamzawi, A.: Comorbidity within mental disorders: a comprehensive analysis based on 145 990 survey respondents from 27 countries. Epidemiology and Psychiatric Sciences. **29**, 153 (2020)
22. Fox, R., Hyland, P., Power, J.M., Coogan, A.N.: Patterns of comorbidity associated with icd-11 ptsd among older adults in the united states. Psychiatry Research. **290**, 113171 (2020)
23. Baranyi, G., Fazel, S., Langerfeldt, S.D., Mundt, A.P.: The prevalence of comorbid serious mental illnesses and substance use disorders in prison populations: a systematic review and meta-analysis. The Lancet Public Health. **7**(6), 557–568 (2022)
24. Plana-Ripoll, O., Musliner, K.L., Dalsgaard, S., Momen, N.C., Weye, N., Christensen, M.K., Agerbo, E., Iburg, K.M., Laursen, T.M., Mortensen, P.B., Pedersen, C.B.: Nature and prevalence of combinations of mental disorders and their association with excess mortality in a population-based cohort study. World Psychiatry. **19**(3), 339–349 (2020)
25. Goodman, R., Ford, T., Richards, H., Gatward, R., Meltzer, H.: The development and well-being assessment: Description and initial validation of an integrated assessment of child and adolescent psychopathology. Journal of Child Psychology and Psychiatry. **41**(5), 645–655 (2000)

Evaluating the Effectiveness of Mitigative and Preventative Actions on Viral Spread in a Small Community Using an Agent-Based Stochastic Simulation

Adrian Chen, Brett Gattinger, Patricia Lively, Kashfia Sailunaz, Ahmed Al Marouf, and Reda Alhajj

Abstract To discover the effects of preventative and mitigative actions on the spread of a virus in a small community, we designed and created an agent-based simulation that incorporates real-world data to simulate agents to investigate how the disease propagates. The community itself is represented as a 2D grid, in which agents move through the simulation, interacting with other agents and transmitting the disease throughout. Locations within the community such as workplaces and homes are abstracted as labelled areas within this coordinate space. The pygame and pygame_menu packages were used to design a graphical interface for the simulation that displays and controls its progress in real-time. Based on different parameters, such as base infection, masked, quarantined, social distancing maintained, the simulation has been performed and graphical user interface shows the impacts. A detail analysis has been presented these different set up to show the variations in the simulation metrics, such as susceptible, incubating, infectious, symptomatic, recovered and deceased.

Keywords Viral spread · Agent-based simulation · Stochastic simulation · Small community based analysis

A. Chen · B. Gattinger · P. Lively · K. Sailunaz · A. A. Marouf
Department of Computer Science, University of Calgary, Calgary, AB, Canada
e-mail: adrian.chen1@ucalgary.ca; brett.gattinger@ucalgary.ca; patricia.lively@ucalgary.ca; kashfia.sailunaz@ucalgary.ca; ahmedal.marouf@ucalgary.ca

R. Alhajj (✉)
Department of Computer Science, University of Calgary, Calgary, AB, Canada

Department of Computer Engineering, Istanbul Medipol University, Istanbul, Turkiye

Department of Heath Informatics, University of Southern Denmark, Odense, Denmark
e-mail: alhajj@ucalgary.ca

M. Kaya et al. (eds.), *Social Network Analysis and Mining Applications in Healthcare and Anomaly Detection*, Lecture Notes in Social Networks,
https://doi.org/10.1007/978-3-031-75204-9_5

1 Introduction

The spread of viral infections within a community is a complex phenomenon that is influenced by various biological, social, and environmental factors. To effectively mitigate and prevent the spread of such viruses, it is crucial to understand the dynamics of viral transmission and the impact of interventions. This study aims to evaluate the effectiveness of mitigative and preventative actions on viral spread in a small community using an agent-based stochastic simulation.

Agent-based modeling has emerged as a powerful tool for simulating the dynamics of disease transmission, as it allows for the incorporation of individual-level interactions and behaviors.[1] By simulating the interactions and movements of individuals within a community, these models can provide insights into the factors that drive viral spread and the potential impacts of interventions.

In the context of the COVID-19 pandemic, the importance of understanding the role of social networks and the impact of non-pharmaceutical interventions, such as physical distancing and contact tracing, has been highlighted. [2] The proposed simulation model will incorporate these elements to evaluate the effectiveness of various mitigation and prevention strategies in a small community setting.

Our topic of research concerns the spread of an infectious virus within a small community. While there is a wealth of data collected for large cities, it is unclear whether the same guide- lines used to mitigate infection will apply to less populous areas. Which preventative actions should be given precedence over others, given limited resources? The importance of this area of study has been made increasingly evident in recent years, particularly with the COVID-19 pandemic that started in March 2020 and continues to be a health risk today.

To answer this question, we have designed a custom simulation with an Agent-Based model to determine which preventative actions and their combinations are most effective at mitigating the spread of a disease within a small community. Our simulation visually displays the simulation and its agents as the virus spreads over time, and is designed to reproduce the statistical and behavioural effects of masking, quarantining, social distancing, and vaccination. Through proper configuration, its outputs can be used to compare and contrast the impact of any combination of these preventative actions on the viral spread in the community.

In this paper, we first examine existing virus simulations in the literature and their details before describing our own created simulation. This covers the infection model chosen, how we manage agents within the simulation, the graphical user interface (GUI), and the output of the simulation.

Afterwards, we use the data generated by our simulation to graphically demonstrate the differences between the chosen preventative/mitigative measures and ultimately answer the research problem.

2 Literature Reveiw

2.1 Overview

In our research, we examined various academic papers that investigate the modelling of infection spread. Within the scope of these studies, two principal approaches have been identified in modelling infection spread: Agent-Based Models and Equation-based Models. An Agent-Based Model assumes a heterogeneous population of agents, each with their own behaviours and patterns. Conversely, an Equation- Based Model assumes a homogeneous population, where each individual has an equal probability of interacting with every other person.

1. Agent-Based Models: The research paper "Prediction of COVID-19 Infection Spread through Agent-Based Simulation" aims to accurately forecast the transmission dynamics of COVID-19 in order to facilitate effective policy planning and resource allocation [3]. To validate the model's accuracy, the authors conducted a rigorous comparison of the predicted outcomes with the observed trends in multiple countries.
2. Equation-Based Models: The book "Mathematical Models in Population Biology and Epidemiology" presents a comprehensive study on mathematical modelling for the spread of infectious diseases [4]. The authors developed SIR (Susceptible-Infectious-Removed) models [5, 6], where removal can be attributed to full immunity or death. Additionally, they formulated SIS (Susceptible-Infectious-Susceptible) models [7, 8], which are applicable to diseases where reinfection is possible. The authors also accounted for demographic effects, such as births and deaths, in their models. Overall, this paper provides valuable insights into the development of mathematical models for the study of epidemiology.

"The Coronavirus Disease (COVID-19) Pandemic: Simulation-Based Assessment of Outbreak Responses and Postpeak Strategies" presents a behavioural dynamic epidemic model that incorporates endogenous virus transmission, social contacts, case testing, and reporting [9].Given its dynamic nature, the model can be adapted to analyze the impact of preventative and mitigative policies. The model's validity is established by utilizing data collected between December 13, 2019 and May 15, 2020, from six countries. The findings demonstrate that increased testing capacity and reduced social contacts are associated with changes in outbreak dynamics, which may explain why different countries have experienced varying levels of virus transmission. The model suggests that individuals who have not received vaccinations will likely continue to maintain social distancing practices below pre-pandemic levels. Finally, targeted interventions may prove effective in increasing the number of social contacts permitted after the outbreak's peak.

The equation-based paper "Modeling of the Small-Scale Outbreak of COVID-19" compared three models to simulate the small-scale outbreaks of COVID-19 in different provinces in China [10]. They used the following models: SIR (Suseptible, Infective, Recovered) [5, 6]; SEIUIDRURD (Susceptible, Exposed, Symptomatic

Infectious, Asymptomatic Infectious, Undetected Recovered, Detected Recovered) [11], and CA (Cellular Automata) [12]. In the analysis, the Cellular Automata model outperformed the other classical compartment models when compared to real data. This suggests that traditional models are no longer suitable for modelling small-scale virus outbreaks.

Most of the work done in the field of epidemiology has been achieved through the use of Compartmental and Agent-Based Models. Both types of models and the curious misnomer that exists between them will be discussed here. A comparison between them will also be made as well as how their pros and cons motivated the decision of which to choose for this paper.

1. Compartmental Models and Agent-Based Models: Compartmental models are a general modelling technique that describes how a collection of objects, treated either homogeneous or heterogeneous, transitions through discrete compartments over time. Compartmental models originate as far back as the 1920's with the Kermack-Mckendrick epidemic model in 1927 and the Reed-Frost epidemic model in 1928 and have been ubiquitous in epidemiology ever since having only relatively recently given ground to other types of models. When researchers and scientists speak about compartmental models they often mean deterministic, equation-based models that assume homogeneity, meaning the people of the model only really manifest as sums in each compartment. This is contrasted by what these same researchers and scientists would refer to as agent-based models. These Agent-based models, in the field of epidemiology at least, also feature discrete compartments but instead simulate individual, heterogeneous agents and their interactions within a limited region. Such agent based models are more recent additions to the field of epidemiology with some of the first not appearing until the 1970's. Since then they have been steadily gaining more and more use and have begun to compete with so-called Compartmental models as the common model in epidemiology [13].
2. Comparing Agent-Based vs "Compartmental" Equation- Based Models: The comparison of Compartmental vs Agent- Based modelling in the field of epidemiology is a misnomer. Both are technically compartmental in that they implement discrete compartments and track transitions between them, the difference is in how they treat the population(s) that moves through these compartments. As mentioned above, compartmental models often refer to deterministic, equation-based models that assume homogeneity, so the comparison is more accurately between Agent-Based vs Equation-Based models. One possible reason for this misnomer is that equation- based models came before agent-based models and so utilised compartments first, thereby making the two synonymous.

The comparison of Agent-Based versus Equation-Based models is summarised in following table [14] (Table 1).

Table 1 Comparison of agent-based and equation-based models

Agent-based model (ABM)	Equation-based model (EBM)
• More computationally intensive	• Less computationally intensive
• Stochastic	• Deterministic
• Treats population as collection of heterogeneous agents. Heterogeneous contact pattern where contact is determined based on each agent's characteristics and behaviours	• Treats population as a Homogeneity Homogeneous contact patterns, each person has an equal probability of coming into contact with every other person.

3 Methodology

After reviewing the existing literature, we determined that the current simulations available were not sufficient to accurately answer our research question. Thus, we have designed and created a custom virus simulation, the details of which will be discussed in this section.

3.1 Data

A virus's ability to propagate throughout a community depends on a variety of factors. The distribution of a community given the population size should be taken into account as the first factor. This would be a breakdown of the community's age distribution and household size. The size of the household is crucial because most infections take place within the home, where an agent spends the majority of their time. Second, an agent's age significantly affects their likelihood of infection. As a result, we want to ensure that the age distribution of our community is accurate. The most current Alberta Census [15], which occurred in 2021, is used to model our community (Table 2).

For the age distribution, we simplify the ages into the following categories: Infant (0–4 years), Youth (5–18 years), Early Adult (19–39 years), Adult (40–59 years) and

Table 2 Household size and number of households for the model

Household size	Number of households
1 person	0.260 * h[a]
2 person	0.338 * h
3 person	0.153 * h
4 person	0.149 * h
5 or more persons	0.101 * h

[a] The variable h is equal to the population size multiplied by 2.6 the average household size of the community

Table 3 Age category, population and death risk for the model

Age category	Population	Death risk
Infant (0–4 years)	0.0587 * [a]	0.00004
Youth (5–18 years)	0.1898 * p	0.00004
Early adult (19–39 years)	0.2783 * p	0.00034
Adult (40–59 years)	0.2633 * p	0.00252
Elder (60+ years)	0.3744 * p	0.04802

[a] The variable p is equal to the total population size of the community. The death risk is the chance of dying if a person becomes infected

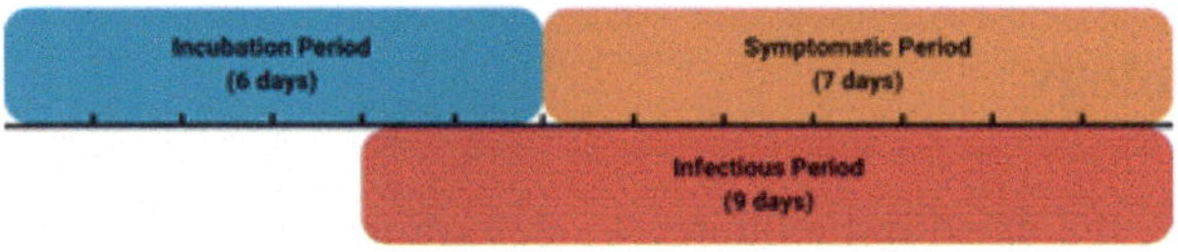

Fig. 1 Visual representation of the agent stages in a simulation

Elder (60+ years). They are grouped together based on the survival rate statistics of COVID-19 according to Alberta statistics [16] (Table 3).

The second factor in virus propagation is the length of various stages related to becoming infected. Our model allows for the possibility of susceptible, infected, recovered, and deceased agents. They might also be symptomatic or asymptomatic. A susceptible agent is one that has not been exposed to an infection in the past 6 months or has never been exposed to one. An infected agent moves through an asymptomatic period and a symptomatic period. The early stage of infection is known as the incubation period, which lasts for 6 days and is characterised by the absence of symptoms. The final 2 days of the incubation phase, before the onset of symptoms, are when they become infectious. After that, agents begin a 7-day symptomatic period during which they are infectious. In the end, they will transition to either be recovered or dead. The recovery phase lasts for 6 months at which point an agent can get reinfected. The reinfection data is collected from a study done by the Emerging Science Group of the Public Health Agency of Canada [17] (Fig. 1).

According to our research, the duration of contact with an infected person affects the risk of contracting the virus. For our simulation, the risk of contracting the virus will be 14% for every hour spent with an infected person. This risk will be further divided into intervals of 0.251% per minute spent within 5 metres of an infected agent. This risk is compounding with each infected agent nearby increasing the transmission risk by 0.251%. Near an infected agent, particles carrying the virus gather. Actions like talking, exercising, coughing and sneezing cause particles to be released in a projectile- like manner. These particles usually fall quickly onto nearby objects or the ground close to the infected person. The longer spent with an infected agent means a longer time exposed to the infectious particles. Many viral particles in a contained area increase the risk of infection. The infection rate is the third factor considered for viral spread in a community.

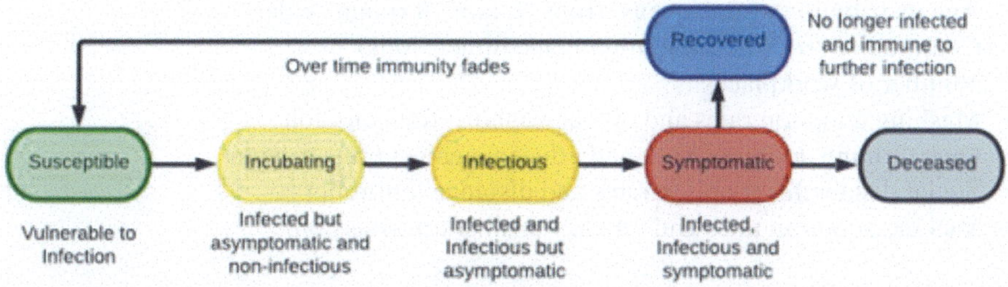

Fig. 2 The compartments in the infection model and their possible transitions

The fourth factor to consider for virus propagation is mitigative and preventative actions. Our simulation uses four different types of actions to control infections in the population. These are quarantining, social distancing, masking, and vaccination. Quarantining impacts the behaviour of the agent. When they become symptomatic they will immediately go home and quarantine. Our research indicates that members of a household have a 50% risk of infection from a quarantined agent in the household. Broken down into a per-minute infection rate is 0.000073859%. Social distancing reduces the risk of infection by 80%. To simulate this reduction the agents will maintain a separation of 2.23 metres. Masking reduces the risk of infection by 34% when using surgical masks. This makes the risk of infection 0.16566% for every minute spent within 5m of an infected agent. Finally, there is vaccination which reduces the risk of infection by 91%. This makes the risk of infection 0.02008% for every minute spent within 5 m of an infected agent (Fig. 2).

3.2 *Simulation*

3.2.1 Overview

Our created simulation takes the form of a Python-based program designed to execute an agent-based simulation with minute-by-minute resolution, with the population placed on a 2-dimensional coordinate plane. Each agent individually decides their behaviour and their destination location, which the simulation takes into account when updating agents' positions while simultaneously orchestrating the calculations required to determine the spread of the virus from one individual to another based on their coordinate positions and the virus' effective transmission radius. The simulation is highly configurable, and allows for modification to:

- Virus transmissibility and infection radius
- Timeline of progression through the infection model states
- Mortality rates for each age class
- Number of agents
- Initial number of infected agents

- Age distribution of the agents, from “infant” through “elder”
- Community size (the simulation plane dimensions)
- Number of workplaces
- Masking adoption rates and efficacy against transmission
- Quarantining adoption rates and efficacy against transmission
- Social distancing adoption rates and distance multiplier
- Vaccine adoption rates and efficacy against transmission.

3.2.2 Infection Model

Agents in our infection model will have 6 states to transition between, they are Susceptible, Incubating, Infectious, Symptomatic, Recovered and Deceased. The simulation will begin with most agents in the Susceptible state while a minority will begin as Infectious to initialise the disease’s spread. Based on gathered data, Susceptible agents that come into contact with Infected or Symptomatic agents have a chance to enter the Incubating state and then, after an Incubation period, progress to Infectious and next to Symptomatic. A Symptomatic agent has a chance, again based on gathered data, to either recover or die. Recovered agents gain a temporary immunity that decreases over time.

3.2.3 Agent Behaviour

Each agent in the simulation is responsible for determining their own behaviour in an agent- based simulation. As our simulation takes place on a 2D plane representing a small community, the primary responsibility of each person is to determine their intended location, using which their x and y coordinates are updated to proceed to the destination. Only the position of each agent is required for the purposes of the research problem, to calculate whether they are in range to infect or be infected by another individual, thus their behaviour within each destination location is not simulated. Once an individual has reached their destination, they will hover around the same position until a new destination is decided.

Every agent uses information about their current state, the time of the simulation, and their pre-programmed locations to determine what to do. Specifically, each agent is assigned a household they belong to, the size of which is chosen using real-world population statistics, and a workplace/school to attend. During weekdays, from the hours of 9am to 5pm, with some random variance, an agent will move towards their workplace or school. Outside of active hours, agents will return to their home to simulate sleep. In addition to this default behaviour, there are certain circumstances that will prompt agents to take unique actions. The current weekday is derived from the internal simulation time, and on weekends agents will randomly choose to either stay at home for the day or wander around the simulation in lieu of going to work (Fig. 3).

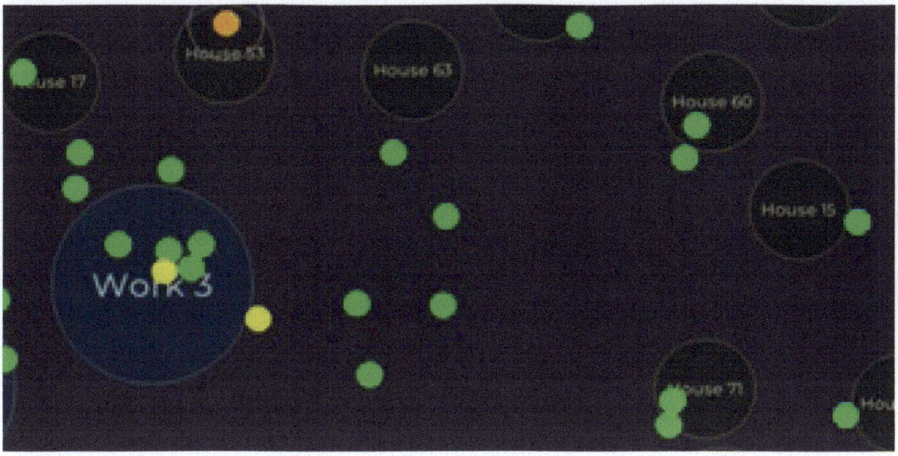

Fig. 3 A number of agents at work, at home, and in transit

The preventative and mitigative measures implemented in the simulation also affect agent behaviour. When executed, the simulation can be configured to set quarantining for an arbitrary percentage of the population. Agents with quarantining behaviour enabled will normally follow their default routines as usual: however, when they are infected with the virus and enter the Symptomatic state of the infection model, the agent will immediately stop their current behaviour to return home and recover until they reach the Recovered or Deceased state. Quarantined individuals will never break quarantine while symptomatic, and their likelihood to transmit the virus to another individual while quarantining is also significantly reduced.

Social distancing is another preventative measure that can be configured to be practised by a portion of the population. Unlike quarantining, social distancing does not change the destination locations chosen by agents: instead, it affects how they interact with other agents while in transit to or at their destination. Normally, agents are fine with being in contact with other agents and will only lightly bounce off when they collide in the simulation plane. When social distancing is active for an individual, they will actively maintain a minimum distance bubble around themselves, effectively reducing the maximum number of individuals they can be in contact with at once (Fig. 4).

Masking and vaccination are implemented in the simulation as modifiers to the base virus transmission change, and do not modify agent behaviour. Infected individuals wearing masks have a reduced chance of spreading the virus proportionally, according to real-world statistics data. In contrast, vaccinated agents have a configurable reduced chance of receiving the virus from a currently infected individual, but their behaviour is otherwise unchanged.

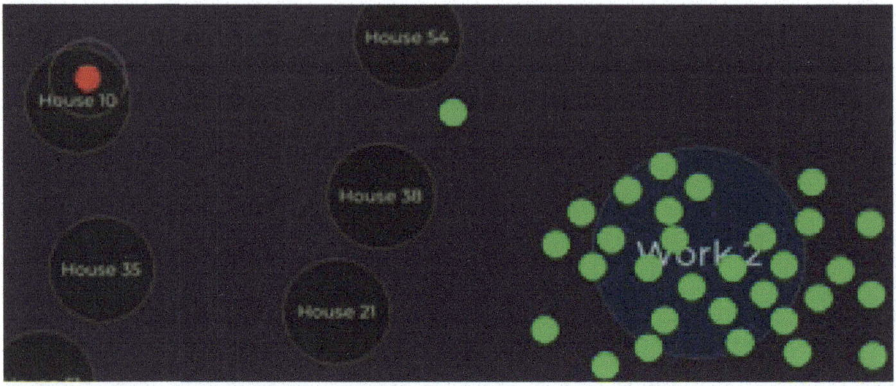

Fig. 4 The leftmost agent is symptomatic and quarantines at home while other agents are at work

3.2.4 The Community

The community is abstracted in the simulation as a collection of homes, workplaces and people. The simulation generates the community layout primarily at random, but obeys general rules which dictate that it concentrates the community's workplaces towards its center and disperses its homes outward to its periphery, all while maintaining a certain distance of separation between them (Fig. 5).

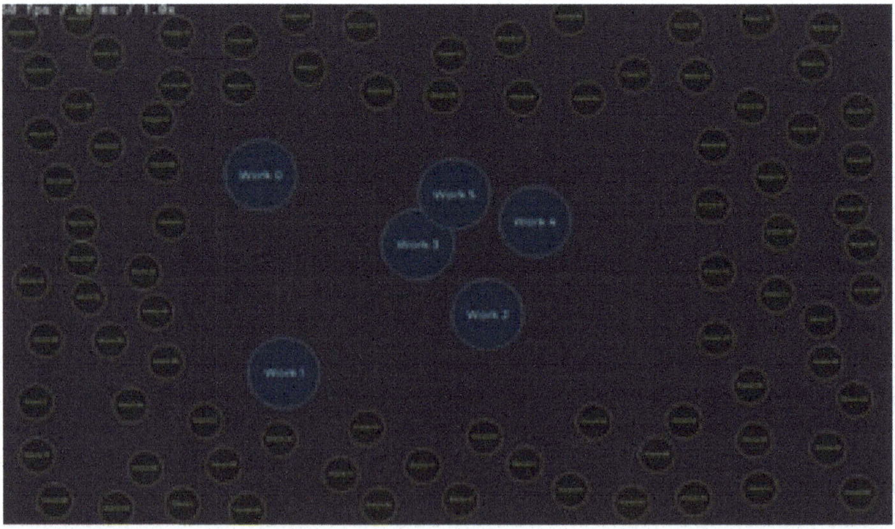

Fig. 5 A view of the community with agents removed. Workplaces are in the center and houses are on the border

In this way the simulation achieves a more realistic depiction of a real-world small community while keeping its representation simplified. The number of homes generated is based on the number of agents in the simulation and gathered statistical census data informing the number of members per home.

3.2.5 Graphical User Interface (GUI)

The GUI is implemented using a combination of pygame [18] and pygame_menu [19]. It is constituted by three main parts:

1. The Simulation Viewport
   (a) Displays the execution of the simulation in real- time, showing the movement and interaction of the agents as they travel about the community and their transition between various states.
   (b) Houses and Workplaces are rendered as labelled transparent circles.
   (c) Agents are rendered as smaller, opaque circles coloured according to their current state in the infection model.
   (d) Features a dynamic camera that allows users to zoom in and pan around the community.
2. The Metrics Menu
   (a) Primarily features an actively updated table that displays, for each state of the infection model, the current number of agents occupying that state.
   (b) A dedicated space to display age- class and infection-state data for an agent selected from the main Simulation Viewport.
3. The Control Menu
   (a) Provides simulation control functions to the user, allowing them to pause or resume the simulation at any time as well as select the speed at which it progresses.

3.2.6 Performance

We display the simulation running in real- time at a stable 60 frames per second, and there are several performance optimizations we have employed to achieve this. Despite the relatively small scale of the simulation, the virus spreading calculations are performed on every step of the simulation, and are based on actual 2D distances between agents. A naive implementation of this algorithm would require comparing the position of each agent to all others, requiring $O(n^2)$ time complexity every simulation tick, which would quickly make maintaining the real-time calculations infeasible at higher populations. To improve this process, we use an implementation of the k-d tree data structure from the scipy package [20], which, after an $O(nlogn)$ initialization, allows for an $O(logn)$ search for neighbours within a certain distance

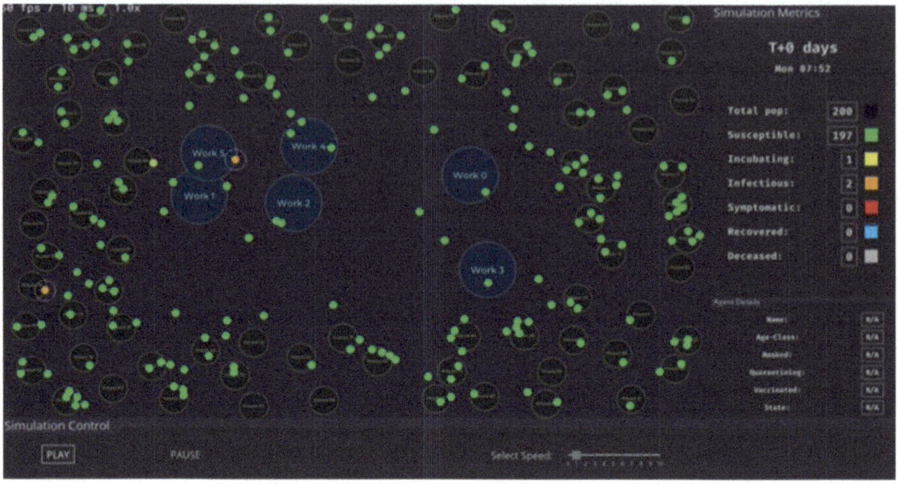

Fig. 6 A full view of the program display, with the simulation and menus visible

of a specific agent, greatly improving simulation performance and scalability [21] (Fig. 6).

For smaller populations, the performance bottleneck comes from the `pygame` [18] GUI. As the simulation is constantly changing, the entire window must be redrawn every frame. However, this can be improved by caching the background of the simulation as a separate surface, as the houses and workplaces do not move: this surface can then be used to repaint the background of every frame, without requiring redraws. In addition, the drawing of the actual agents and locations are performed using the `gfxdraw` package [22] from `pygame` [18], which allows for hardware-accelerated shape drawing. As the size of the simulation is configurable, the individuals in the community can become difficult to see when the simulation area increases, as their size is fixed. To allow for closer inspection of each household, our program includes a custom- built camera system that provides the ability to zoom and pan a viewport over the normal simulation surface as well as track a specific individual throughout the simulation, keeping them centered in the viewport. However, `pygame` performance drops significantly when scaling surfaces to higher dimensions, and scaling up using transforms cannot preserve fine details of the simulation, causing pixelation and blurriness. As a result, we instead apply the camera position before drawing the base simulation, scaling the size of objects and offsetting their draw position appropriately. This also allows us to cull objects that are off-screen by comparing their centre coordinates and radius to the visible viewport rectangle, skipping expensive draw operations for significant portions of the simulation when zoomed in (Fig. 7).

Although the `pygame`-based GUI is useful for visualising the spread of the virus through the community and ensuring the accuracy of the simulation, there is a fair amount of performance sacrificed to maintaining the display and drawing

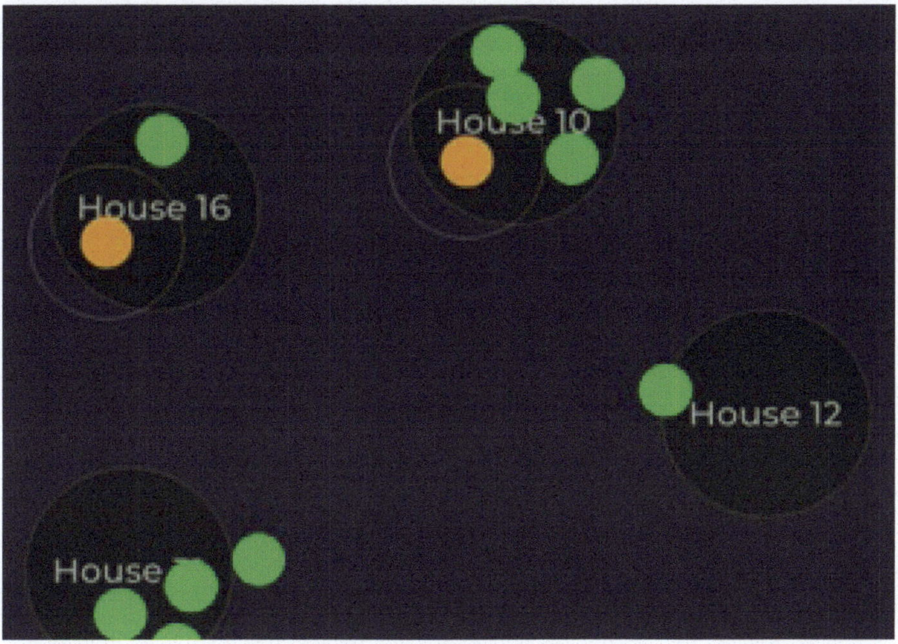

Fig. 7 Agents grouped in their respective households

the objects. In order to efficiently gather the data required from running the simulation in varying configurations multiple times, our program can also be run as a command-line interface (CLI) [23, 24]. In CLI mode, no GUI is displayed, and the simulation is instead manipulated through text-based commands that allow for stepping through the simulation, printing of population details to the console, and others. For the purposes of gathering data, an "auto-complete" option is also implemented, which runs the simulation to its end without requiring any additional input: that is, it continues stepping the simulation until every agent is either susceptible, recovered, or deceased, at which point the virus has effectively been eliminated from the community. This allows for the simulation to be quickly executed with different configurations to gather data, when a visual display is not required.

```
Simulation initialized with 72 houses.
<SIMULATION READY>

Outbreak: T+0

[p]lay/[p]ause [d]isplay [a]uto-complete [s]et-sim-speed [i]nfo
[h]elp
[w]rite and quit [q]uit

Begin Simulation? (y/n) >> y
```

```
<BEGINNING SIMULATION>

>>>
Sim Running @ x1 speed [In-Sim date: Day 1, Mon
13:56]

Sim Running @ x1 speed [In-Sim date: Day 5, Fri
12:53]

Sim Running @ x1 speed [In-Sim date: Day 9, Tue
13:14]

Sim Running @ x1 speed [In-Sim date: Day 13, Sat
01:19]
p

>>>
<SIMULATION PAUSED>
d

>>>
<DISPLAYING SIM METRICS>

Susceptible:
============
      total: 60
      infant: 2
      youth: 9
      young adult: 14
      adult: 23
      elder: 12

Incubating:
============
      total: 69
      infant: 2
      youth: 12
      young adult: 19
      adult: 15
      elder: 21

Infectious:
============
      total: 43
      infant: 0
      youth: 3
      young adult: 16
      adult: 16
      elder: 8

Symptomatic:
============
      total: 26
      infant: 1
```

```
        youth: 4
        young adult: 4
        adult: 9
        elder: 8

Recovered:
============
        total: 2
        infant: 0
        youth: 1
        young adult: 0
        adult: 0
        elder: 1

Deceased:
============
        total: 0
        infant: 0
        youth: 0
        young adult: 0
        adult: 0
        elder: 0
```

3.2.7 Output

While running, the simulation periodically writes its current state to a CSV file, containing the current simulation time and the current totals of the population in each infection model state, grouped by age class. This data allows for visualizations to be created that chart the progression of the virus through the community over time, from which we can infer the accuracy of the simulation and draw conclusions about the effectiveness of each preventative or mitigative measure. The program uses functionality from the `matplotlib` python package [25] to automatically generate line graphs from the output CSV file, saved as a PDF (Fig. 8).

3.3 Challenges and Constraints

3.3.1 Simulation Details

Although the simulation is designed to be configurable for many use cases and simulation models, there are certain areas that could be further developed for increased accuracy and flexibility. In particular, the initialization of the community currently randomly places all houses in a zone around the border of the simulation, while grouping the workplaces at the center. More research can be done to determine realistic infrastructure patterns and general routines in small communities, allowing

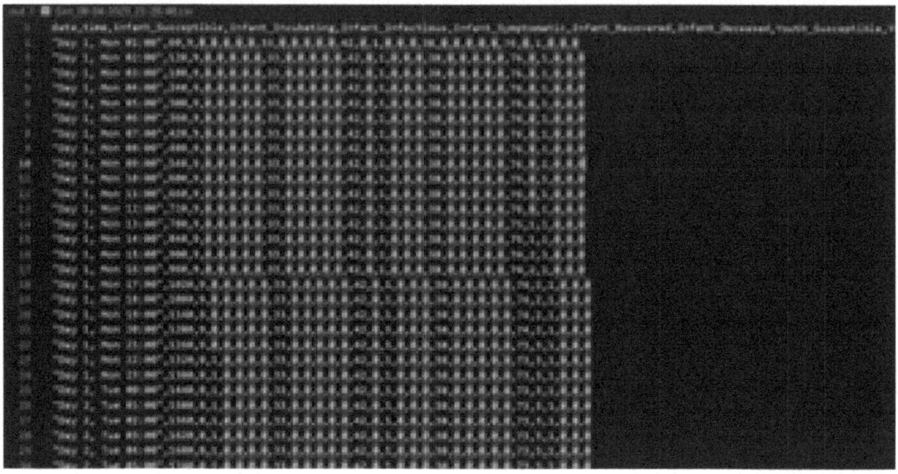

Fig. 8 The CSV output file generated by the simulation, the text of which is too long to reasonably fit in this report

for increased precision in modelling agent behaviour and consequently interactions between individuals.

Currently, agents only have two predefined destinations, excluding wandering on weekends: their house and their workplace. Adding additional locations such as parks and other recreational places will better reflect the actions of real-world people, and have the additional benefit of introducing new infection paths the virus can take to reach the populace. Any additional virus data found during research can also be used to accurately determine transmission and infection parameters. Apart from the duration of each state, the agents' progression through the infection model is currently non-configurable and could be improved by including options to provide a custom weighted-edge graph-based infection model. Despite these drawbacks, the simulation program is highly extensible and can be updated to add these features. In addition, additional preventative or mitigative actions that alter agent behaviour can be added to expand the scope of the project.

3.3.2 GUI

The Control Menu's simulation speed selection can be expanded to offer users not only a wider range of simulation speeds but also provide them with more comprehensive simulation speed settings. For instance, users could be given the ability to program simulation speed changes based on when the population achieves certain conditions such as slowing down once members of the population begin dying or a certain number become symptomatic. The control menu could also be loaded with new options to change how the simulation is rendered, like options for highlighting certain agents if they belong to a particular age-class or live in a certain house. The Main application menu could also be further developed to allow users to view the initial simulation configuration and adjust it before the simulation is executed.

3.3.3 Data

Our simulation tracks the number of agents occupying each state of our infection model at any given time and records this data for each in-sim hour that elapses. The simulation records this data in a basic CSV file which is then subsequently used to generate a collection of line charts for data visualisation. The limitation of this data collection and presentation is its narrow scope. For example, a future expansion of the application could replace the CSV file with a relational database to allow for a more custom and fine- toothed analysis of the data via relational queries. The data visualisation could also be expanded beyond just line charts and allow users to choose the kinds of graphics they want to use to display the data.

4 Discussion

As discussed, the problem at hand is to determine the efficacy of certain preventative and mitigative measures within a small community, for which our custom simulation was designed to find the solution. To provide an adequate answer, we ran the simulation over various configurations and permutations of certain preventative/mitigative actions to obtain output CSV data of the virus' progression throughout the community and compared it against the baseline results when no actions are taken. In particular, we are interested in the relative curve of the infected population in the community, how long it takes for the virus to be eliminated, and the total number of agents infected. The following sections will show the results of these simulations, visualized as graphs, and discuss our findings.

4.1 Simulation Data

The following pages contain graphs depicting the data generated by running our simulation on a variety of different infection cases. For all the test cases, we chose to have 200 agents in the simulation, with six workplaces that they transit to. The "Base" case shows the simulation running without any preventative or mitigative actions active and is the baseline for comparison against other configurations.

Note that because the simulation is inherently stochastic, the output data is unlikely to be the same even with the same configuration: however, there are similar trends that can be observed across multiple executions of the program. The data in the graphs shown here were selected as generally representative of an average simulation with the given parameters, after comparing the results from multiple executions (Figs. 9 and 10).

4.2 Interpretations

To determine the efficacy of a particular preventative or mitigative action against the spread of the virus, the graphs are used to determine three metrics:

- *Maximum symptomatic population* In the graph visualisations, this is the global maximum value of the red line. This value is important as it represents the potential number of individuals that may need to be hospitalized at once. Lower numbers are better.
- *Total number of infected people* Naturally, it is preferable for as few people as possible to be infected during the virus' spread. As our small community is modelled such that most people will come into contact with each other fairly often, generally every individual in the simulation will be infected eventually. However, some preventative actions, as seen in the graphs, allow for a portion of the population to escape infection for the duration of the simulation.
- *Duration before the virus subsides* The differences between the data sets must be considered in relation to the timeline of the virus' progression: as the simulation was configured to terminate immediately once the virus was eliminated, the x-axes on the graphs above do not match. Unexpectedly, it is generally prefer- able for a virus to subsist for a longer duration in a small community, as it implies that the infection curve is flatter and the virus will be more manageable. This is not always the case, however, as in some of the simulations the virus is eradicated early due to effective preventative measures.

4.2.1 Individual Measures

As a baseline for comparison, the "Base" graph shows that the virus lasts for approximately 30 days in the simulation, and has a peak of approximately 150 symptomatic people at approximately the 19 day mark. All people are eventually infected, and there are a few individuals for who the virus is fatal.

Looking at the "Masked" graph, although the shape of the infection is similar, the longer duration of 35 days means that the curve is slightly flatter, with a peak of about 125 people symptomatic at the 24 day mark.

Examining the "Quarantine" graph we can see that it follows a similar trend to the baseline however the shape of its Symptomatic trend is changed. We observe in the baseline case when no one is quarantining that the number of symptomatic people begins climbing exponentially after around 6 days, peaking around 16 days and then exponentially declining over the next 20 days. In the Quarantining case, however, we see that the increase is not exponential but is broken up more into a jagged

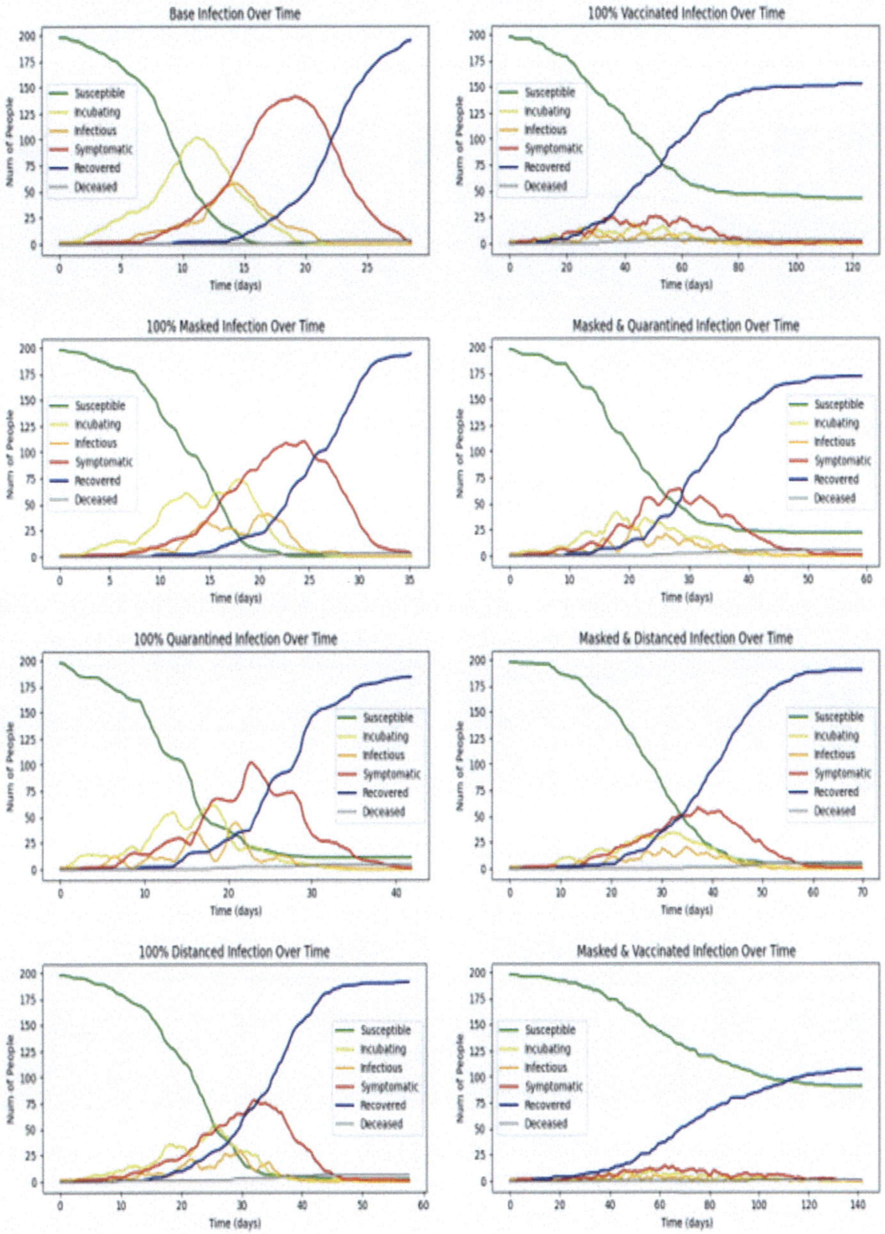

Fig. 9 Simulation in different set up

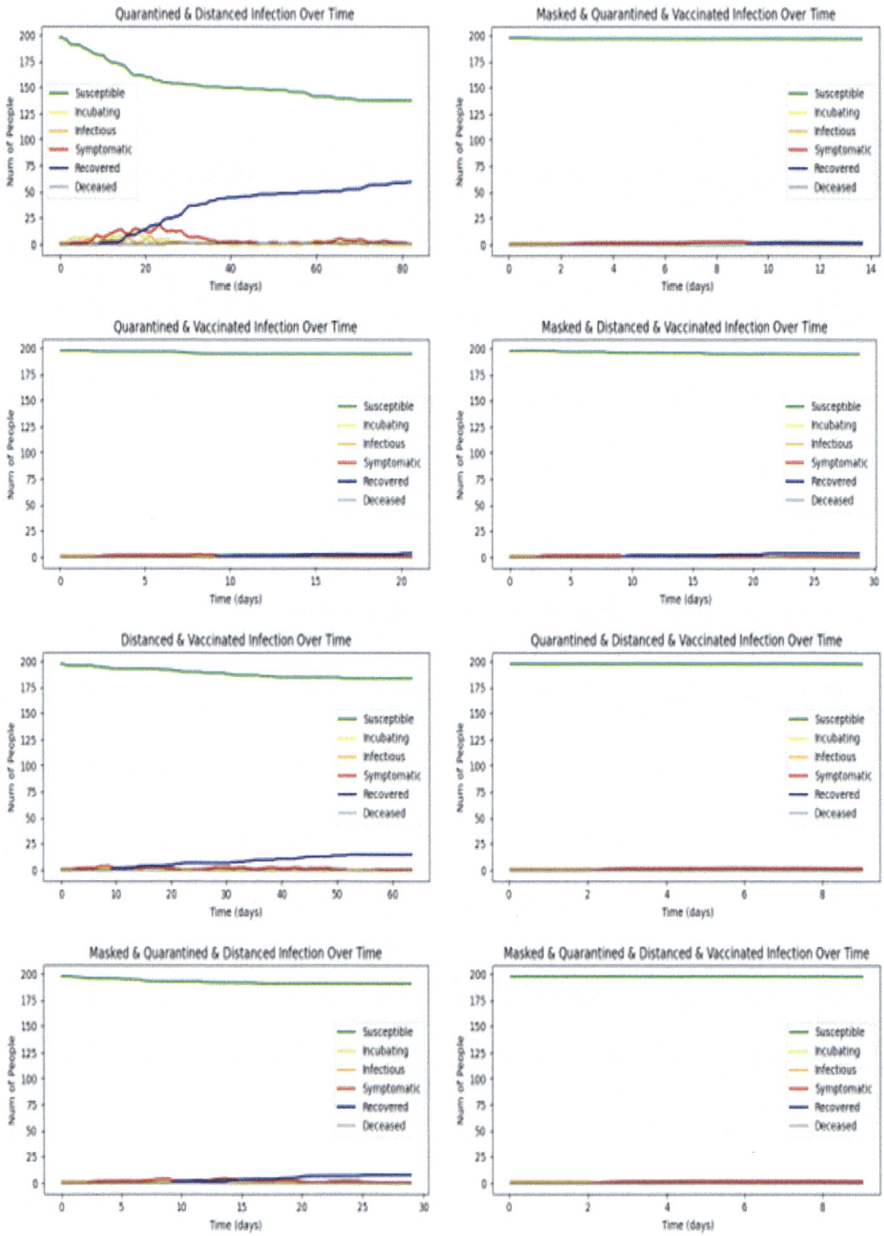

Fig. 10 Simulation in different set up

"staircase". This is a result of the number of symptomatic people increasing causing an increase in the rate of quarantining. More people begin spending less time near symptomatic agents and so the rate of increase in symptomatic agents "stalls" in the quarantine case where it would otherwise continue growing in the baseline case. It does not stop however as quarantining does not entirely eliminate contact with infectious agents due to the stochastic nature of the simulation, meaning incubating agents are still being produced and developing into symptomatic agents, usually at and over the same periods of time. This results in the jagged leaps we see in the number of symptomatic agents after each stall.

For the simulation that included social distancing, the peak number of symptomatic individuals is drastically lower than the "Base" simulation, as well as the "Masked" and "Quarantined" simulations, at only 75 individuals. While the graph extends to 60 days, the virus has effectively subsided by day 50, with only a few stragglers left to progress through each state of the infection.

However, the "Vaccination" simulation graph clearly shows that it is the most effective preventative measure: the peak symptomatic population never exceeds 30, and approximately 25% of the population is able to escape infection entirely, demonstrating the significant impact a well-vaccinated pop- ulation can have on the spread of a virus in a community. Thus, when comparing the effects of individual preventative and mitigative measures, vaccination is the most effective.

4.2.2 Combination Measures

The preventative and mitigative measures are not mutually exclusive: it is not only feasible but recommended for multiple measures to be taken together. After the individual measures data, graphs are displayed which visualise the spread of the virus with two or more preventative actions active.

Among the six permutation of two-groups of actions, it is clear that those including vaccination are the most effective, with the "Quarantined & Vaccinated" and "Distanced & Vaccinated" simulations having nearly the entire population avoid infection entirely. It is notable, however, that "Quarantined & Distanced" is the best two-group that does not involve vaccination. For outbreaks where a vaccine has not yet been developed, our results would suggest that recommendations for quarantining and social distancing, with high enough adoption rates, will be the most effective way to flatten the infection curve.

Looking at the 4 permutations of three-groups of actions we can see whenever the number of preventative actions implemented is 3 or more a peak of mitigation is reached that prevents almost anyone beyond the initial infected from becoming infected initially. That is, the choice of any three out the four actions becomes irrelevant, implementation of any three or more of them renders the population effectively immune to the infectious disease.

4.3 Partial Measures

While the data discussed thus far is useful in determining which measures are preferable when implemented perfectly across all individuals in a community, reality has shown there will always be those who refuse to adopt these measures. By comparing the impact of each preventative measure to its corresponding adoption rate, we can determine the level of effectiveness of the measure (Figs. 11 and 12).

Based on the simulation results, the shapes of the graphs remain consistent despite a greater implementation of masking by the population. The number of symptomatic cases peaks at 125. However, when the masking percentage reaches 75% or more, the simulation duration stretches out by 5 days. This suggests a slight reduction in the severity of the spread due to a significant proportion of the population adopting masking.

Quarantine measures have demonstrated a significant impact on the peak number of symptomatic individuals, as well as the duration of the simulation. The immediate implementation of quarantining, results in a plateau effect in the number of newly infected individuals, as infected individuals remain at home. This mitigative action has been found to have the greatest impact at an adoption rate of 75% or greater.

Although distancing was only second to vaccination when comparing the single measures, it quickly drops in efficiency when adoption rates decrease. At 100% adoption, the max symptomatic population is only 75 individuals, but increases to over 100 at 75% adoption and 125 at the 50% rate. This suggests that distancing must be well-enforced to maintain its preventative capacity, as a few bad actors will quickly spread the virus throughout the community.

Among all the singular preventative measures, vaccination was the only one with a significant reduction with an adoption rate of 25% or higher. At this level, the peak symptomatic agents reach only 125, and the duration is extended by 5 days from the baseline. At 50 and 75% efficacy, the peak symptomatic agents are 75, and the duration is extended by 30 days from the baseline. At 100% efficacy, we observe the most effective flattening of the curve among all the single preventative measures, with peak symptomatic agents under 25 and the simulation extending 90 days past the baseline. Additionally, we saw a linear increase in the number of susceptible agents remaining at the end of the simulation.

Using the data from our simulation, we conclude vaccination is undoubtedly the most effective preventative measure that can be taken to reduce the total spread of a virus in a small community. In all scenarios where vaccination was involved, there was always an uninfected portion population being maintained. In contrast, masking appears to be the least effective as the trends observed in the masking-only scenario match those observed in the baseline case more than any of the other actions when implemented separately. However, it did appear to enhance the effectiveness of both vaccination and quarantining, reducing the number of people infected overall and the number of symptomatic agents, respectively.

In the absence of a readily available vaccine, our data indicates that distancing is the next best single option to employ. When taking multiple preventative measures

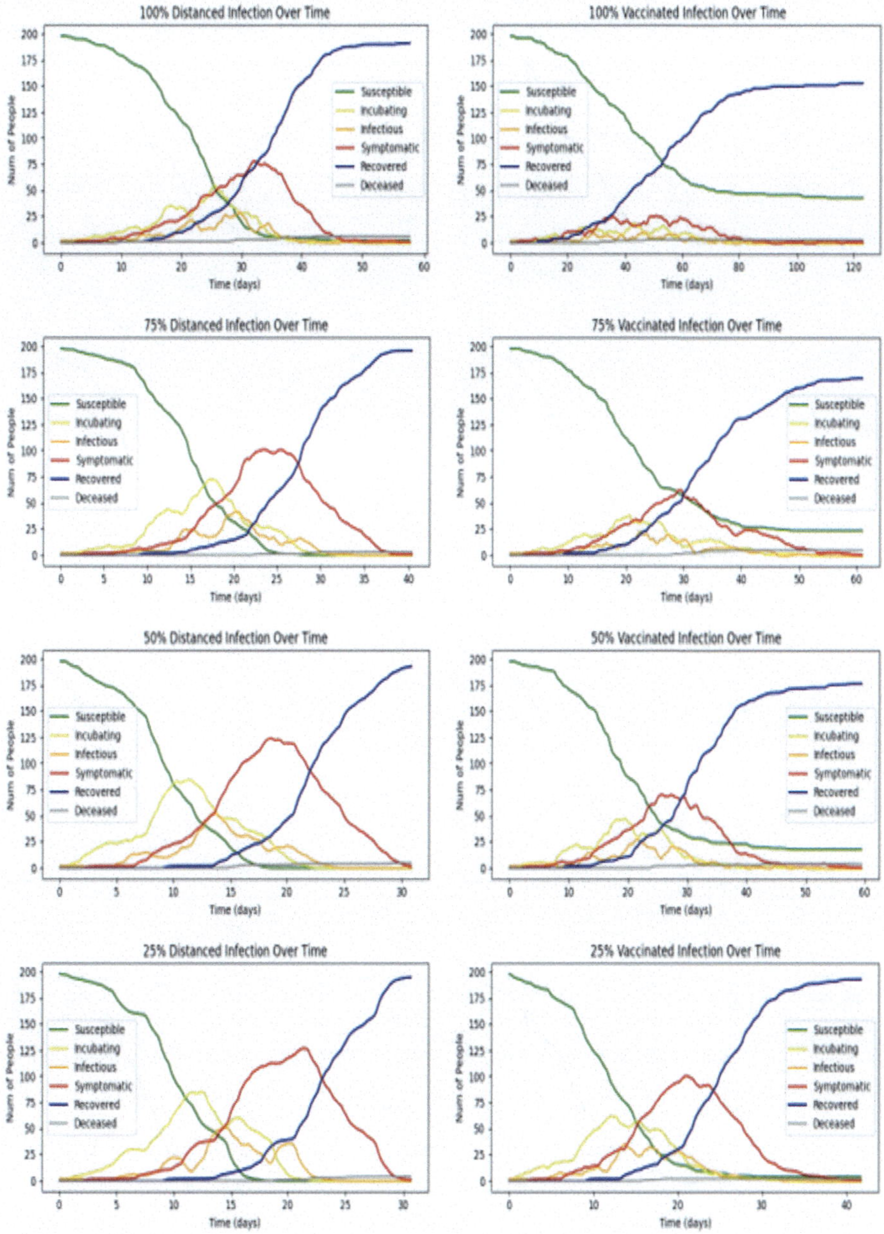

Fig. 11 Simulation in different set up

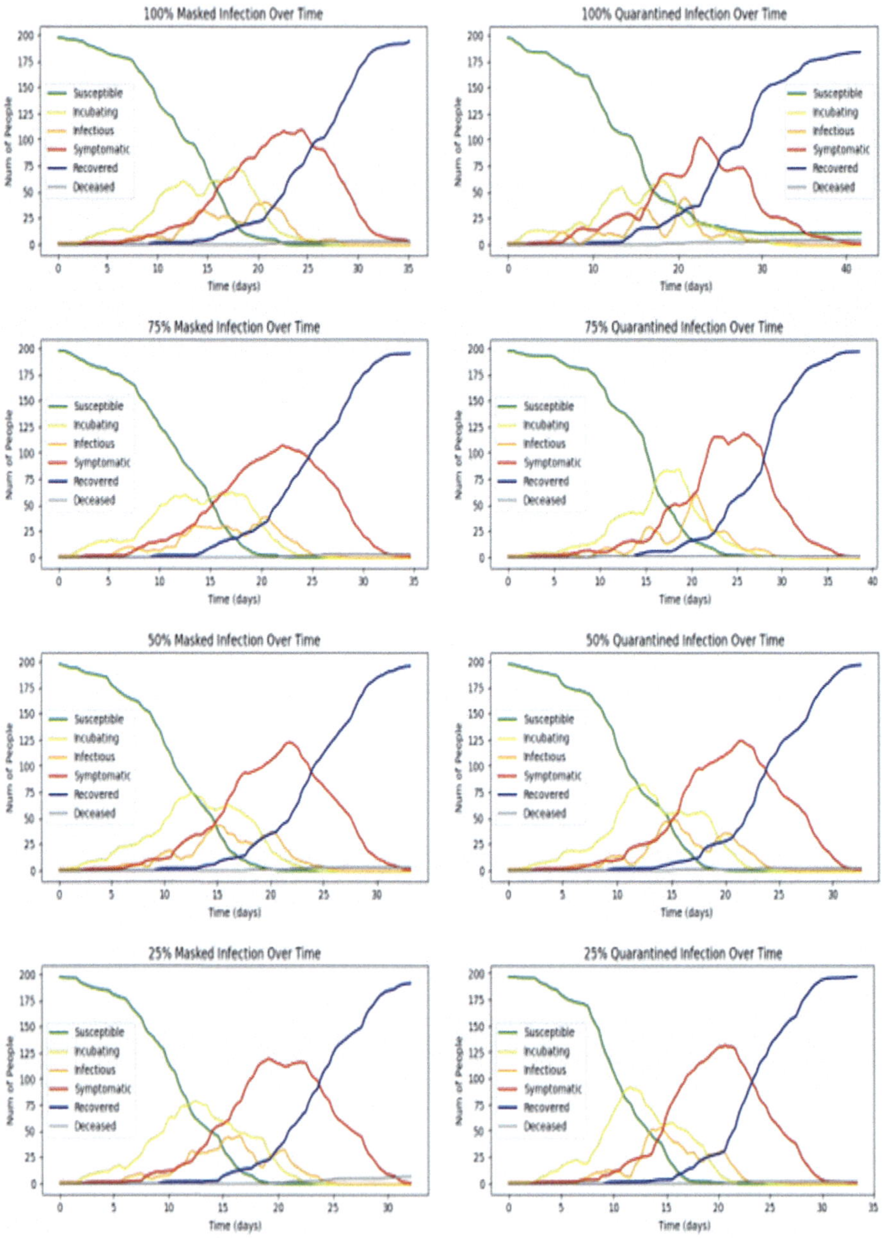

Fig. 12 Simulation in different set up

into account, it is preferable to include both quarantining and distancing for increased prevention. However, it is noteworthy that distancing in particular is implemented properly as its efficacy decreases quickly as adoption rates drop.

5 Conclusion

This study has successfully developed and implemented an agent-based simulation model to explore the impact of various preventative and *mitigative* strategies on the spread of infectious diseases within a small community. By simulating agent interactions, movement, and disease transmission, we have gained valuable insights into the dynamics of disease outbreaks.

The model's flexibility allows for the exploration of different scenarios, including varying levels of social distancing, mask usage, and quarantine measures. The results demonstrate the significant impact of these interventions on disease spread, highlighting the importance of timely and effective public health responses.

The graphical user interface provides a visual representation of the simulation, making it easier to understand and interpret the results. This tool can be used to educate the public and *policymakers* about the potential consequences of different actions and to inform decision-making during future outbreaks.

While this study provides valuable insights, further research is needed to refine the model by incorporating more complex factors, such as environmental conditions, population demographics, and healthcare system capacity. Additionally, exploring the impact of different vaccination strategies and emerging variants would be beneficial.

References

1. Kirkeby, C., Brookes, V.J., Ward, M.P., Dürr, S., Halasa, T.: A practical introduction to mechanistic modeling of disease transmission in veterinary science. Frontiers in veterinary science **7**, 546651(2021)
2. Karaivanov, A.: A social network model of covid-19. Plos one **15**(10), 0240878 (2020)
3. An, T., Kim, H., Joo, C.: Prediction of covid-19 infection spread through agent-based simulation. In: Proceedings of the Twenty-Third International Symposium on Theory, Algorithmic Foundations, and Protocol Design for Mobile Networks and Mobile Computing, pp. 247–252 (2022)
4. Brauer, F., Castillo-Chavez, C., Castillo-Chavez, C.: Mathematical Models in Population Biology and Epidemiology vol. 2. Springer, New York (2012)
5. Shapiro, M.B., Karim, F., Muscioni, G., Augustine, A.S.: adaptive susceptible-infectious-removed model for continuous estimation of the covid-19 infection rate and reproduction number in the united states: Modeling study. Journal of Medical Internet Research **23**(4), 24389 (2021)
6. Ajbar, A., Alqahtani, R.T., Boumaza, M.: Dynamics of an sir-based covid-19 model with linear incidence rate, nonlinear removal rate, and public awareness. Frontiers in Physics **9**, 634251 (2021)

7. Dobie, A.P.: Susceptible-infectious-susceptible (sis) model with virus mutation in a variable population size. Ecological Complexity **50**, 101004 (2022)
8. Pont, M.T.S., Mora, H.M., Castillo, A.C.: A discrete approach of the susceptible-infectious-susceptible (sis) model of disease expansion. International Journal of Computers **2** (2017)
9. Struben, J.: The coronavirus disease (covid-19) pandemic: simulation-based assessment of outbreak responses and postpeak strategies. System Dynamics Review **36**(3), 247–293 (2020)
10. Wu, Z.-Y., Zhang, H.-B., Zhao, H.-F.: Modeling of the small-scale outbreak of covid-19. Frontiers in Public Health **10**, 907814 (2022)
11. Okhuese, A.V., *et al.*: Estimation of the probability of reinfection with covid-19 by the susceptible-exposed-infectious-removed-undetectable-susceptible model. JMIR Public Health and Surveillance **6**(2), 19097 (2020)
12. Codd, E.F.: Cellular Automata. Academic press, Orlando (2014)
13. Gallagher, S., Baltimore, J.: Comparing compartment and agent-based models. In: Joint Statistical Meeting, Baltimore, pp. 1–21 (2017)
14. Hunter, E., Mac Namee, B., Kelleher, J.D.: A comparison of agent-based models and equation based models for infectious disease epidemiology (2018)
15. Profile Table, Census Profile, 2021 Census Of Population - Alberta [Province]". www12.statcan.gc.ca. www12.statcan.gc.ca/census-recensement/2021/dp-pd/prof/details/page.cfm?Lang=E&SearchText=Alberta&DGUIDlist=2021A000248&GENDERlist=1,2,3&STATISTIClist=1&HEADERlist=0. [Accessed 01-07-2024] (2023)
16. Respiratory virus dashboard — alberta.ca. https://www.alberta.ca/stats/dashboard/respiratory-virus-dashboard.htm. [Accessed 01-07-2024]
17. Canada, S.: Protective Immunity Post-COVID-19 Infection, Canada Communicable Disease Report. https://www.canada.ca/en/public-health/services/reports-publications/canada-communicable-disease-report-ccdr/monthly-issue/2021-47/issue-4-april-2021/post-covid-19-immunity.html. [Accessed 03-07-2024]
18. pygame news — pygame.org. https://www.pygame.org/news. [Accessed 03-07-2024]
19. pygame-menu; pygame-menu 4.4.2 Documentation — pygame-menu.readthedocs.io. https://pygame-menu.readthedocs.io/en/4.4.2/. [Accessed 03-07-2024]
20. scipy.spatial.KDTree – SciPy v1.10.1 Manual, SciPy documen- tation. https://docs.scipy.org/doc/scipy/reference/generated/scipy.spatial.KDTree.html. [Accessed 03-07-2024]
21. Wald, I., Havran, V.: On building fast kd-trees for ray tracing, and on doing that in o (n log n). In: 2006 IEEE Symposium on Interactive Ray Tracing, pp. 61–69 (2006). IEEE
22. pygame.gfxdraw; pygame v2.6.0 documentation — pygame.org. https://www.pygame.org/docs/ref/gfxdraw.html. [Accessed 03-07-2024]
23. Command-line interface - Wikipedia — en.wikipedia.org. https://en.wikipedia.org/wiki/Command-line_interface#. [Accessed 03-07-2024]
24. Sampath, H., Merrick, A., Macvean, A.: Accessibility of command line interfaces. In: Proceedings of the 2021 CHI Conference on Human Factors in Computing Systems, pp. 1–10 (2021)
25. Matplotlib; Visualization with Python — matplotlib.org. https://matplotlib.org/. [Accessed 03-07-2024]

Predicting Donor Behavior Using the Dynamics of Event Co-Attendance Networks

Shwetha K. M. Srikanta, Katie L. Pierce, Joshua E. Introne, Chilukuri K. Mohan, and Sucheta Soundarajan

Abstract This study investigates the dynamics of charitable donor co-attendance networks to help understand fundraising outcomes. We analyze a multi-year network of co-attendance at fundraising events, examining topological structure, node characteristics, and network properties. Key findings include a 76% increase in giving value for donors with increased centrality rank and a positive peer effect indicated by increased co-attendance with high-capacity donors, among donors who increased or maintained their giving levels. Additionally, we observe assortativity in giving patterns among co-attending donors, and identify interlinked cliques of communities with varying sizes, with larger communities having a higher proportion of wealthy donors. Furthermore, we develop a Long Short-Term Memory (LSTM) network to predict donor propensity, considering node-level features such as assortativity, centrality, clustering coefficient, and exposure to high-capacity donors. Our results demonstrate that a multi-variate model outperforms baseline statistical models, enabling outcome assessment before events. These findings have implications for budget allocation strategies and maximizing fundraising effectiveness.

Keywords Charitable donations · Co-attendance network · Deep learning · Multivariate forecasting model

1 Introduction

For non-profit organizations, fundraising events serve as platforms for donors and staff to strengthen or form new connections. The outcomes of such events have been observed to be influenced by similarities between donors, their relationships with

S. K. M. Srikanta (✉) · K. L. Pierce · J. E. Introne · C. K. Mohan · S. Soundarajan
Syracuse University, Syracuse, NY, USA
e-mail: smanchin@syr.edu; klpierce@syr.edu; jeintron@syr.edu; ckmohan@syr.edu; susounda@syr.edu

M. Kaya et al. (eds.), *Social Network Analysis and Mining Applications in Healthcare and Anomaly Detection*, Lecture Notes in Social Networks,
https://doi.org/10.1007/978-3-031-75204-9_6

the recipient organization, and interactions with the soliciting individuals [11, 27]. We propose a network-theoretic perspective on analyzing such events, exploring the extent to which the event co-attendance network influences giving behaviors of donors.

This chapter expands on our study presented in [31], analyzing multi-year data (from a large private research university) that includes donations made by individuals and events attended by those individuals (Sect. 2). Using this data, we construct a co-attendance network, where nodes represent donors and edges indicate whether donors have attended at least one fundraising event together. We recognize that other factors beyond the co-attendance network also influence giving behavior, such as undocumented personal relationships, mutual interactions, influence networks, and recommendations.

Our analysis reveals low-moderate positive assortativity, indicating a tendency for donors with similar giving behaviors to co-attend events. We observe a positive correlation between centrality and the amount of giving, consistent with prior studies [19] in this area. More importantly, our findings indicate that co-attendance with high-capacity donors correlates with increased donation amounts. We also explore other network properties that may influence giving behavior, discovering that larger communities have a greater proportion of above-median and high-giving donors.

In addition to the work presented in [31], this chapter includes the following additional results.

1. We enhance our formulation for updating edge weights in the network construction that captures the potential strength of interactions between individuals while co-attending events with emphasis on event size.
2. We predict donor propensity using node-level features extracted from the co-attendance network, including assortativity with neighbors, centrality rank, clustering coefficient, and exposure to donors within the local neighborhood and community.
3. We extend our analysis beyond donors retained between non-overlapped windows ($S = 456$) to include all (including irregular) donors, significantly increasing the sample size ($S = 99{,}431$). This facilitates exploring a wider range of donor behaviors, so that we can identify patterns in donations across different donor segments.

We propose a multivariate forecasting model that significantly outperforms the baseline in predicting the giving class of an individual in the current time window based on the co-attendance network node properties in preceding time windows. The AUC for our model exceeds that of the baseline for both the donor segments. The node features are perfectly separable in our multi-year analysis, indicated by an AUC of 1.0 for all three classes. Learning from the network snapshots enhances the model prediction capability because it incorporates the dynamic nature of the network and its influence on donor behavior.

The proposed multivariate model outperforms all statistical baselines in terms of median absolute error (MAE) for both regular and irregular event attendee segments.

Although the performance of statistical models in predicting the donation amount for regular donors is comparable to that of the proposed multivariate model (in terms of RMSE), the latter demonstrates superior performance for a filtered set of donors (i.e., excluding very high donors). In this segment, the multivariate model achieves a lower test RMSE of $16,874.49 compared to the statistical model's RMSE of $22,428.29.

Thus, our research presents a new approach to predicting donor propensity by incorporating network properties, specifically event co-attendance networks, unlike previous models that have focused on personal traits and other properties. Our analysis can be useful to nonprofit organizations in identifying potential donors and donor segments, understanding donation patterns, and optimizing their resource allocation to various donor segments such as retained donors, new donors, and donors who changed their behaviors. This helps in improved targeting and thus improves fundraising outcomes.

Section 2 describes the properties of the dataset. Section 3 discusses prior work related to network analysis in fund-raising efforts, as well as the baseline statistical approach and relevant neural network models. This is followed by Sect. 4, which describes our methodology and parameters of the multi-variate model. Next we present our analysis in Sect. 5 followed by discussion in Sect. 6. Conclusions are presented in Sect. 7.

2 Dataset Description and Statistics

The dataset used for our study contains over 46,175 (including staff) unique donors who contributed varying amounts to events and non-event-associated donations. The data spans over 3000 events organized by a large private research university from 2014 to 2021. These events include meetings, fundraising campaigns, alumni engagement programs, networking events, and lectures and donations received by the university are utilized for endowments, scholarships, and funding various university facilities.

Figure 1 shows the retained (existing) donors and newly joined donors for each year, from 2014 to 2021. We see that each year the events draw a similar number of new donors and with time there is an increase in the number of retained donors. Figure 1 also provides the number of unique events organized each year, which increases with time. The donors have varying primary constituencies with the University, including alumni, students, parents or spouses of students/alumni, and staff. For this analysis, we focus on two types of giving: promised lifetime giving (which includes amounts that have not yet been given), and the actual amount given each year.

Figure 2 illustrates the yearly totals, the actual data points that represent the totals for each years. The moving average curve helps to smooth out short term fluctuations and shows an upward trend. To enhance the prediction capabilities, we have augmented our previous dataset with new fields, such as first campaign gifts.

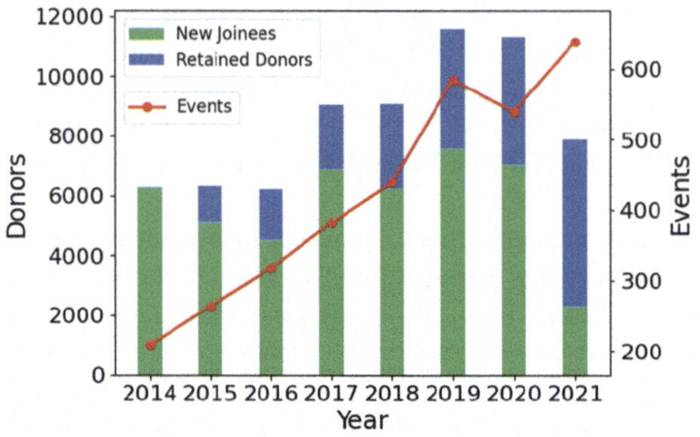

Fig. 1 Growth of donors and events organized in period 2014–2021 [31]

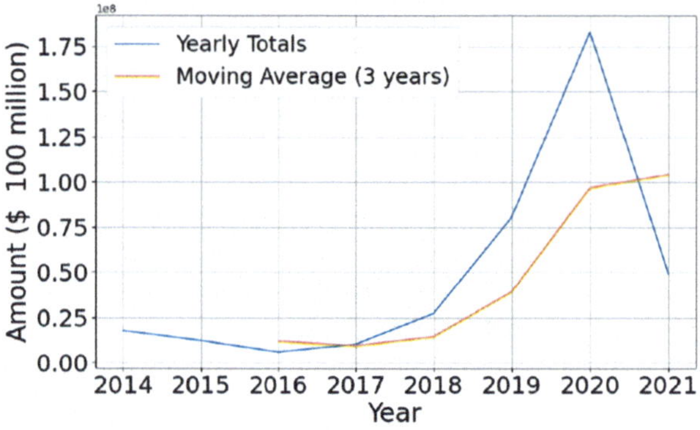

Fig. 2 Yearly totals and 3-year moving averages for all donors in period 2014–2021

We perform various analyses to forecast donor propensity. Initially, we utilize the annual co-attendance network to examine two distinct donor segments. The first segment comprises consistent donors who consistently attend events over the course of 8 years. The second segment consists of both regular and irregular donors who attend small-sized events.

Additionally, we conduct a multi-year analysis to evaluate the multivariate model's performance on donor activities within a rolling window of 3 years. This investigates how the network dynamics potentially influence donor propensity. The sample sizes representing time series data of individuals attending events and contributing amounts for all dataset types are listed in Table 1.

Table 1 Sample size for dataset

Analysis	Attendee type	Individual donors	Sample size
Yearly	Regular attendee (all events)	57	456
Yearly	All attendees (small events)	175	5578
Multi-year	All attendees (all events)	44,385	99,431

3 Background

In this section, we discuss prior research in three areas related to our work. First, we summarize network analytics work addressing donation data. We then describe the baseline statistical approach used to evaluate our proposed approach. We then discuss the use of recent neural network models for forecasting.

3.1 Donation Data Analysis

Prior analyses have shown that effective communication with donors can increase charitable donations, with people more likely to donate when they perceive similarities with fundraisers [7, 30]. Donors also give more often to organizations to which they feel connected, such as their *alma mater* [4]. Overall, research suggests a positive social influence among similar individuals in donor-solicitor and donor-recipient dyads, while the effects of social influence on charitable giving in donor-donor dyads can be both positive and negative [25, 29]. Existing research has found that donor-donor dyads exhibit assortativity, meaning individuals tend to donate similar amounts as their peers [15, 20]. Studies have also examined the extent to which giving behavior is influenced by similarities in personal characteristics, such as gender, location, income, age, and relationships with others [32].

Network properties have been used to detect donor influence, particularly on social media [8, 27, 34]. Studies have found that a Twitter campaign network's size, decentralization, and cultural norms are positively correlated with the average donation amount per day [33]. Authority and centrality within internal social connections also impact success in fund-raising [12]. Additionally, social connection variables have been found to improve the performance of algorithms that predict funding outcomes, with external social connections having a stronger impact compared to internal connections.

Numerous studies have focused on constructing predictive models to enhance the effectiveness of fundraising efforts within charitable organizations [23]. These research endeavors have attempted to predict a donor's giving likelihood (propensity) [28], and to forecast the specific amount a donor might contribute, based on historical data. The influence of organizational connections on individuals' donation propensities has been studied based on the preceding 3 years of donations, considering age, gender, race/ethnicity, and relational characteristics as features [2].

Research has also focused on identifying individuals who change their giving behavior over time [1, 26]. Previous research has also explored donor segmentation based on various factors, including altruism, belief in mission clarity, and susceptibility to external influences [18].

In this study, we extract individual (node)-level features from the co-attendance network to predict donor propensity. We segment donors based on event attendance frequency and compare this against baselines. Our approach includes conducting a multi-year network analysis to study the potential influence of network dynamics on donor behavior, aiming to predict donor propensity. For classification tasks, we use simple time series-dependent baselines, while for regression tasks, we employ more complex statistical methods such as ARIMA modeling. This work contributes to the limited research on associating fundraising outcomes with longitudinal network analysis and on predicting donor propensity using such data. The following subsections describe our baselines in more detail.

3.2 Baseline

For our classification task we employ a baseline that predicts the giving class of each individual for the next time window to be the same as their most recent value. This is a simple approach based on the assumption that the future behavior of an entity will be similar to its past behavior.

We also use two baseline methodologies for regression tasks: Exponential smoothing [10] and Auto-Regressive Integrated Moving Average (ARIMA) models [22]. These approaches offer complementary techniques to tackle the complexities of forecasting. While exponential smoothing models focus on the seasonal patterns and trends in the data, the ARIMA model captures the autocorrelation structure inherent in the dataset. In an autoregressive model **(AR (p))** of order p, the variable of interest is forecast using a linear combination of past values of the variable. A moving average model of order q **(MA (q))**, on the other hand, uses past forecasting errors in a regression-like model. If we combine differencing with autoregression and a moving average model, we obtain a non-seasonal ARIMA model, expressed as follows.

$$y'_t = c + \phi_1 y'_{t-1} + \ldots + \phi_p y'_{t-p} + \phi_1 \epsilon_{t-1} + \ldots + \phi_{t-q} \epsilon_{t-q} + \epsilon_t. \tag{1}$$

3.3 Neural Network Models for Forecasting

Artificial neural networks provide forecasting algorithms that use mathematical models inspired by biological neural networks and capture nonlinear relationships between the response variable and its predictors [21]. They were first used for forecasting in the early 1990s [3, 16] but the recent introduction of well-designed recurrent neural network (RNN) modules has resulted in extraordinary successes in forecasting for several practical applications [17]. For our multivariate time series model, we employ Long Short-Term Memory (LSTM) [14] and Gated Recurrent Unit (GRU) networks [5].

An LSTM is a type of recurrent neural network (RNN) module designed to learn long-term dependencies. Unlike traditional RNNs, LSTMs have a cell state to facilitate remembering information over extended periods, and use gates to control the flow of information into and out of the cell state, enabling learning of complex temporal relationships. GRU networks are similar, but use a simpler recurrent network module. The key differences between LSTM and GRU lie in their architectures and associated trade-offs. LSTM networks have more gates and parameters, providing greater flexibility and expressiveness, but requiring higher computational cost and overfitting risk. GRU networks are simpler and faster since they have fewer gates and parameters, but don't always perform as well as LSTM networks. LSTM networks maintain separate cell state and output channels, hence storing and outputting different information, unlike GRUs whose single hidden state may limit its capacity. Both models exhibit varying sensitivities to hyperparameters such as learning rate, dropout rate, and sequence length [24].

4 Methodology

Our primary objective is to understand the relationship between the network properties of an individual in the dataset and that individual's giving (propensity and level) by analyzing longitudinal network data. This information can be valuable in evaluating the potential effectiveness of fund-raising campaigns. To achieve this, we construct weighted network snapshots at the end of each specified time window and measure the co-attendance network properties, using them to predict donors' giving propensity for the subsequent time window.

4.1 Network Construction

The usefulness of events for predicting donor behavior declines with time, and donor participation in recent events is more important than in older events. One possible way to represent this fact in our updated co-attendance network is by halving the weight in every successive time slice [31].

$$W_{ij}^{t} = N_{ij}^{t} + \frac{W_{ij}^{t-1}}{2^{d}} \tag{2}$$

Event size matters: in smaller events, individuals have a higher chance of engaging in conversations and interacting with one another, while in larger gatherings, one-on-one interactions between two co-attendees is less likely. Equation (3) shows how we may use the relative strength of possible interactions between two co-attending individuals to update edge weights, using a slower decay function than Eq. (2), capturing long term dependencies for our multivariate models (Sects. 5.5–5.7).

$$W_{ij}^{t} = \sum \frac{k}{|E^{t}(i, j)|} + \frac{W_{ij}^{t-1}}{d} \tag{3}$$

4.2 Node Features

To predict donor propensity, we leverage network structural characteristics. Since we focus on individual donations, we consider properties at the node (individual) level. Our analysis reveals similarity in giving behavior among neighbors of a node, indicating the impact of assortativity on donor propensity. We observe a positive peer effect, with increased giving levels among donors who showed increased co-attendance with high-capacity donors. We hence investigate the influence of an individual's local neighborhood and their community (identified using the Louvain community detection algorithm [1]) on donor propensity. Additionally we consider centrality, as more central individuals tend to have higher giving levels supported by prior studies and our analysis. We also take into account the clustering coefficient, which measures the extent to which nodes cluster together into well-knit sub-networks.

4.2.1 Assortativity

This property indicates the preference for nodes to attach to others that have similar characteristics, i.e., whether individuals with similar giving behaviors are more likely to co-attend the same events. To capture the local assortativity property, we use the simple and well-known *EI homophily index*, a measure of in-group (internal) and out-group (external) preference [6] whose value ranges from -1 (*complete homophily*) to 1 (*complete heterophily*), using Eq. (4).

$$EI = \frac{External - Internal}{External + Internal} \tag{4}$$

4.2.2 Centrality

The centrality of an individual in a network impacts their access to resources and opportunities. Central individuals are invited to more events, meet more people, and benefit from these resources, fostering a sense of gratitude and a desire to give back to the community. Also, highly influential donors may be specifically invited to larger gatherings, further increasing their centrality in the network [27]. Here we consider weighted Eigenvector centrality as well as degree centrality [13].

4.2.3 Clustering Coefficient

This measures the extent to which nodes from tightly knit clusters, providing insights into the structure of the co-attendance network [13].

4.2.4 Local Exposure

This refers to the percentage of neighbors of a node that represent donors, and is important since the effect of co-attending donors may be diluted by the presence of many co-attending non-donors. Co-attending events with a higher number of donors can create a greater positive peer effect and increase the likelihood of donating.

4.2.5 Community Exposure

Membership in a community (obtained using the Louvain method) with more donors may be more meaningful than local exposure which may be merely coincidental in a co-attendance network. We also expect giving behaviors to be positively influenced if the community to which a node belongs has a greater proportion of high-capacity donors, who may exert greater influence [11]. Hence we consider two variants of *Community Exposure*, respectively referring to the percentage of a node's community members that represent (i) donors, and (ii) high-capacity donors.

4.3 Multivariate Forecasting Model

We split the data into training and testing as described in Sect. 4.3.1. Then we train neural network models with the LSTM and GRU modules, using the node features extracted for each individual based on their previous time window of co-attendance. The models predict the giving class or donation amount for the test data.

4.3.1 Model Parameters

During model training, we incorporate lagged input features along with other node features. Specifically, we include lagged EI homophily index, which is positively correlated with donation likelihood, as shown in Fig. 3, and lagged exposure to high-capacity donors, considering the observed correlation between increased giving and increased co-attendance with high-capacity donors. By incorporating assortativity

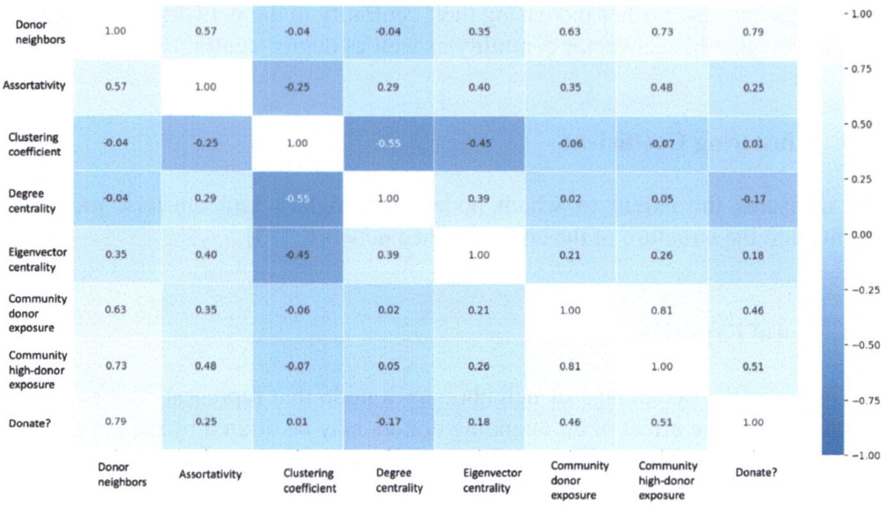

Fig. 3 Correlation heatmap

as a lagged feature, we capture the dynamic nature of this similarity and its influence on donor behavior. Additionally, we include a lagged output feature, i.e., giving class or amount.

We perform cross-validation on time series data, training the model for each time window and testing it on the subsequent window to prevent leakage of future data during training [9]. For binary classification, we employ *binary cross-entropy* loss with a *sigmoid* activation function, while for multi-class classification, we use *categorical cross-entropy* loss with a *softmax* activation function. For the regression task we minimize *mean squared error* using the *ADAM* optimizer.

4.3.2 Donor Segments

Different parts of the donor dataset have different characteristics in event attendance and donor behavior, and are best understood separately. Hence we segment donors based on event attendance frequency (regular and irregular donors attending small events), identifying patterns related to co-attendance and giving.

4.3.3 Multi-Year Analysis

In order to identify network characteristics that drive changes in donor behavior, it is essential to analyze a multi-year network. To achieve this, we construct weighted network snapshots for a rolling window of 3 years using Eq. (3). By extracting the aforementioned features from these network snapshots, we can test

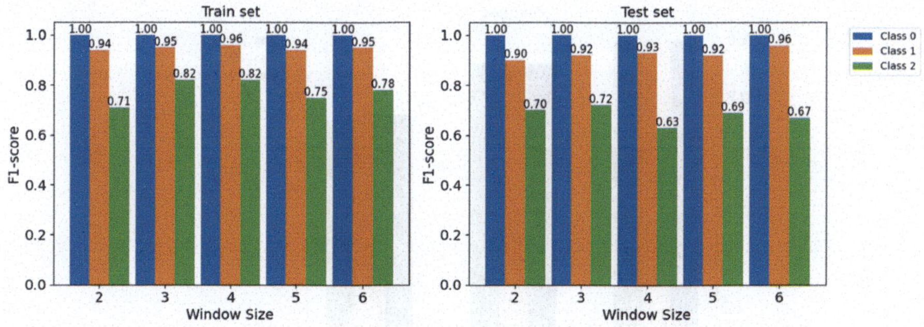

Fig. 4 Comparison of f1-score for the three classes for varying window sizes

the multivariate model and investigate how network dynamics potentially influence donor propensity.

4.3.4 Choice of Time Window

We perform sensitivity analysis for various time windows ranging from very short $w = 2$ to $w = 6$ and record the F1-score. The bar plot in Fig. 4 shows the optimal window (3 years). A small window size is appropriate for our dataset as it spans over only 8 years. A very short 2-year window is more sensitive to rapid changes in donor activity and captures the rapid fluctuations in yearly totals as seen in Fig. 2, whereas more smoothing occurs with a 3-year moving average window.

4.3.5 Balancing Classes

The time-series data for all donor segments exhibits class imbalance due to unequal numbers of donors and non-donors. The regular attendee segment has a larger set of donors (23% non-donors and 77% donors), while the irregular attendee segment shows a contrast (65% non-donors and 35% donors). To address this, we assign higher weights to the minority class compared to the majority class during loss function calculation using the inverse class frequency method indicated in Eq. (5).

$$W_j = \frac{|S|}{(|N_c| * |S_j|)} \tag{5}$$

Here, the weight for each class w_j is computed using the sample size $|S|$, $|N_c|$ represents the number of classes for the target, and $|S_j|$ is the number of samples in class j. This approach prevents over-fitting and mitigates the impact of class imbalance, and is preferable to resampling or generating synthetic samples.

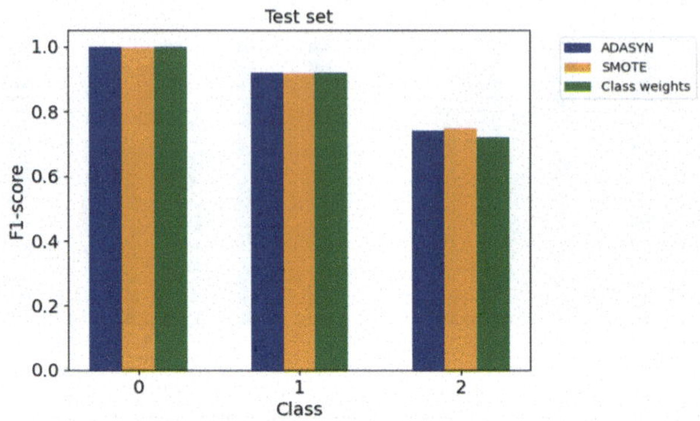

Fig. 5 Comparison of F1-scores obtained using various class balancing methods

Figure 5 illustrates that our model's performance is invariant to the method used for balancing data of different classes.

4.3.6 Donor Propensity and Evaluation

We employ LSTM and GRU models to make predictions for the current time window based on the data from the previous window. The binary classification models predict whether an individual will make a donation (Target=1) or not (Target=0), whereas multi-class classification models predict the giving class of that individual, and regression models predict the amount that individual is likely to donate. For classification tasks, we utilize precision, recall, and F1-score as evaluation metrics, while for regression we use root-mean-squared-error (RMSE) and median-absolute-error (MAE) to compare the predicted donation amounts with the actual donation amounts.

5 Analysis

In this section, we present key findings from our study that provide insights for assessing fundraising based on event participation and structural properties of the co-attendance network. We gain insights about factors that may influence increased giving behavior. Furthermore, we leverage node-level features extracted from the co-attendance network to predict donor propensity for different donor segments. Further, we utilize a multi-year network to study the influence of network dynamics on donor behavior.

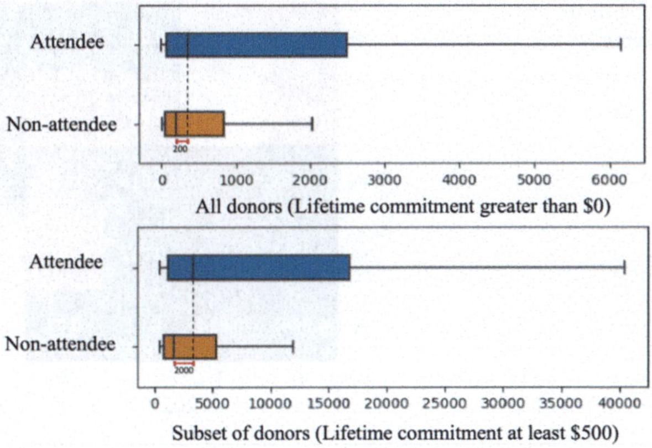

Fig. 6 Box plots for event attendees and nonattendees [31]: the upper subplot represents the distribution of donations > $0 and the lower subplot represents donations >= $500 in the second subplot

5.1 *Impact of Event Attendance*

We first examine the impact of event attendance on the donor giving amount and compare it to the data for non-attendees. The box plot in Fig. 6 demonstrates that attendees have a higher giving average and median than non-attendees, particularly for larger donation amounts, as seen in the second subplot with donations of at least $500. We confirm that our results are statistically significant by performing Mann-Whitney U test [18] on the bootstrapped samples.

Having established that participation has an impact on the effectiveness of fundraising, we identify similarities in donor characteristics in this network.

5.2 *Evolving Assortativity at Network Level*

We search for similarities among event co-attendees by measuring the assortativity of the network, which indicates the preference for nodes to attach to others that have similar characteristics. We perform our tests on overlapped windows of 3 years, using the decay function described in [31]. In all cases, assortativity is consistently small but positive, indicating that individuals have a slight tendency to attend events with others of similar giving status.

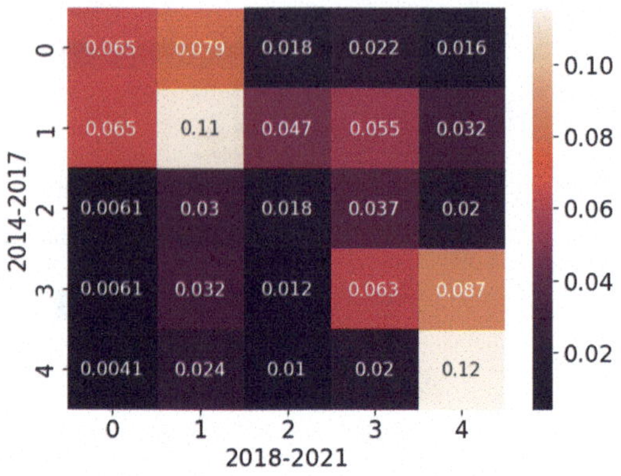

Fig. 7 Fraction of shift in donors between giving classes [31] listed in Sect. 5.2

5.3 *Changes in Behavior at Node Level with Time*

Next, we examine variations in donor behavior from the 2014–2017 period to the 2018–2021 period. We observe that more than half the donors retained between the two periods showed an increase in centrality and 76% of donors that had an increased centrality exhibited increased giving. Additionally, *more than half* of the donors (54%) that had a decreased or equal rank displayed a decrease in giving. Next, we examine the extent to which these donations amplify between the two periods. We label each node based on their donation band [$500, $1000], ($1000, $5000], ($5000, $10,000], ($10,000, $50,000], ($50,000, . . .) discussed with the fundraising team [31].

From Fig. 7 we observe that 41% of people shifted from a lower class to a higher class. Moreover, 35% of those who shifted to a higher giving class or remained in the same class exhibited increased co-attendance with high-capacity donors. *None* of the donors that shifted to lower classes exhibited increased co-attendance.

5.4 *Changes in Group-Level Behavior with Time*

We apply the Louvain community detection algorithm [1] on the weighted co-attendance networks for a 5-year overlapping window. Figure 8 shows a clique of communities that marks strong participation; we observe that community sizes are moderate to large. In the visualization, node size represents community size, green color intensity reflects average donation amounts (lighter shades indicate lower donations), while the edges are unweighted. We observe that community sizes

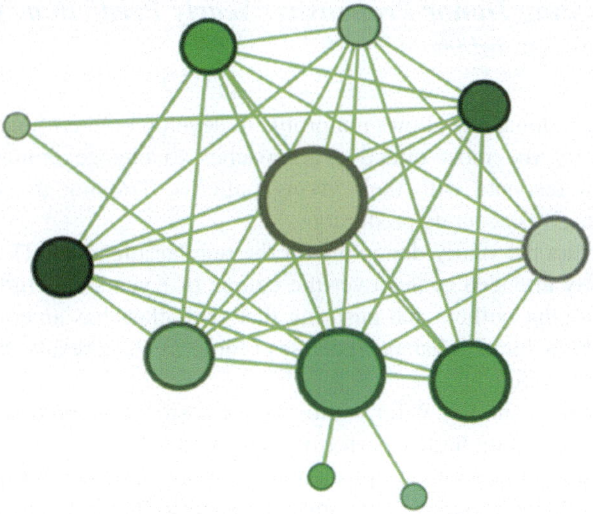

Fig. 8 Communities for a snapshot of 5 years (2017–2021) [31]; color intensity indicates average donation amounts, and circle size represents the community size (number of co-attendees)

increase over time, larger communities tend to have higher giving levels and the correlation becomes stronger over time [31]. Here community size represents the number of co-attendees who attend.

Leveraging the structural attributes of the network, we develop our multivariate model and evaluate its performance on different donor segments and conduct a multi-year analysis. While binary classification yields poor results for both the baseline and multivariate models, multi-class classification results in better performance for our model compared to the baseline. The regression results for multivariate model outperformed the baselines for both regular and irregular donors in terms of MAE. Although the test RMSE values were similar for the baseline and multivariate models, however, when trained on a filtered dataset excluding high donors, performance in terms of test RMSE was significantly better for the multivariate model than the baseline models.

In the multi-class prediction problem, we follow a separate class split for each case individually. This is necessary because the ratio of donors to non-donors differs between the sets, and a uniform approach of maintaining equal class sizes is not suitable. The irregular dataset consists of a higher proportion of smaller donors compared to very high donors, unlike the regular attendee segment. By adapting the class splits to the characteristics of each dataset, we can account for the variations in donor distribution and achieve more effective predictions.

5.5 *Forecasting Donor Propensity: Yearly Predictions for Regular Attendees*

Predicting yearly donations allows nonprofits to develop tailored fundraising strategies and identify the most effective approaches to engage donors and design campaigns that resonate with their giving patterns. Training the model on the segmented data gives accurate predictions.

We first predict the yearly donations for the regular attendees. These are donors who consistently attended events over the course of 8 years. We further refine the dataset by removing outliers and ensuring that each class has an equal number of samples, thereby achieving balanced classes (Table 2). As a result, the sample size decreases to $S = 456$.

The ROC curves in Fig. 9 for multi-class classification predict One-Vs-Rest classes, and demonstrate higher performance (greater AUC) for the LSTM model across all classes. The precision, recall, and F1-scores indicate that the classes are relatively separable for classes 0, 1, and 3 as seen in Table 3. The LSTM model outperforms the baseline model, with a significant difference in F1-score for class 0 and class 3. However, this difference is smaller for class 1 and 2. Notably, the precision and F1-score remain low for class 2 in both models. Meanwhile,the GRU multivariate model performs better than the others in the cases with lowest test RMSE and MAE values, as seen in Table 4.

Table 2 Equal size class segments for regular attendees

Donor classes	Giving range	Class label
Non donors	\$0	0
Low capacity donors	[\$10, \$145)	1
Medium capacity donors	[\$145, \$900)	2
High capacity donors	[\$900, \$45k]	3

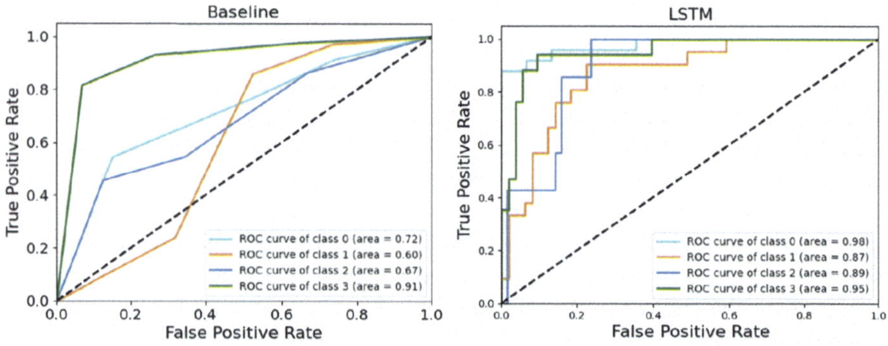

Fig. 9 Comparison of AUC for the Receiver Operating Characteristic for LSTM vs Baseline Sect. 3 for Regular event attendee

Table 3 Classification report

Model	Class	Precision	Recall	F1-score
Regular attendee baseline	0	0.68	0.54	0.60
	1	0.54	0.62	0.58
	2	0.43	0.45	0.44
	3	0.71	0.81	0.76
Regular attendee LSTM	0	0.94	0.89	0.92
	1	0.75	0.46	0.57
	2	0.33	0.75	0.46
	3	0.83	0.88	0.86
Irregular attendee baseline	0	0.78	0.46	0.58
	1	0.54	0.77	0.63
	2	0.56	0.77	0.65
Irregular attendee LSTM	0	**1.0**	**1.0**	**1.0**
	1	0.75	0.81	0.78
	2	0.74	0.67	0.70
Network snapshot baseline	0	0.96	0.89	0.92
	1	0.60	0.78	0.68
	2	0.65	0.85	0.74
Network snapshot LSTM	0	**1.0**	**1.0**	**1.0**
	1	0.92	0.93	0.92
	2	0.73	0.71	0.72

The bold faced numbers indicate highest prediction performance

5.6 *Forecasting Donor Propensity: Yearly Predictions for Small-Sized Event Attendees*

We employ the same approach as Sect. 5.5 on a different segment that includes individuals who do not attend events consistently (irregular attendees). We focus on filtering donor attendees of small-sized events, as these events are indicative of their co-attendance behavior. Based on discussions with the fundraising team, events with 20 or fewer attendees are classified as small-sized events. Class 0 represents non-donors who attend events, Class 1 represents donors who donate between $0 and $1000, and Class 2 represents donors who donate more than $1000. These particular bands are chosen because irregular donors typically contribute lower amounts, often influenced by spontaneous decisions or witnessing fellow donors' contributions. Given the significantly larger number of samples in classes 0 and 1, and the relatively smaller number in class 2, further dividing them would result in fewer samples for the model to learn from, inhibiting the model's ability to capture patterns and make accurate predictions. The LSTM model outperforms the baseline model because its network properties effectively handle the temporal irregularities present in the data.

Table 4 Regression results

Type	Model	Train RMSE	Test RMSE	Train MAE	Test MAE
Regular event attendee	MA	3560.24	9221.99	200.0	78.12
	ARIMA	**3255.10**	7979.89	1053.31	280.46
	ES	3412.78	8438.86	365.39	280.46
	LSTM	6937.15	7873.73	209.59	211.05
	GRU	6922.49	**7858.51**	**111.79**	**90.03**
Irregular event attendee	MA	184,480.33	33,462.85	925.0	100.0
	ARIMA	**108,452.34**	69,808.79	20,488.89	20,994.67
	ES	118,368.10	58,727.36	16,089.77	42,077.67
	LSTM	110,686.14	35,487.12	**222.10**	**222.26**
	GRU	109,775.15	**24,239.65**	433.69	94.26
All attendee (Multi-year)	ARIMA	**73,111.46**	150,637.36	**0**	**0**
	ES	84,824.18	145,089.20	**0**	**0**
	LSTM	88,213.66	103,038.07	**0.20**	**0.16**
	GRU	88,198.64	**103,027.14**	**0.87**	**0.79**
Filtered attendee (Multi-year)	ARIMA	**9652.80**	22,428.29	**0**	**0**
	ES	10,857.28	20,687.33	**0**	**0**
	LSTM	18,891.85	16,874.49	2.09	1.63
	GRU	18,867.08	**16,857.38**	4.12	4.29

The highlighted numbers represent the minimum MAE/RMSE values

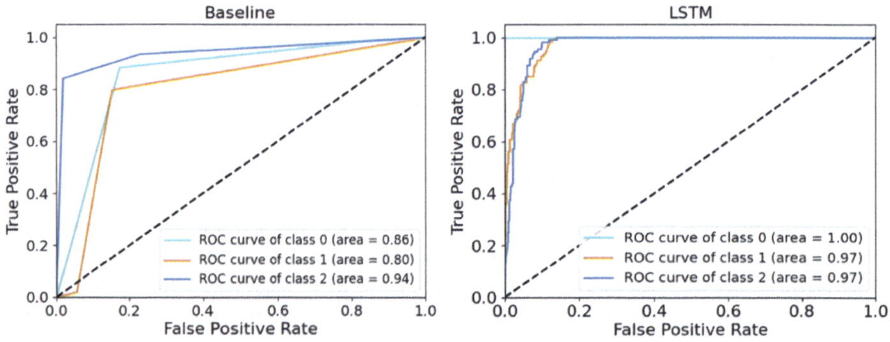

Fig. 10 Comparison of AUC for the Receiver Operating Characteristic for LSTM vs Baseline for irregular event attendees

When considering all donors ($S = 5578$) including those with more irregular attendance patterns, the baseline model's precision and F1-score decrease to 0.20 and 0.31 for class 1, and 0.22 and 0.33 for class 2, respectively. In contrast, the LSTM model significantly outperforms the baseline, achieving precision and F1-scores of 0.75 and 0.76 for class 1, and 0.74 and 0.72 for class 2. However, when we focus on a subset of donors who have attended events consecutively for over 2 years ($S = 589$), we observe an improvement in the baseline model's performance.

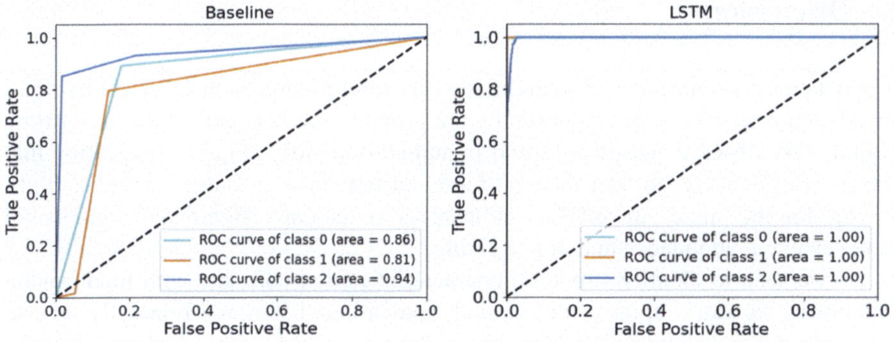

Fig. 11 Comparison of AUC for the receiver operating characteristic for LSTM vs Baseline for network snapshots for a rolling window of 3 years

Nevertheless, the LSTM model still outperforms the baseline for all classes as seen in Fig. 10 and Table 3. With respect to the regression task, LSTM multivariate model outperformed all the other models with lowest train and test MAE values (222.10 and 222.26).

5.7 Multi-Year Analysis: Learning from Network Snapshots for Long-Term Trends

Rolling window network characteristics provide insights into the evolving relationships and interactions among donors and nonprofits can identify long-term trends and seasonal trends in donor behavior. We observe improved model performance when trained with weighted network snapshots and an increased sample size ($S = 99{,}431$). The LSTM model achieves complete separability for the classes, as illustrated in Fig. 11, outperforming the baseline model.

From Table 4 we observe lowest test RMSE for the multivariate GRU model, and the MAE values are fairly close to 0. We observe improved performance for the regression task, and the LSTM and GRU models outperform the statistical models in terms of test RMSE, despite having comparable training losses. This pattern persists when the donors are filtered by removing extremely high donors (those who donate more than a million dollars) with test RMSE significantly reduced.

6 Discussion

The data we examine suggests that the relevant fund-raising team successfully organized engaging events, as evidenced by the growth in donor participation over time (Fig. 1). We observe an upward trend in annual donations (Fig. 2), suggesting that the team effectively utilized their professional networks and attracted more high-giving donors, since our analysis indicates a statistically significant relationship between event attendance and donor giving.

As we seek to identify structural characteristics that correlate with fund-raising outcomes, we draw upon prior research indicating that donor-donor dyads can influence donor behavior. We identify similarities in individual characteristics for our dataset, observing positive assortativity of co-attendees with respect to their giving values. A low-to-moderate assortativity in co-attendance is beneficial for fund-raising networks and suggests the success of event organization and attendee placement. In contrast, a high assortativity value would hinder new connections and diminish the positive peer pressure effect. This is backed by studies that show individuals being influenced to match or exceed the generosity of their fellow attendees, resulting in higher overall donation amounts [20, 30].

It is important to assess how donor characteristics change with time. We find that 76% of donors that had increased centrality also showed increase in giving amounts, and more than half of the donors that displayed an equal or lesser centrality decreased their giving. Increased centrality indicates that donors are actively co-attending more events or are co-attending with other high-centrality donors. Figure 7 shows the shift in giving class (of a donor) and its relationship with co-attendance. Overall, 41.37% donors increased their giving class, 37.53% maintained the same class, and the remaining decreased their giving level. Moreover, we observe that 35% that remained in the same class or shifted to an upper giving class showed an increased co-attendance with high-giving donors, while none of the donors that shifted to a lower class exhibited increased co-attendance.

In addition to individual characteristics associated with increased giving, we also analyze group-level characteristics that may contribute to this change. Figure 8 provides a structural visualization of communities of co-attendees, showing a clique of communities that mark active participation of donors. The donor-attendee community analyses enable organizations to examine donor engagement and identify major donor prospects. This information can be used to strengthen relationships and maximize event impact. We further observe:

- Increased community sizes over the years;
- Larger and more tightly-knit participation of donors over time; and
- Increase (with time) in the correlation between fraction of above-median donors and community size.

Our results are partially explained by the fact that larger communities have many donors that benefit from resources such as business opportunities, and professional networks. Individuals who have gained from these resources may feel a sense of gratitude and a desire to give back to the community that provided them with such advantages [15].

Having gained insights into the network characteristics associated with fundraising outcomes, we construct a multivariate model by extracting features from the network. These features include assortativity (similarity) at the individual level, exposure to high-capacity donors, exposure to donors who can potentially influence non-donors, the structural positions of individuals in the network, and their levels of potential interactions with their local neighborhoods.

Our multivariate model outperforms baselines for both classification and regression tasks across various donor segments. Notably, the multivariate models' precision, recall, and F1-score are significantly better than the baselines when tested on irregular event attendees, and using multi-year analysis, as seen from Table 3. Figures 9, 10, and 11 show that the AUC for our model is consistently higher than the baseline for all three analysis. Moreover, the node features become perfectly separable when considering network snapshots for a window size of 3 years, as indicated by an AUC of 1.0 for all three classes.

When predicting the donation amount for regular donors, we find that the multivariate model performs better than the baselines, as evidenced by test RMSE and, train and test MAE(median absolute error) for the two donor segments in Table 4. Significant differences in test RMSE and MAE values are observed for the irregular attendee segment and the multi-year network.

The enhanced performance of the multivariate model can be attributed to the following factors. First, statistical baselines encounter difficulties in handling missing data, which is prevalent in cases where users have donated in the past few years and may donate in the future. Second, there is a scarcity of known data about new donors, making it challenging for statistical models to draw accurate inferences. Third, donors who attend events regularly tend to be more loyal to the recipient organization. Their donation behavior may be influenced by external factors such as donor-solicitor and donor-recipient dyads, including communication with the fundraising team, beyond just donor-donor dyads. While these donors contribute annually, their giving potential may primarily reflect their long-term commitments.

Our analysis predicting donor propensity can be highly valuable for fund-raisers, as it enables them to identify potential donors and donor segments well in advance. By understanding the regularity in donation patterns and optimizing resource allocation to various donor segments, such as retained donors, new donors, and donors who have changed their behavior, fund-raisers can improve targeting and ultimately improve fund-raising outcomes.

One of the limitations of our work is the inability to model causal relationships linking network properties to giving outcomes. With respect to predicting donor propensity, our dataset appears to be insufficient for accurate binary classification as both the baseline model and the multivariate model failed to effectively identify the non-donors. The best performance was achieved using cross-validation, suggesting that the models do not necessarily benefit by learning from extensive historical data.

7 Conclusion

This study highlights the potential of utilizing donor co-attendance networks for understanding fund-raising outcomes and how network features can be harnessed for donor propensity prediction. Our analyses show that people who attended more events donated more often and greater amounts. We identified that there is a low-to-moderate similarity in the giving characteristics of co-attendees. We also observe that donors who occupied central positions had increased giving as well as increased co-attendance with high-capacity donors over the periods increased their giving class membership. The community structure also revealed strong connections that are beneficial for maximizing the effectiveness of their resource allocation strategies. By incorporating these network features into our multivariate model, we achieve accurate predictions of the giving class and donation amount, outperforming baseline models for all three analyses.

This study contributes to the body of knowledge on assessing fundraising outcomes by utilizing the dynamics of the co-attendance network. Our research demonstrates the enhanced predictive capability of incorporating event co-attendance networks in predicting donor propensity. This can be used by fundraisers in assessing outcomes, making informed decisions and develop tailored strategies to enhance fundraising outcomes.

Our results have relied on limited information readily available from the donor history database. With access to more data, we can consider interactions influenced by co-location, organizational co-affiliation, and other factors. Future work can also attempt to distinguish between correlation and causation in the relationships between network properties and fundraising outcomes. Finer-grained analysis is also needed to explain the divergence of behaviors of subsets of individuals that are initially similar, identifying the extent to which co-attendance may explain the divergence.

Acknowledgments Srikanta and Soundarajan were funded by NSF 2047224.

References

1. Thomas Aynaud. Community detection for networkx's documentation, 2018.
2. Victor MH Borden, Genevieve G Shaker, and Brittany L Kienker. The impact of alumni status on institutional giving by faculty and staff. *Research in Higher Education*, 55:196–217, 2014.
3. Kanad Chakraborty, Kishan Mehrotra, Chilukuri K Mohan, and Sanjay Ranka. Forecasting the behavior of multivariate time series using neural networks. *Neural networks*, 5(6):961–970, 1992.
4. Cassandra M Chapman, Barbara M Masser, and Winnifred R Louis. The champion effect in peer-to-peer giving: Successful campaigns highlight fundraisers more than causes. *Nonprofit and Voluntary Sector Quarterly*, 48(3):572–592, 2019.

5. Kyunghyun Cho, Bart Van Merriënboer, Caglar Gulcehre, Dzmitry Bahdanau, Fethi Bougares, Holger Schwenk, and Yoshua Bengio. Learning phrase representations using rnn encoder-decoder for statistical machine translation. *arXiv preprint arXiv:1406.1078*, 2014.
6. James Samuel Coleman et al. Introduction to mathematical sociology. *Introduction to mathematical sociology.*, 1964.
7. Rod Duclos and Alixandra Barasch. Prosocial behavior in intergroup relations: How donor self-construal and recipient group-membership shape generosity. *Journal of Consumer Research*, 41(1):93–108, 2014.
8. Harmonie Farrow and Y Connie Yuan. Building stronger ties with alumni through facebook to increase volunteerism and charitable giving. *Journal of Computer-Mediated Communication*, 16(3):445–464, 2011.
9. Soledad Galli and Kishan Manani. Feature engineering for time series forecasting.
10. Everette S Gardner Jr. Exponential smoothing: The state of the art. *Journal of forecasting*, 4(1):1–28, 1985.
11. Elizabeth M Gerber, Julie S Hui, Pei-Yi Kuo, et al. Crowdfunding: Why people are motivated to post and fund projects on crowdfunding platforms. In *Proceedings of the international workshop on design, influence, and social technologies: techniques, impacts and ethics*, volume 2, page 10, 2012.
12. Lihuan Guo, Wei Wang, Yenchun Jim Wu, and Mark Goh. How much do social connections matter in fundraising outcomes? *Financial Innovation*, 7(1):79, 2021.
13. Aric Hagberg and Drew Conway. Networkx: Network analysis with python. URL: https://networkx.github.io, 2020.
14. Sepp Hochreiter and Jürgen Schmidhuber. Long short-term memory. *Neural computation*, 9(8):1735–1780, 1997.
15. Nicola Lacetera, Mario Macis, and Angelo Mele. Viral altruism? charitable giving and social contagion in online networks. *Sociological Science*, 3, 2016.
16. Ming Li, K Mehrotra, Chilukuri Mohan, and Sanjay Ranka. Sunspot numbers forecasting using neural networks. In *Proceedings. 5th IEEE International Symposium on Intelligent Control 1990*, pages 524–529. IEEE, 1990.
17. Bryan Lim and Stefan Zohren. Time-series forecasting with deep learning: a survey. *Philosophical Transactions of the Royal Society A*, 379(2194):20200209, 2021.
18. Henry B Mann and Donald R Whitney. On a test of whether one of two random variables is stochastically larger than the other. *The annals of mathematical statistics*, pages 50–60, 1947.
19. Kevin R McClure, Leah Frierson, Adam W Hall, and Kara L Ostlund. Philanthropic giving by foundations to higher education institutions: A state-level social network analysis. *Philanthropy & Education*, 1(1):1–28, 2017.
20. Jonathan Meer. Brother, can you spare a dime? peer pressure in charitable solicitation. *Journal of public economics*, 95(7–8):926–941, 2011.
21. Kishan Mehrotra, Chilukuri K Mohan, and Sanjay Ranka. *Elements of artificial neural networks*. MIT press, 1997.
22. Brian K Nelson. Time series analysis using autoregressive integrated moving average (arima) models. *Academic emergency medicine*, 5(7):739–744, 1998.
23. Albert A Okunade and Robert L Berl. Determinants of charitable giving of business school alumni. *Research in higher education*, 38:201–214, 1997.
24. Anton Pudikov and Alexander Brovko. Comparison of lstm and gru recurrent neural network architectures. In *International Scientific and Practical Conference in Control Engineering and Decision Making*, pages 114–124. Springer, 2020.
25. Peter H Reingen. Test of a list procedure for inducing compliance with a request to donate money. *Journal of Applied Psychology*, 67(1):110, 1982.
26. Adrian Sargeant. Using donor lifetime value to inform fundraising strategy. *Nonprofit Management and Leadership*, 12(1):25–38, 2001.
27. Gregory D Saxton and Lili Wang. The social network effect: The determinants of giving through social media. *Nonprofit and voluntary sector quarterly*, 43(5):850–868, 2014.

28. George B Schreiber, UK Sharma, DJ Wright, SA Glynn, HE Ownby, Y Tu, G Garratty, J Piliavin, T Zuck, R Gilcher, et al. First year donation patterns predict long-term commitment for first-time donors. *Vox sanguinis*, 88(2):114–121, 2005.
29. Jen Shang, Rachel Croson, and Americus Reed. "i" give, but "we" give more: the impact of identity and the mere social information effect on donation behavior. *ACR North American Advances*, 2007.
30. Sarah Smith, Frank Windmeijer, and Edmund Wright. Peer effects in charitable giving: Evidence from the (running) field. *The Economic Journal*, 125(585):1053–1071, 2015.
31. Srikanta, Shwetha Koushik Manchinahalli, Katie L. Pierce, Joshua E. Introne, Chilukuri K. Mohan, and Sucheta Soundarajan. Structure and dynamics of a charitable donor co-attendance network. In *Proceedings of the International Conference on Advances in Social Networks Analysis and Mining*, pp. 514–521, 2023.
32. Yuan Tian and Sara Konrath. The effects of similarity on charitable giving in donor–donor dyads: A systematic literature review. *Voluntas: International Journal of Voluntary and Nonprofit Organizations*, 32:316–339, 2021.
33. Tijs A van den Broek, Ariana Need, Michel L Ehrenhard, Anna Priante, and Djoerd Hiemstra. The influence of network structure and prosocial cultural norms on charitable giving: A multilevel analysis of movember's fundraising campaigns in 24 countries. *Social networks*, 58:128–135, 2019.
34. Shengsheng Xiao and Qing Yue. The role you play, the life you have: Donor retention in online charitable crowdfunding platform. *Decision Support Systems*, 140:113427, 2021.

Analyzing the Impact of COVID-19 on Portuguese Social Media

Richard Adolph Aires Jonker, Roshan Poudel, Olga Fajarda, Sérgio Matos, José Luís Oliveira, and Rui Pedro Lopes

Abstract The COVID-19 pandemic has had a widespread global impact, with social media platforms such as Twitter serving as a key source of communication and information sharing. In this study, we present the first large-scale Portuguese Twitter dataset on COVID-19, providing a unique perspective on the impact of the pandemic on Portuguese-speaking communities on social media. The dataset includes over 31 million Tweets from 2020 and 2021. We conducted sentiment analysis using the LeIA (Lexicon for Adapted Inference) model to examine the relationship between spikes in Tweet count and sentiment scores with news articles and government announcements in Portugal and Brazil. Additionally, we employed manual data clustering, providing more insights into the data and understanding of its composition. We perform a comparative analysis among different groups to understand how the dataset's composition changes over time and compare this between Portugal and Brazil. This research offers valuable insights into the pandemic's impact on Portuguese-speaking communities on social media. The dataset is available on https://github.com/bioinformatics-ua/Portuguese-Covid19-Dataset.

Keywords COVID-19 · Sentiment Analysis · Twitter · Dataset

R. A. A. Jonker (✉) · O. Fajarda · S. Matos · J. L. Oliveira
University of Aveiro, IEETA- Institute of Electronics and Informatics Engineering of Aveiro, Aveiro, Portugal
e-mail: richard.jonker@ua.pt; olga.oliveira@ua.pt; aleixomatos@ua.pt; jlo@ua.pt

R. Poudel · R. P. Lopes
Polytechnic Institute of Bragança, Research Centre in Digitalization and Intelligent Robotics, Bragança, Portugal
e-mail: roshan@ipb.pt; rlopes@ipb.pt

M. Kaya et al. (eds.), *Social Network Analysis and Mining Applications in Healthcare and Anomaly Detection*, Lecture Notes in Social Networks,
https://doi.org/10.1007/978-3-031-75204-9_7

1 Introduction

The COVID-19 pandemic, without a doubt, stands as the most significant crisis of the twenty-first century. According to the World Health Organization (WHO), the global tally of confirmed COVID-19 cases has exceeded 761 million, resulting in a staggering loss of over 6.8 million lives to date [3]. This pandemic has triggered a series of cascading effects, influencing every facet of our lives, from public health and economic stability to social and psychological well-being [28].

Governments across the globe resorted to drastic measures to curb the spread of the virus, implementing widespread home-based quarantines and lockdowns. While these measures were vital for controlling the virus, they also brought about several unintended consequences, particularly among the youth. Studies have highlighted the adverse social and psychological costs incurred by young individuals during extended lockdowns [28]. Furthermore, the pandemic's pervasive uncertainty and isolation have contributed to soaring levels of stress, anxiety, and depression within the general population [9, 29, 31].

Amid such crises, people turned to social media platforms as vital channels for communication, information sharing, and expressing their thoughts and emotions. It has been shown that news frequently arrives on social media before it is reported by mainstream news reporters [19] and that individuals also respond swiftly to these events. Twitter[1] is a very popular social media platform worldwide and the primarily used platform to collect large volumes of social media data for research purposes, due to its accessible openly available Application Programming Interface (API). Twitter datasets have proven to be helpful in many applications, including the detection of influenza outbreaks [5, 26], disaster management assistance [22], public health surveillance [21], and the identification of misinformation flows [11]. Moreover, sentiment analysis on Twitter datasets offers insightful information about user reactions to specific events [30] which can be utilized to improve the public's perception of similar future events.

Over the past 2 years, numerous COVID-19 Twitter datasets have been made available to researchers, allowing them to explore public sentiment and responses to the pandemic [6, 10, 13, 14, 16, 23–25, 27]. However, the majority of these datasets primarily consist of English-language tweets or multilingual collections. Only a limited number are dedicated to non-English languages [6, 14, 16]. Given the behavioral differences among Twitter users from various linguistic backgrounds [17], it is crucial to have non-English, language-specific COVID-19 Twitter datasets to provide a comprehensive understanding of global sentiments. Multilingual datasets inherently include fewer tweets in a given language due to limitations imposed by the Twitter API.

Notably, Portuguese has emerged as one of the dominant languages on Twitter, as evidenced by Alshaabi et al. [8], who analyzed language use trends on the platform

[1] Twitter Social Media Platform: www.twitter.com.

from 2009 to 2020. Despite the prevalence of Portuguese on Twitter, the availability of Portuguese COVID-19 Twitter datasets for research remains limited. To date, only one such dataset has been released [14], encompassing approximately 4 million tweets collected during the early stages of the pandemic, from January to May 2020.

In this paper, we present an extensive Portuguese COVID-19 Twitter dataset, which has been expanded to encompass over 31 million tweets [20]. Additionally, we integrated sentiment analysis into our work to explore the emotional landscape of the Portuguese-speaking Twitter community during the pandemic. Leveraging the LeIA model, we applied sentiment analysis to each tweet, yielding sentiment scores that encompass measures of positivity, negativity, and compound sentiment. This enhanced dataset enables a more nuanced exploration of public sentiment in response to the pandemic within the Portuguese-speaking population.To gain deeper insights into the data, we conducted cluster analysis, allowing us to categorize and identify specific topics within this extensive dataset. The cluster analysis provides valuable insights into the prominent discussions on Twitter within the Portuguese-speaking community during the COVID-19 pandemic.

The remainder of the paper is organized as follows: the methodology used to collect the dataset, including tools and software used, is covered in Sect. 2. Section 3 presents an in-depth breakdown of the dataset with various exploratory items investigated, including a breakdown of the peaks of the Tweet counts in the dataset and various news articles that appeared during the same time. In Sect. 4, we present the clusters we obtained by manually filtering the dataset, and Sect. 5 analyzes the clusters. Finally, Sect. 6 concludes the paper.

2 Methodology

This section presents the methodology and several tools used to collect the Tweets regarding the COVID-19 pandemic, as well as the techniques used to perform sentiment analysis on each Tweet.

As depicted in Fig. 1, our system pipeline centers around the ELK stack (Elasticsearch, Logstash, and Kibana) and the Twitter API. Initially, data is collected from the Twitter API with the assistance of Tweepy, and the results are periodically stored on a local server, enabling us to resume data retrieval in the event of a failure. Subsequently, the files are indexed into Elasticsearch, enhancing our ability to analyze tweets efficiently. For sentiment analysis, we utilized LeIA, a derivative of VADER. LeIA operates as its standalone service, ingesting tweets from the Elastic API, conducting sentiment analysis, and returning the scores to Elasticsearch. We leveraged the Elastic API and Kibana dashboard for additional clustering and exploratory analysis.

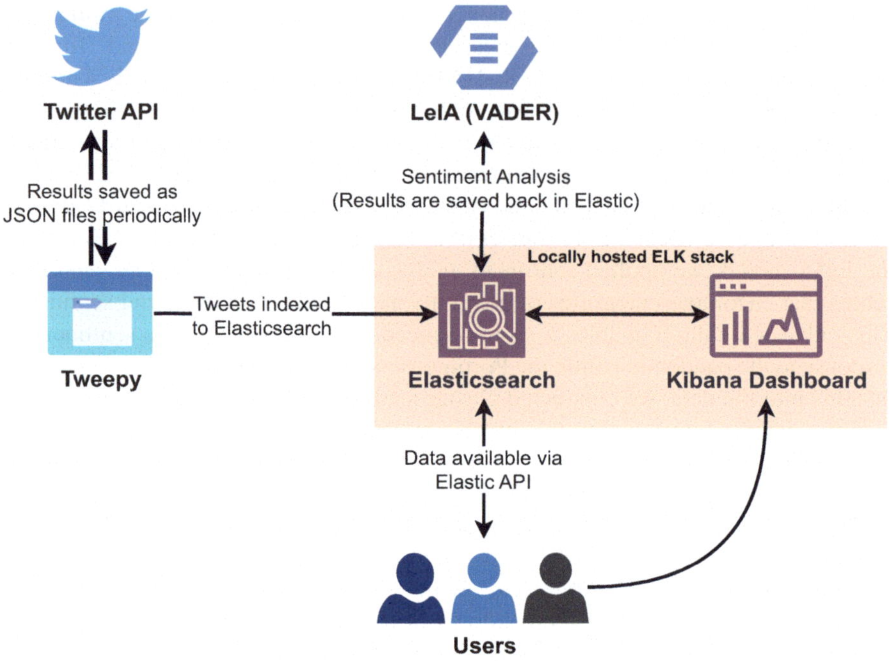

Fig. 1 Overall architecture of system used

Table 1 Query terms used to collect the dataset

Keywords
covid OR covid19 OR #covid19pt OR #novocoronavirus OR coronavirus OR pandemic OR pandemia OR confinamento OR desconfinamento OR (corona virus)

2.1 *Dataset Collection*

The Python library Tweepy [2] was used to gather the Tweets. The library provides a flexible and easy-to-use interface for gathering Tweets and dumping them into a text file. The library works with Twitter's official API. The Twitter Search API V2[2] was accessed through a Twitter academic research account. This enables retrieving all Tweets that match a query over the whole archive of Tweets going back to the first Tweet in 2006. Tweets were collected for the years 2020 and 2021, starting on January 1, 00:00 2020, and ending on December 31, 23:59 2021. The keywords used to collect the Tweets can be seen in Table 1.

[2] Twitter Search APIv2: https://developer.twitter.com/en/docs/twitter-api/tweets/search/introduction.

Retweets were not included in the data collected because they contain the same text and would add unnecessary data to the dataset. All Tweets were tagged by Twitter as Portuguese and contain words relevant to COVID, the pandemic, and confinements. From the keywords used to collect the Tweets in this dataset, the keywords *#covid19pt*, *novocoronavirus*, *pandemia*, *confinamento*, and *desconfinamento* were not used by any of the multilingual datasets [10, 13, 24]. Consequently, this dataset contains different Portuguese Tweets than the Portuguese Tweets retrieved by these multilingual datasets.

Due to the large scale of the dataset, the ELK (Elasticsearch, Logstash, and Kibana) stack was used to store, process, and manage the data [1]. Using ELK allows to load and process the data efficiently, as well as generate visualizations that summarize the data easily.

To perform sentiment analysis and more complex data manipulations, we used Python and the Elasticsearch library to connect to and stream the data from the ELK server.

2.2 Sentiment Analysis

To perform sentiment analysis, we used the model LeIA - Lexicon for Adapted Inference [7]. LeIA is a Portuguese lexicon fork for VADER (Valence Aware Dictionary for sEntiment Reasoning), which is used for sentiment analysis on social media [18]. VADER is a lexicon-based sentiment analysis tool, meaning that linguists have decided on a set of words with sentiment values that will act as a dictionary from which the sentiments for documents are calculated. The main advantage of using a lexicon-based sentiment analyzer is that it is very fast and does not need to be trained. VADER is designed for use on social media, as it accounts for various internet slang-related acronyms, words, and symbols. It uses various heuristics to further influence the sentiment. These heuristics include punctuation - type and count, use of capitalization, degree modifiers, such as adverbs, the use of contrastive conjunctions, and the use of certain tri-grams. LeIA further builds upon this model by providing a lexicon that is based on Portuguese social media.

VADER outputs a dictionary of four values: positive, negative, neutral, and compound. Positive, negative, and neutral refer to the proportion of words in the text that are positive, negative, and neutral, respectively. The compound score is the heuristic-adjusted cumulative score for the sentence. This score ranges from -1 to 1, with -1 being a negative sentiment and 1 being a positive sentiment. The dataset provides the positive, negative, and compound scores for each Tweet. Neutral is not provided as it can be calculated with $1 - (pos + neg)$. To determine if a Tweet is positive, negative, or neutral, the same thresholds recommended by the original VADER authors are used:

- negative: $compound < -0.05$
- neutral: $-0.05 \leq compound \leq 0.05$
- positive: $compound > 0.05$

3 Dataset

The dataset is arranged by day, and in compliance with Twitter's Terms of Service, we only publish the Tweet IDs, sentiment scores, and summary statistics. The dataset contains 31,260,897 Tweets, coming from 4,009,842 different users. We collected 21,278,917 Tweets in 2020, and 9,981,980 Tweets in 2021. According to the entity tags assigned by Twitter (tags based on what content is written in the Tweet), around 1.7 million of the Tweets are tagged to be about Brazil, and around 140,000 are tagged to be about Portugal. Just under 700,000 Tweets are associated with a Place ID (a user-defined location assigned to their Tweet), most of which are associated with locations in Brazil. Only 78,514 Tweets have been tagged with geo-location coordinates.

In terms of users, a Brazilian news agency shared 64,485 Tweets, making it the most active user in the dataset. Figure 2 displays the cumulative percentage of the number of Tweets for the ten most active users. Table 2 summarizes the Top 10 user types, most of which are news agencies.

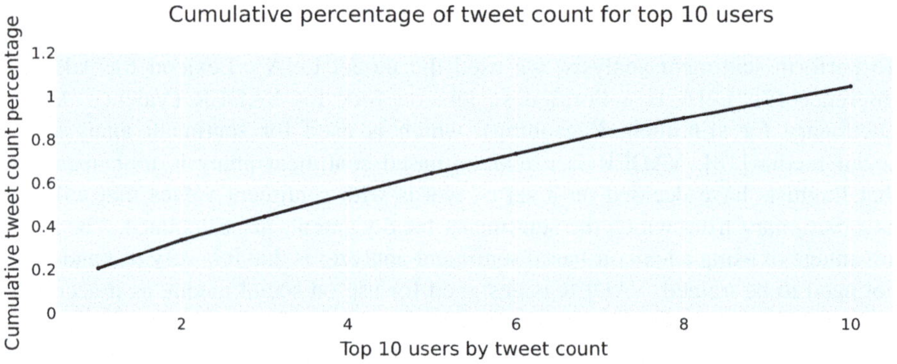

Fig. 2 Cumulative percentage of tweet count for the top 10 users

Table 2 Top 10 posting user types

User type	Count of records
Brazilian news	64,485
Portuguese journalist	41,027
Brazilian journalist	33,730
Portuguese news	32,138
Portuguese news	30,213
Portuguese news	28,126
Bot	27,984
Brazilian news	23,378
Portuguese news	23,323
Portuguese journalist	22,766

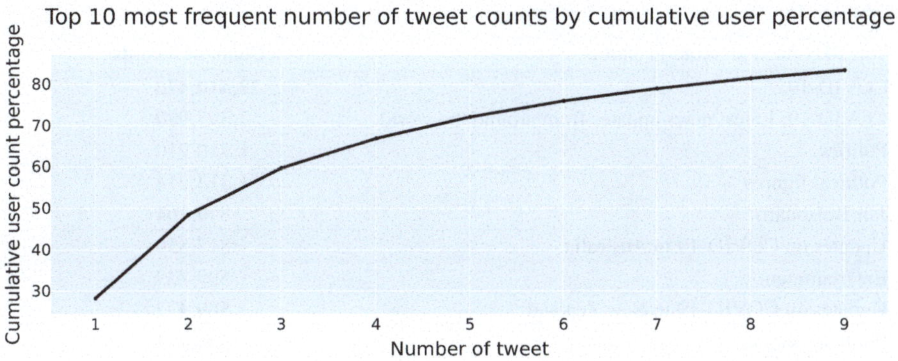

Fig. 3 Ten most frequent number of tweet counts by cumulative user percentage

Table 3 Top 10 hashtags not related to COVID

Top 10 hashtags not related to COVID	Count of records
ForaBolsonaro	96,296
FiqueEmCasa	68,231
Brasil	58,256
Stop	51,997
Quarentena	48,308
G1	43,492
BolsonaroGenocida	37,701
Vacina	36,865
FicaEmCasa	35,716
Saúde	33,547

Just over a quarter of the users, 884,069 (28%), have only 1 Tweet and 2,662,090 users (1%) have ten or fewer Tweets, which is shown in Fig. 3. The users which have ten or fewer Tweets make up for 84.9%.

Table 3 lists the top trending hashtags that are not COVID related. We can observe that most of the top hashtags are related to Brazil, either being related to the Brazilian president Jair Bolsonaro, news agencies, or other COVID-related terms such as quarantine and vaccine.

The top ten context annotations for the dataset are listed in Table 4. Context annotations are the people, places, products, and organizations mentioned in the Tweet, which are automatically tagged by Twitter. COVID-19 is the most common context annotation. This is followed by politics and Jair Bolsonaro. There are then updates on COVID-19 in Australia and New Zealand, and some general topics. The updates on COVID-19 in Australia and New Zealand were attributed to their strong zero COVID policies during March 2020.

Figure 4 shows a line chart summarizing the statistics of the Tweet count. The figure contains the total Tweet count aggregated per week as well as a Moving average of the Total Tweets with a lag of 5. The 95% confidence interval is generated from the moving average. Peaks are identified if the value is outside the previous

Table 4 Top 10 Context annotation entities

Top 10 context annotation entities	Count of records
COVID-19	28,410,476
COVID-19: Latest news updates from around the world	2,397,920
Politics	1,710,910
Political figures	1,313,214
Jair Bolsonaro	879,164
Updates on COVID-19 in Australia	817,850
Entertainment	599,839
Updates on COVID-19 in New Zealand	569,472
Political issues	496,714
Soccer	491,717

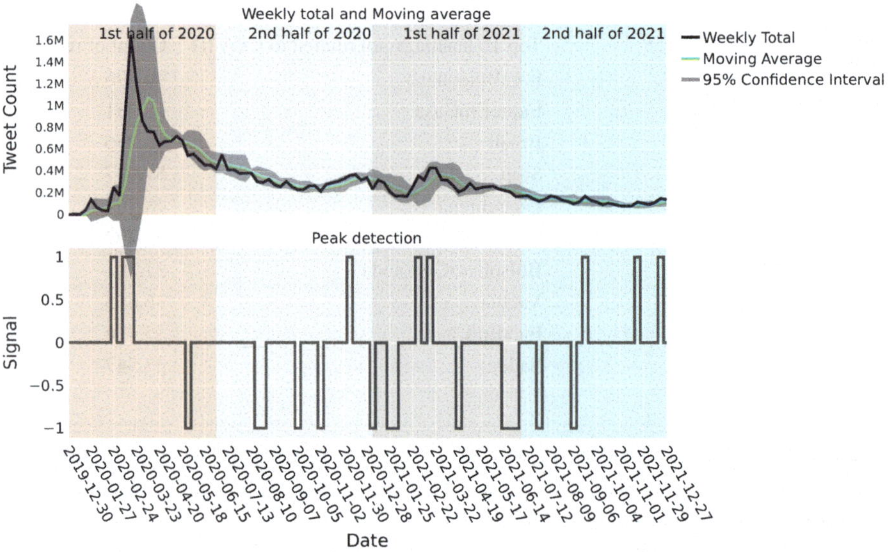

Fig. 4 Rolling weekly average of total Tweets and peaks detected by peak detector

95% confidence interval. This approach is suggested by Brakel [12] for peak signal detection, with **lag** = 5, **threshold** = 1.96, and **influence** = 1. Using these parameters, separate peaks can be observed, which we will analyze, in conjunction with the number of positive, negative, and total Tweets, as well as the number of COVID cases and deaths for both Brazil and Portugal. Data regarding the number of cases and deaths were taken from the WHO [4]. In order to make the graphs comparable, the plots containing the deaths and cases use a percentage relative to the maximum value. Due to the nature of the data, we investigated modeling the number of Tweets with time series models, however, there did not appear to be any visible seasonal components and the models did not fit the data well.

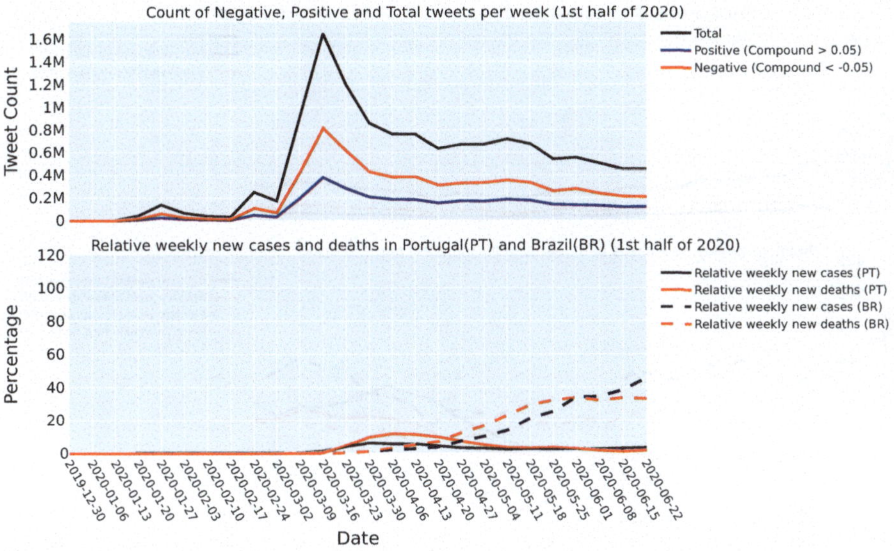

Fig. 5 Count of negative, positive, and total Tweets per week and Weekly new cases and deaths of PT and BR for the first half of 2020

Inspecting the first half of 2020 in Fig. 5, the initial peak happened between the end of February 2020 and mid-March 2020. On 2020-03-16, the first death due to COVID-19 appeared in Portugal, and lockdown measures began taking place, namely restricting travel to Spain. On 2020-03-18, Portugal declared its first state of emergency. Analyzing the sentiment values for this time period, it can be seen that the number of positive Tweets is relatively constant, with fluctuations in the number of negative Tweets matching those of the total Tweet counts. Generally, the number of negative Tweet counts was almost double that of the positive Tweet count. Looking into the statistics regarding the number of cases and deaths, we see a large peak of deaths around the first 2 weeks of April, and at the same time, we see Brazil's cases and deaths begin to increase, with a very large amount of relative deaths by the end of June.

Moving onto the second half of 2020, seen in Fig. 6, the only peak occurs during December 2020, which is to be expected, as people are generally on holiday and will have more time to use social media. The Portuguese government also announced special restrictions for the holiday time on 2020-12-17, including the banning of movement on public roads and limiting the operational hours of restaurants. All these restrictions did not manage to reduce the growing number of cases in Portugal. The negative sentiments also further increase during November. This could be due to either the rise in Portuguese or Brazilian cases during that time period.

Looking at the first half of 2021, Fig. 7, two peaks occurred close to each other during March. These peaks were difficult to attribute to any major event. There was a record for the number of deaths caused by the virus in Brazil, as well as very large moving averages for the number of deaths caused by COVID. Upon

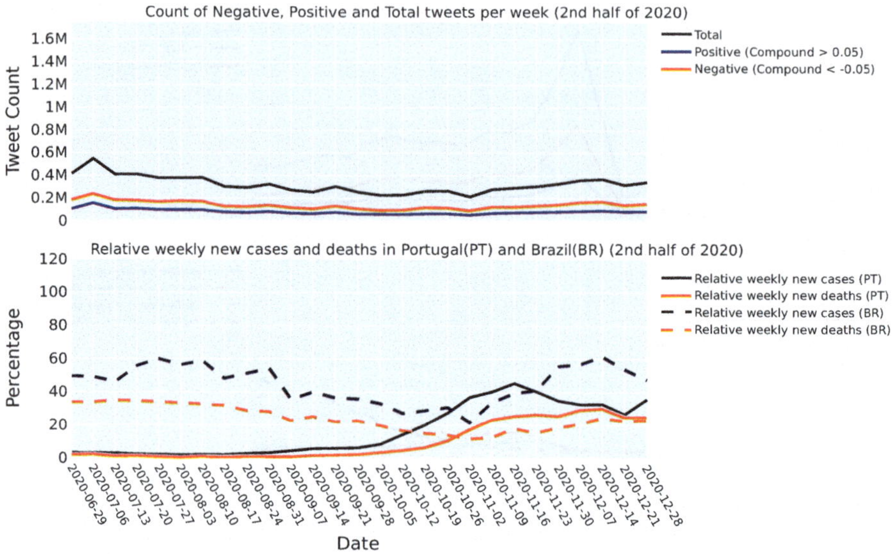

Fig. 6 Count of negative, positive, and total Tweets per week and Weekly new cases and deaths of PT and BR for the second half of 2020

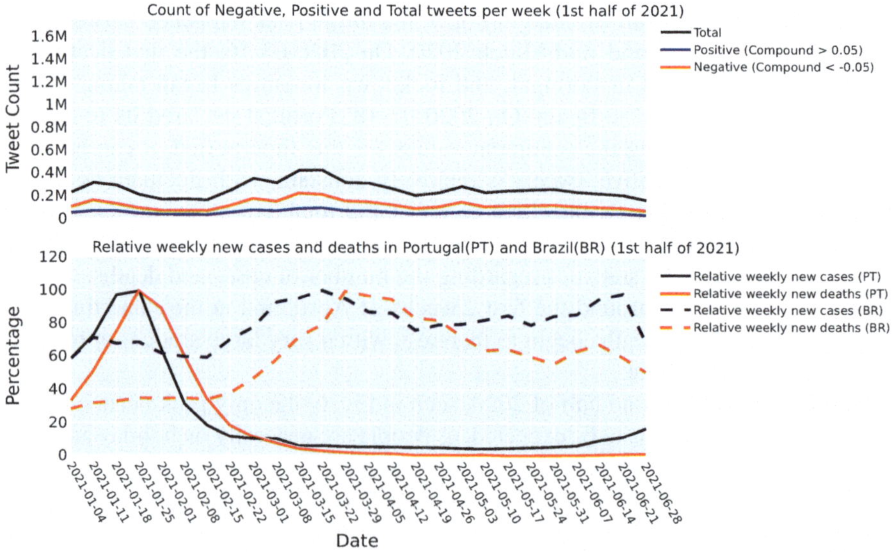

Fig. 7 Count of negative, positive, and total Tweets per week and Weekly new cases and deaths of PT and BR for the first half of 2021

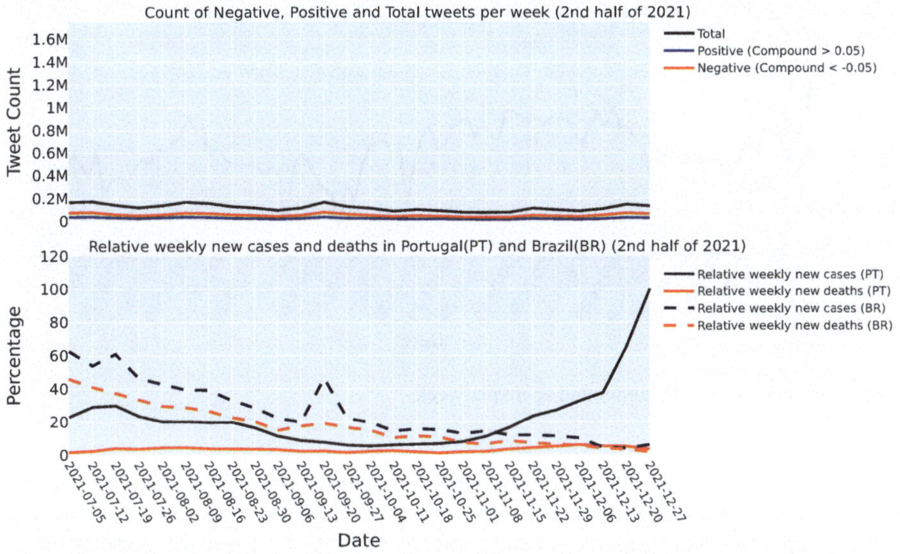

Fig. 8 Count of negative, positive, and total Tweets per week and Weekly new cases and deaths of PT and BR for the second half of 2021

investigating the Twitter data during this time, some Tweets mention the deaths of loved ones and people grieving, as well as complaints about the Brazilian President. The high number of negative Tweets further supports this. This trend continues for the next 2 weeks, where we see the next spike on 2021-03-15, which is also attributed to the rising number of deaths and cases in Brazil, with shortages of vaccines and the eventual replacement of the Brazilian health minister on 2021-03-15. In Portugal, various alleviations to the state of emergency were announced on 2021-03-11, including the resuming of face-to-face schooling on 2021-03-15.

Moving onto the final part of our dataset, in the second half of 2021, Fig. 8, the first spike occurred during 2021-09-20, the same time we see a spike in the number of cases in Brazil. On 2021-09-23, the Portuguese government declared a situation of alert as of October 1, as well as the last stage of deconfinement with the opening of bars. The next spike occurred on 2021-11-22. On 2021-11-25, the Portuguese government announced a state of calamity as of 2021-12-01, with teleworking between 2022-01-02 and 2022-01-09, as well as the mandatory use of masks in closed places. The final peak of the dataset occurred on 2021-12-20. As mentioned previously, it is expected to have an increase in the number of cases during the holiday season. Besides that, on 2021-12-22, the Portuguese government announced the closure of bars and nightclubs, as well as mandatory telework between 2021-12-25 and 2022-01-09. In Brazil, there was a cyberattack on the system whereby the states report their statistics for COVID. The attack was on 2021-12-10 and was still affecting certain states by 2021-12-20. This attack prevented states from reporting their cases.

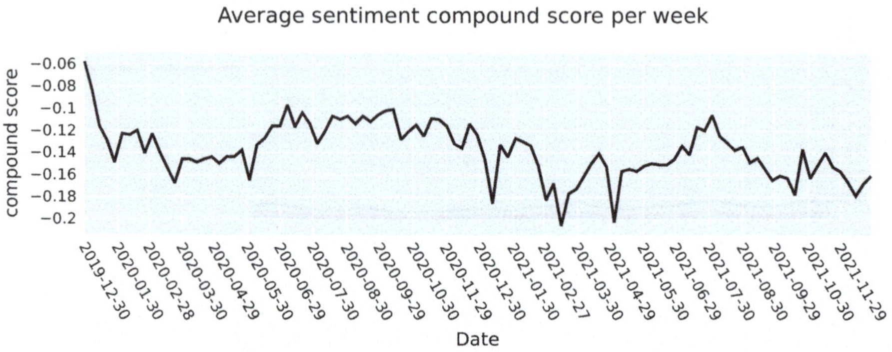

Fig. 9 Average sentiment compound score per week

In Fig. 9, we can see the average compound sentiment per week. Generally, we can see that the average sentiment is always negative, ranging from −0.05 to around −0.21, reflecting the negative attitude toward COVID-19 from the population as a whole. We do see some fluctuations in the sentiment, which inversely correlate to that of the Tweet count. In general, when there is a peak in Tweet count, the average sentiment decreases. This is evident in the previous sentiment figures, where generally the number of positive Tweets stays relatively constant with spikes in the number of negative Tweets.

As shown in Fig. 10, the dataset was used to generate wordclouds for each sentiment category. These exclude covid, covid19 and various Portuguese abbreviations. Generally, all the wordclouds show the same most frequent words. This is to be expected, as the Tweets should speak about the same topics, namely, vaccination, friends, people, and death. Words associated with the positive wordcloud include God, hospital, world, and father. Words associated with the negative wordcloud include governor, Bolsonaro, and virus. This tells us that people had negative feelings toward the virus, as well as governors and the Brazilian president Jair Bolsonaro. In the neutral wordcloud no word of interest appears.

4 Clusters

As a further investigation of the data we present, we decided to categorize and cluster the data to better understand what people are talking about. Due to the large size of the dataset, any kind of manual clustering is not feasible. Although unsupervised clustering techniques such as Latent Dirichlet Allocation (LDA) exist, these techniques may not provide sufficient insight into the data. As a different approach, we propose a more heuristic analysis of the data by manually filtering the dataset. Manual filtering uses keyword-based filtering to select the data belonging to

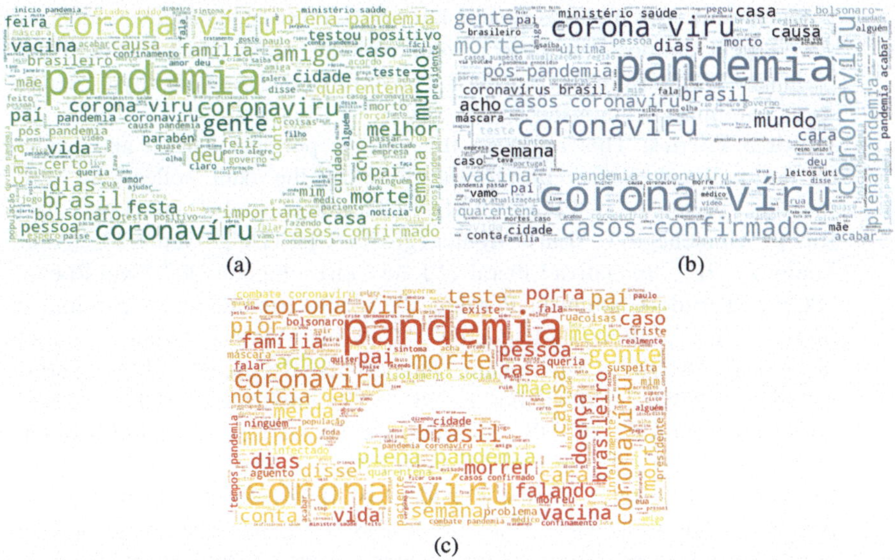

Fig. 10 Wordclouds for different sentiment categories (covid and covid19 are excluded). (**a**) Positive; (**b**) Neutral; (**c**) Negative

the clusters , which allows for a more descriptive analysis of the data by identifying Tweets related to certain topics.

A description of the various keyword-based analyses is as follows.

- **Discussion of impact**: This cluster is aimed at identifying the impact of COVID on the society, including economic, medical, and social impacts. The list of words used to filter this cluster is as follows: "econômico", "econômica", "demitidos", "demitido", "desemprego", "trabalho remoto", "zoom", "escola", "hospital", "quarantena", "isolamento", "confinamento". These words translate to: "economical", "economic", "dismissed", "fired", "unemployment", "remote work", "zoom", "school", "hospital", "quarantine", "isolation", "confinement". For the economic impact, we considered that including the keyword "economic" was sufficient. The goal of this specific keyword is to obtain Tweets in which people openly discuss the economic impact directly. For the medical impact, we considered it interesting to see what is being said about the hospital system. Finally, for the social impact, we considered it interesting to discuss how COVID affected the work field and other social impacts, such as schooling and more general confinement.
- **Opinion towards the government**: This cluster is aimed at identifying people's opinions towards the government and various government entities. Due to the larger number of ways possible to discuss the government, further division of this cluster was considered to be the best.

- **Government**: This includes generic keywords referring to the government and government entities: "governo", "município", "departamento", "ministra", "ministro", "ministério". Translated: "government", "municipality", "department", "minister", "minister", "ministry".
- **Political Parties**: This refers to the various political parties and leaders of the political parties during the time of the data collection: "PS", "Partido Socialista", "PPD", "PSD", "Partido Social Democrata", "Rui Rio", "Montenegro", "Luis Montenegro", "CHEGA", "Ventura", "André Ventura", "IL", "Iniciativa Liberal", "João Cotrim Figueiredo", "Rui Rocha", "PCP", "Partido Comunista Português", "Paulo Raimundo", "Jerónimo de Sousa", "B.E.", "Bloco de Esquerda", "Catarina Martins", "Marcelo Rebelo de Sousa", "MDB", "Movimento Democrático Brasileiro", "PL", "Partido Liberal", "PODE", "Podemos", "PP", "Progressistas", "PT", "Partido dos Trabalhadores", "PSDB", "Partido da Social Democracia Brasileira", "UNIÃO", "PSB", "Partido Socialista Brasileiro", "Republicanos".
- **Bolsonaro**: This refers to the President of Brazil during the time of the pandemic, Jair Bolsonaro. This cluster was separated because of the large number of hits it received, to reduce bias in the cluster statistics.
- **Costa**: This refers to the prime minister of Portugal during the time of the pandemic, Antonio Costa.

- **Origin of the virus**: Due to the large debate surrounding the origin of the pandemic, especially during the early stages of the pandemic, we considered it interesting to see the actual impact of this on the public. The keywords used were: "origem", "Wuhan", "morcego", "laboratório", "lab", "arma biológica", "criado", "5G". Translated: "origin", "Wuhan", "bat", "lab", "lab", "bioweapon", "created", "5G". The idea is to discuss many of the original theories about the origin of the virus, mainly that the virus came from a bat, was a biological weapon, or stemmed from 5G technology.
- **Vaccines**: The aim is to identify discussions about vaccines. This cluster was divided into two separate clusters.

  - **Vaccines**: In this cluster, the idea is to use the generic words "vacina" (vaccine) and "vacinação" (vaccination) to obtain general discussions of vaccinations.
  - **Vaccine names**: This cluster targets specific vaccines used in both Portugal and Brazil: "moderna", "omnicron", "pfizer", "biontech", "janssen", "johnson", "astrazeneca", "sputnik", "coronavac", "sinovac".

- **International**: The idea behind this discussion is to identify debates about other countries to assess the political influence of countries outside the study area and how they influence Portugal and Brazil. This cluster comprises a list of Portuguese-language countries, excluding Portugal and Brazil.

5 Cluster Analysis

The total number of Tweets existing among the sets is 6,461,964. This is only a small portion of the entire dataset collected; however, it still contains useful information. In Table 5, we can see a summary of the amount of data in each cluster, as well as the number of items unique to each cluster. What is of interest is that the general topic of vaccines has a much higher number of items than expected, especially considering that this cluster has only two search terms. The next interesting analysis is that most of the data are contained only in one of the clusters, whereas in most clusters, approximately 60-80% of the data are unique to a cluster. This was much higher than what was originally anticipated. It was assumed that because a dictionary search was used, there would be a much larger overlap between clusters, and most of the data would be repeated between clusters.

Only three clusters have fewer than 1 million items, and all the others contain a sizeable number of items. Among the clusters, the economic impact cluster has the highest percentage of items exclusive of the set (79.54%). We initially expected that this cluster would exhibit the highest degree of overlap with the largest cluster, which is centered on vaccines. However, the Venn diagram presented in Fig. 11 reveals a small overlap of 33,433 items between the vaccines and economic impact clusters. Based on these findings, we hypothesized that the economic cluster would have a large overlap with the government cluster and the political parties cluster because governments tend to comment on large economic crises and announce many regulations regarding rules and laws. Analyzing the upset graph in Fig. 12, we can see that the overlap between the economic impact and the other two sets accounts for 128,560 items, which is roughly half of the total overlapping data of the set. Furthermore, we assumed that with the discussion of economic impacts, various other countries beyond Portugal and Brazil would be mentioned, considering the global impact of the pandemic. Figure 13 shows that the overlap between the sets is 65,448. These last two overlaps make up for most of the overlap between the sets, however, we cannot establish that the overlap results from the large set size or shared common factors and discussions.

Table 5 Table summarizing the set of Tweets in each cluster

Cluster	Items in the set	Items exclusive to the set
Vaccines	1,804,966	1,309,420
Political parties	1,519,008	1,152,117
Government	1,435,224	974,505
International	1,433,155	1,031,226
Economic impact	1,258,674	1,001,252
Bolsonaro	1,116,208	815,453
Vaccine names	191,440	59,904
Origin of virus	157,411	91,755
Costa	42,818	26,332

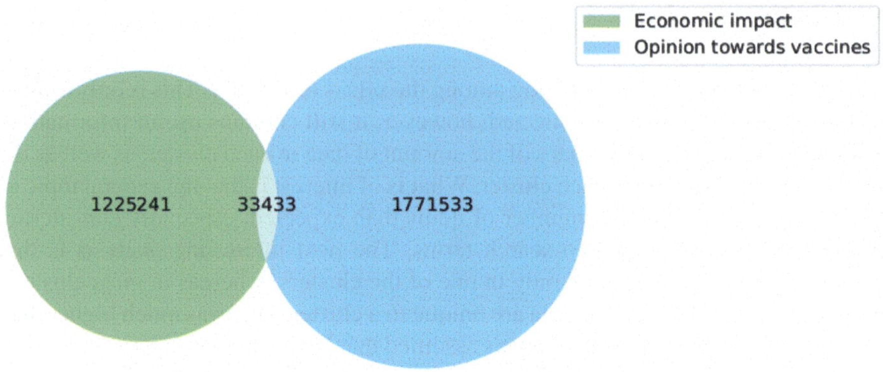

Fig. 11 Venn Diagram comparing the sets of economic impact and opinions towards vaccines

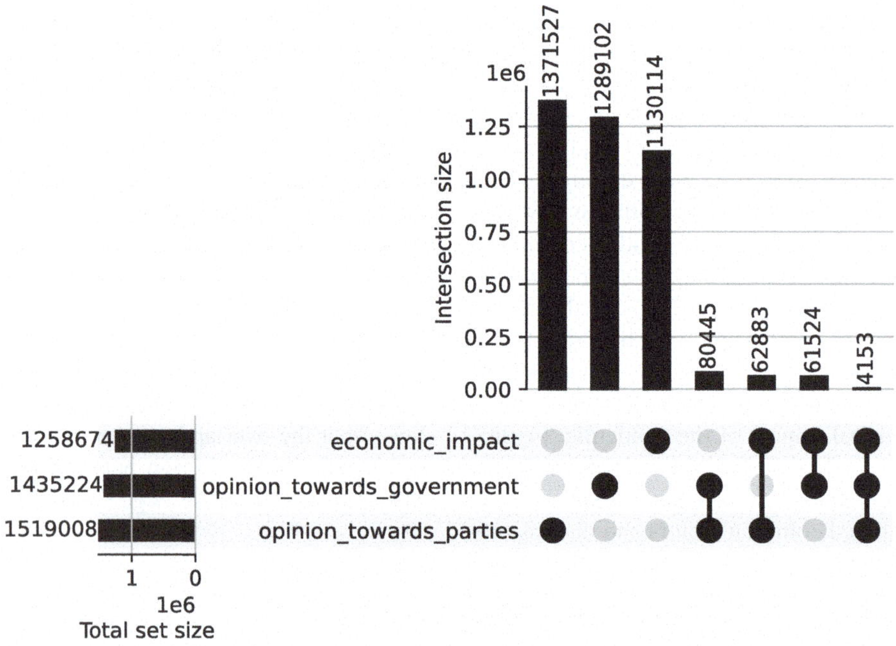

Fig. 12 Upset Graph comparing the sets of economic impact with the opinion towards the government and political parties

The next set of interests to investigate is the overlap between Bolsonaro, political parties, and the government. Looking at the upset plot in Fig. 14, the first notable observation is the large overlap between Bolsonaro and government clusters. However, this is expected given that discussions involving the government often mention Bolsonaro. This is also the largest overlapping set in the clusters. Interestingly, the degree of overlap between government and political parties is not

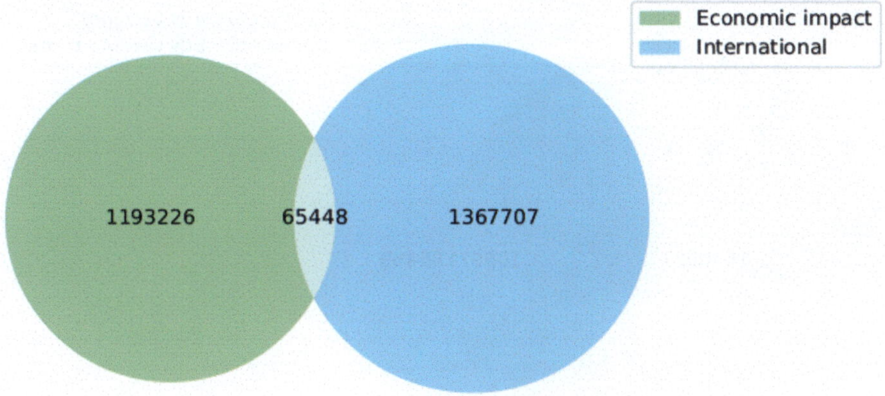

Fig. 13 Venn Diagram comparing the sets of economic impact and international

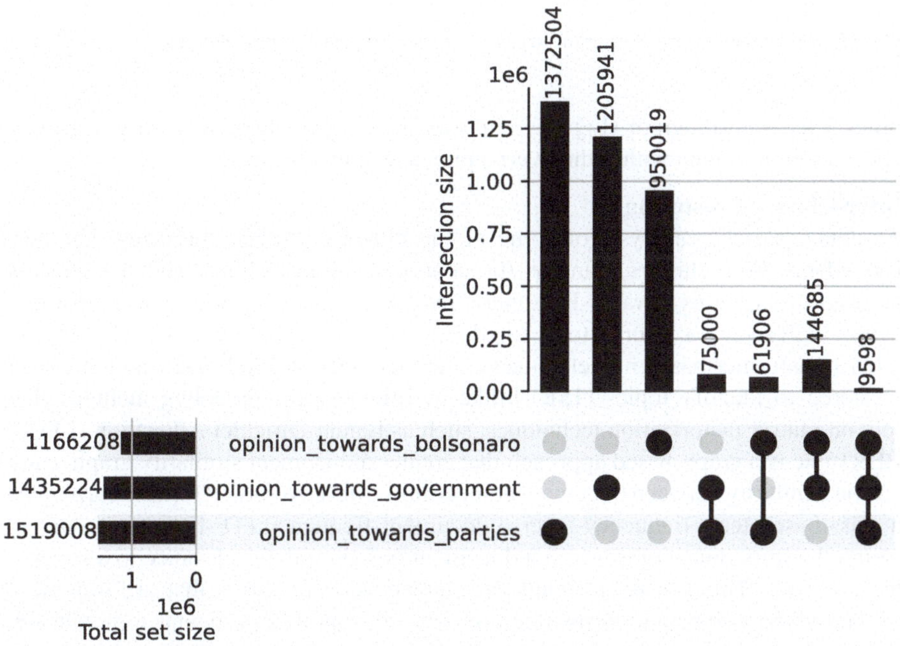

Fig. 14 Upset Graph comparing the sets of Bolsonaro, political parties, and government

as extensive as anticipated; however, a sizable intersection still exists between these two clusters.

One of the main intersections expected was between the vaccines and vaccine names clusters because they refer to the same subject matter. Additionally, the mention of a vaccine name involves referencing the word vaccine most of the

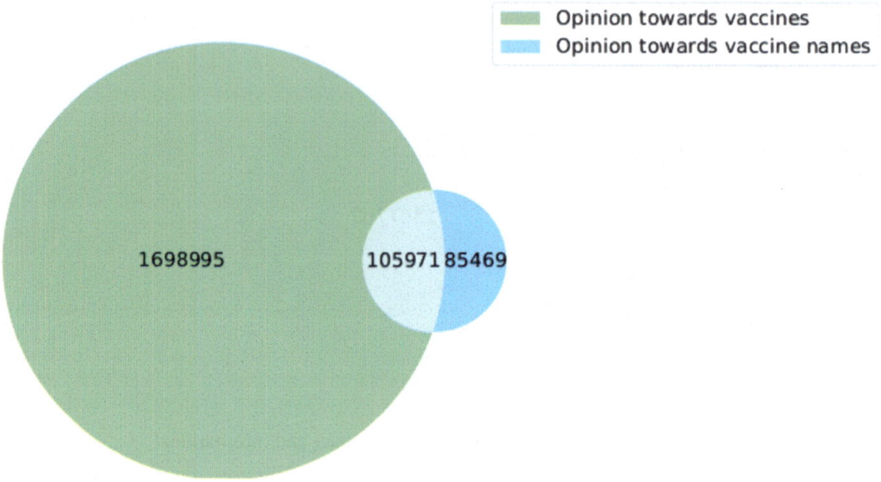

Fig. 15 Venn Diagram comparing the sets of economic impact and international

time. The Venn diagram (Fig. 15) confirms this expectation, revealing a greater concentration of data within the overlapping sets than outside.

Inter-Cluster Clustering

To obtain a richer analysis of some of the clusters, further clustering was performed on three clusters, namely, the economic impact cluster and the clusters focused on opinions towards Bolsonaro and Costa. Sub-clustering was performed using BERTopic, a neural topic modeling approach that uses BERT (or any other transformer-based model) to generate document embeddings, which are then clustered to identify topics [15]. Unlike traditional topic modeling methods that rely on matrix factorization techniques, such as Latent Dirichlet Allocation (LDA), BERTopic is a graph-based approach that creates a document similarity graph using cosine similarity between document embeddings. Moreover, BERTopic incorporates a class-based term frequency-inverse document frequency (TF-IDF) procedure to weigh the importance of terms in a document based on their relevance to a specific topic cluster. This procedure helps distinguish between terms that are important to the overall corpus and terms that are only relevant to a particular topic cluster. BERTopic is also modular and allows the selection of the algorithm to be used in each step.

In this work, the following methods were used in each step :

1. **Embedding extraction**: As our Tweets were in Portuguese, we used a multilingual transformer-based model **paraphrase-multilingual-MiniLM-L12-v2**[3]

[3] https://huggingface.co/sentence-transformers/paraphrase-multilingual-MiniLM-L12-v2.

with SentenceTransformers[4] to create text embeddings. SentenceTransformer models are optimized for semantic similarity, which is helpful for clustering the documents.

2. **Dimensionality Reduction**: Clustering models usually have a difficult time handling high dimensional data and so it is better to reduce the dimension of the data. We used UMAP(with n_neighbors=15, n_components=5, min_dist=0.0, metric='cosine') because it retains some of the dataset's local and global structures when reducing dimensions.
3. **Clustering**: To cluster the documents in reduced dimensions, we decided to use HDBSCAN as it does not force documents into clusters and it simplifies the removal of the edge case tweet documents. We used a minimum cluster size of 500 with Euclidean distance as the metric for cluster size and Excess of Mass to select flat clusters from the cluster-tree hierarchy.
4. **Tokenizer**: We used countVectorizer with Portuguese stop words (PT stopwords from NLTK, slangs, search terms for original Twitter query, and some more general Portuguese phrases) to tokenize text at a cluster level and get the representation topic for each cluster.
5. **Weighting Scheme**: To actually use the vectorized documents, we needed some algorithms to know what makes one cluster different from another. We used the ClassTfidfTransformer, which modifies TF-IDF and considers topics (i.e., clusters or classes) instead of documents.
6. **Representation Tuning**: Using KeyBERT[5] inspired model, we can fine-tune the generated topics further to polish the topic modeling. This basically means treating the previously generated topics as candidate topics and then fine-tune a new model on the representative documents.

The results of the inter-cluster clustering are summarized in Tables 6, 7, and 8, where the top 10 clusters are presented. Only clusters containing at least 1000 samples were considered as cluster. Among the cluster related to opinions about Costa, there were only two that contained more than 1000 samples: the first is about COVID and the second is about schools. Regarding the Bolsonaro clusters, a broad range of terms emerged, the most interesting being medication, death, and Bolsonaro testing positive. Analyzing the economic impact clusters, those related to the medical sector and schools are more prominent, followed by discussions related to Brazil, social problems, Bolsonaro, athletes, confinement, the virus, and vaccines.

Following this, we decided to investigate the frequency of the top 10 economic impact topics over time as shown in Fig. 16. The cluster related to patients and doctors peaked in April and May of 2020 when the pandemic started to take off and lockdowns were in place. The second peak occurred in March 2021. The topic related to school remained prevalent throughout most of the pandemic period. The cluster related to Brazil peaked during the first quarter of 2020. Cluster 8, which

[4] https://www.sbert.net/.

[5] https://github.com/MaartenGr/KeyBERT.

Table 6 Top keywords for Bolsonaro cluster

Rank	Frequency	Keywords
1	122,970	coronavírus, coronavirus, vírus, virus
2	69,376	Brasil, brasileiro, brasileiros, brasileira
3	56,969	Vacina, vacinar, vacinada, vacinado
4	26,326	Coronavírus, coronavirus, vírus, virus
5	22,389	Bolsonaro, porra, covid, vc
6	17,742	Remédios, medicação, medicamentos, medicamento
7	14,058	Bolsonaro, porra, dia, sei
8	13,514	Pegou, desse, morreu, matar
9	10,786	Pandemia, merda, pior, presidente
10	10,480	Positivos, positivo, positiva, bolsonaro

Table 7 Top keywords for costa cluster

Rank	Frequency	Keywords
1	35,265	Covid19, costa, covid, bolsonaro
2	1080	Escolas, escolar, escola, educação

Table 8 Top keywords for economic impact cluster

Rank	Frequency	Keywords
1	215,207	Paciente, pacientes, médica, médico
2	75,216	Escolar, escola, escolas, ensino
3	41,459	Brazil, brasil, brasileiros, brasileira
4	20,527	Pandemia, causa, social, existe
5	17,318	Bozo, bolsonaro, brasil, disse
6	16,476	Atletas, equipe, jogador, futebol
7	15,951	Confinamento, confinado, deixa, vão
8	14,405	Confinamento, durante, fiquei, aguento
9	13,463	Coronavírus, coronavirus, vírus, virus
10	12,134	Vacinada, vacinar, vacinação, vacina

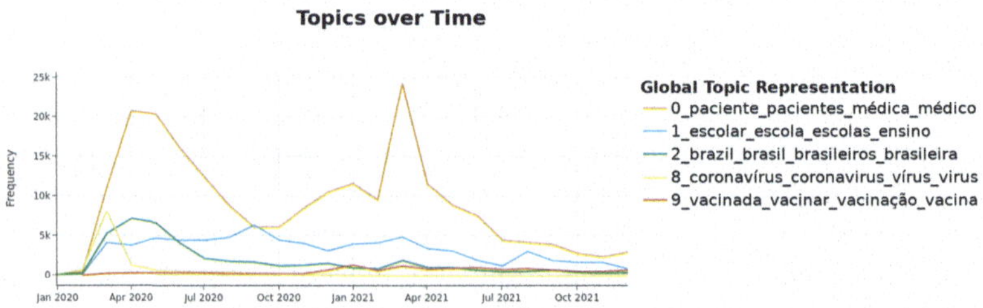

Fig. 16 Count of topics over time for the economic impact cluster

relates to the virus in general, also reached its peak in March 2020. Most of the clusters peaked during this time because this was the time when the peak of the dataset occurred.

6 Conclusions

This paper describes a large-scale COVID-19 Twitter dataset containing over 31 million Portuguese Tweets from 2020 and 2021. We conducted sentiment analysis on every Tweet and the scores were included in the dataset. This provides insightful information on user reactions to specific events that can be utilized to improve public perception of similar future events.

Furthermore, an in-depth analysis of the dataset was performed, where peaks in Tweet counts and sentiment scores could be correlated with government announcements and relevant events related to Covid-19 happening in Portugal and Brazil. Additionally, we performed clustering on the dataset and analyzed the resulting clusters, providing valuable insights into the composition of the dataset and how it changes over time.

While this paper presents a vast dataset of COVID-19-related Portuguese Tweets from 2020 and 2021, along with sentiment analysis, it has limitations and suggests areas for future research. The dataset's focuses on a set of keywords and hashtags which may not capture the full picture of public sentiment during the pandemic. Expanding the dataset to include more keywords and hashtags would provide a broader perspective. Additionally, sentiment analysis, while useful, is limited in capturing the complexity of public opinion. Future research could explore advanced natural language processing techniques and predictive modeling to better understand and anticipate public reactions to similar events in the future. Analysis of user and tweet clusters was limited in this research and deeper analysis can provide interesting results. This study serves as a starting point for more comprehensive and nuanced research on public sentiment during crisis and highlights the significance of language-specific Twitter datasets for social analysis.

Acknowledgments This work was supported by FCT—Fundação para a Ciência e Tecnologia within project DSAIPA/AI/0088/2020.

References

1. The ELK Stack: From the Creators of Elasticsearch.
2. Tweepy Documentation — tweepy 4.10.0 documentation.
3. WHO Coronavirus (COVID-19) Dashboard.
4. WHO COVID-19 Dashboard. publisher: Geneva: World Health Organization, 2020.
5. ALKOUZ, B., AL AGHBARI, Z., AL-GARADI, M. A., AND SARKER, A. Deepluenza: Deep learning for influenza detection from twitter. *Expert Systems with Applications 198* (2022), 116845.

6. ALLÉS-TORRENT, S., DEL RIO RIANDE, G., BONNELL, J., SONG, D., AND HERNÁNDEZ, N. Digital narratives of covid-19: A twitter dataset for text analysis in spanish. *Journal of Open Humanities Data 7* (2021).
7. ALMEIDA, R. J. Leia - lexicon for adapted inference. https://github.com/rafjaa/LeIA, 2018.
8. ALSHAABI, T., DEWHURST, D. R., MINOT, J. R., ARNOLD, M. V., ADAMS, J. L., DANFORTH, C. M., AND DODDS, P. S. The growing amplification of social media: Measuring temporal and social contagion dynamics for over 150 languages on twitter for 2009–2020. *EPJ data science 10*, 1 (2021), 15.
9. ASSOCIATION, A. P., Mar. 2020.
10. BANDA, J. M., TEKUMALLA, R., WANG, G., YU, J., LIU, T., DING, Y., ARTEMOVA, E., TUTUBALINA, E., AND CHOWELL, G. A Large-Scale COVID-19 Twitter Chatter Dataset for Open Scientific Research—An International Collaboration. *Epidemiologia 2*, 3 (Sept. 2021), 315–324.
11. BOVET, A., AND MAKSE, H. A. Influence of fake news in twitter during the 2016 us presidential election. *Nature communications 10*, 1 (2019), 1–14.
12. BRAKEL, J. V. Robust peak detection algorithm using z-scores. https://stackoverflow.com/questions/22583391/peak-signal-detection-in-realtime-timeseries-data/22640362, 2014.
13. CHEN, E., LERMAN, K., AND FERRARA, E. Tracking Social Media Discourse About the COVID-19 Pandemic: Development of a Public Coronavirus Twitter Data Set. *JMIR Public Health and Surveillance 6*, 2 (May 2020), e19273.
14. DE MELO, T., AND FIGUEIREDO, C. M. S. A first public dataset from Brazilian twitter and news on COVID-19 in Portuguese. *Data in Brief 32* (Oct. 2020), 106179.
15. GROOTENDORST, M. BERTopic: Neural topic modeling with a class-based TF-IDF procedure, Mar. 2022. arXiv:2203.05794 [cs].
16. HAOUARI, F., HASANAIN, M., SUWAILEH, R., AND ELSAYED, T. ArCOV-19: The First Arabic COVID-19 Twitter Dataset with Propagation Networks. *arXiv:2004.05861 [cs]* (Mar. 2021). arXiv: 2004.05861.
17. HONG, L., CONVERTINO, G., AND CHI, E. Language matters in twitter: A large scale study. In *Proceedings of the international AAAI conference on web and social media* (2011), vol. 5, pp. 518–521.
18. HUTTO, C., AND GILBERT, E. VADER: A Parsimonious Rule-Based Model for Sentiment Analysis of Social Media Text. *Proceedings of the International AAAI Conference on Web and Social Media 8*, 1 (May 2014), 216–225.
19. IMRAN, M., OFLI, F., CARAGEA, D., AND TORRALBA, A. Using AI and Social Media Multimodal Content for Disaster Response and Management: Opportunities, Challenges, and Future Directions. *Information Processing & Management 57*, 5 (Sept. 2020), 102261.
20. JONKER, R. A. A., POUDEL, R., FAJARDA, O., MATOS, S., OLIVEIRA, J. L., AND LOPES, R. P. Portuguese Twitter Dataset on COVID-19. In *2022 IEEE/ACM International Conference on Advances in Social Networks Analysis and Mining (ASONAM)* (Nov. 2022), pp. 332–338.
21. JORDAN, S. E., HOVET, S. E., FUNG, I. C.-H., LIANG, H., FU, K.-W., AND TSE, Z. T. H. Using twitter for public health surveillance from monitoring and prediction to public response. *Data 4*, 1 (2018), 6.
22. KARIMIZIARANI, M., JAFARZADEGAN, K., ABBASZADEH, P., SHAO, W., AND MORADKHANI, H. Hazard risk awareness and disaster management: Extracting the information content of twitter data. *Sustainable Cities and Society 77* (2022), 103577.
23. LAMSAL, R. Design and analysis of a large-scale COVID-19 tweets dataset. *Applied Intelligence 51*, 5 (May 2021), 2790–2804.
24. LOPEZ, C. E., AND GALLEMORE, C. An augmented multilingual Twitter dataset for studying the COVID-19 infodemic. *Social Network Analysis and Mining 11*, 1 (2021), 102.
25. MEMON, S. A., AND CARLEY, K. M. Characterizing COVID-19 Misinformation Communities Using a Novel Twitter Dataset. *arXiv:2008.00791 [cs]* (Sept. 2020). arXiv: 2008.00791.
26. MOLAEI, S., KHANSARI, M., VEISI, H., AND SALEHI, M. Predicting the spread of influenza epidemics by analyzing twitter messages. *Health and Technology 9*, 4 (2019), 517–532.

27. Naseem, U., Razzak, I., Khushi, M., Eklund, P. W., and Kim, J. COVIDSenti: A Large-Scale Benchmark Twitter Data Set for COVID-19 Sentiment Analysis. *IEEE Transactions on Computational Social Systems 8*, 4 (Aug. 2021), 1003–1015.
28. Owens, M., Townsend, E., Hall, E., Bhatia, T., Fitzgibbon, R., and Miller-Lakin, F. Mental Health and Wellbeing in Young People in the UK during Lockdown (COVID-19). *International Journal of Environmental Research and Public Health 19*, 3 (Jan. 2022), 1132.
29. Sameer, A. S., Khan, M. A., Nissar, S., and Banday, M. Z. Assessment of Mental Health and Various Coping Strategies among general population living Under Imposed COVID-Lockdown Across world: A Cross-Sectional Study. *Ethics, Medicine and Public Health 15* (Oct. 2020), 100571.
30. Saroj, A., and Pal, S. Use of social media in crisis management: A survey. *International Journal of Disaster Risk Reduction 48* (Sept. 2020), 101584.
31. Sønderskov, K. M., Dinesen, P. T., Santini, Z. I., and Østergaard, S. D. The depressive state of Denmark during the COVID-19 pandemic. *Acta Neuropsychiatrica 32*, 4 (Aug. 2020), 226–228.

SegSkin: An Effective Application for Skin Lesion Segmentation Using Attention-Based VGG-UNet

Anwar Jimi, Hind Abouche, Nabila Zrira, and Ibtissam Benmiloud

Abstract Skin cancer is a worldwide health problem with high morbidity and mortality rates. To successfully diagnose skin lesions, computer-aided automatic diagnostic systems are required. It offers dermatologists a reliable approach to assessing skin lesions. The segmentation is difficult because of the artifacts in dermoscopic images like hair and the low contrast. In this paper, we present a new model that integrates two architectures, the U-Net and the VGG-19, as well as the attention mechanism. Furthermore, to improve the segmentation results, we also employ image preprocessing, including the Dull-Razor algorithm for hair removal and Contrast Limited Adaptive Histogram Equalization (CLAHE) to improve the image quality. We implement our approach as an online application to help the dermatologist segment the skin lesion for further diagnosis; this application is named SegSkin. Moreover, we evaluate our model on four datasets: ISIC 2016, ISIC 2017, ISIC 2018, and PH2. The proposed model has obtained satisfactory results compared to the state-of-the-art.

Keywords Skin lesion segmentation · U-Net · Deep learning · VGG-19 · Attention · SegSkin

1 Introduction

The most prevalent type of cancer in the world is skin cancer. It happens when skin cells start to grow out of control and develop into a tumor. Melanoma, squamous cell carcinoma, and basal cell carcinoma are the three most common types of skin cancer.

A. Jimi (✉) · H. Abouche · N. Zrira · I. Benmiloud
National Superior School of Mines, Rabat, Morocco
e-mail: anwar.jimi@enim.ac.ma; hind.abouche@enim.ac.ma; zrira@enim.ac.ma; benmiloud@enim.ac.ma

M. Kaya et al. (eds.), *Social Network Analysis and Mining Applications in Healthcare and Anomaly Detection*, Lecture Notes in Social Networks,
https://doi.org/10.1007/978-3-031-75204-9_8

Melanoma, a form of skin cancer, has a high mortality rate and is highly metastatic. Melanoma is the primary cause of skin cancer mortality, even though it accounts for only 1% of all skin cancer cases. By 2021, 106,110 new cases of melanoma were predicted to be found in the United States, resulting in 7180 deaths [14]. When diagnosed at an advanced stage, melanoma has a survival rate of just 14%, compared to an estimated five-year survival rate of over 99% when it is diagnosed early [15]. Therefore, early detection is crucial for both treatment and preventing metastases, which improves the prognosis.

Dermoscopy is a typical non-invasive imaging procedure. It amplifies the brightness and size of the skin image to highlight skin spots more prominently [16], by reducing the surface reflex, which provides more details about the skin issue, can enhance the visual effect of deep skin. Even though dermoscopy has been demonstrated to be more accurate [17], correct interpretation of dermoscopy images is often time-consuming, challenging, and vulnerable to observer bias. As a result, to help dermatologists diagnose dermoscopy images more quickly and accurately, computer analysis techniques have been created [30].

In computer-aided diagnosis (CAD), automatic segmentation of skin lesions is crucial [31, 40]. Nevertheless, because skin lesions differ significantly in form, size, and color, this task is still challenging, in addition to the many artifacts in image dermoscopy such as markers, body hair, body fibers, air bubbles, reflections, uneven illumination, rolling lines, shadows, and uneven vignetting. Figure 1 illustrates a few of these artifacts in the dermoscopic images. Furthermore, some lesions have fuzzy and irregular edges. Thus, dermoscopy is being improved using computer vision and image processing techniques to develop tools that are capable of correctly diagnosing lesions, with the aim of improving access to reliable data to assist doctors. There are several ways to accomplish this improvement, including the

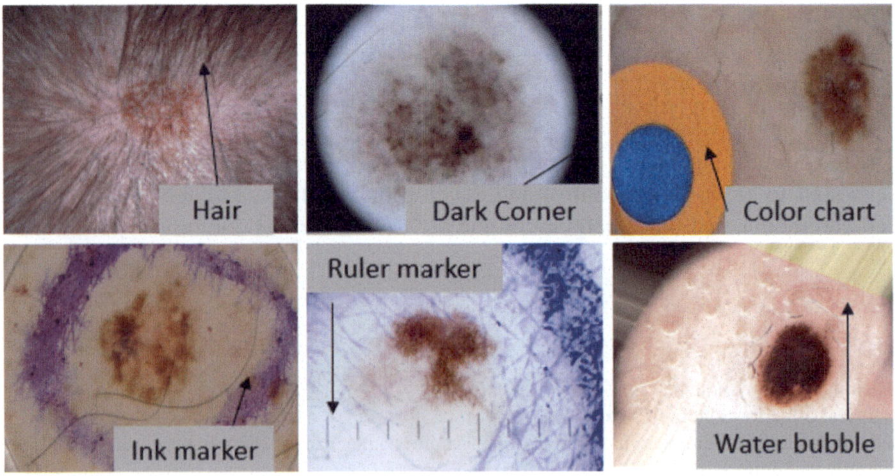

Fig. 1 Skin lesions with artifacts such as hair, dark corner, color chart, link marker, ruler marker, and water bubble

detection of lesions, their colors, and their borders, as well as the segmentation of several types of lesions.

Deep learning based on Convolutional Neural Networks (CNNs) has gained prominence recently in machine learning and computer vision, especially in semantic image segmentation [18, 38, 42–44]. In the context of skin cancer segmentation, Deep learning algorithms can be applied to skin lesion images to precisely segment and identify cancer areas. In this paper, we propose a novel automatic method for skin lesion segmentation using the VGG-19 pre-trained model combined with U-Net and the attention mechanism. In addition, we used image inpainting for hair removal and the CLAHE method to enhance the contrast of the image, to improve the segmentation result.

The following is a description of our paper's main contributions:

1. We propose a VGG-Unet deep neural network that combines the VGG-19 and U-Net architectures to excel at extracting intricate features from medical images for accurate segmentation of skin lesions and The introduction of the attention mechanism to suppress the irrelevant feature.
2. In order to enhance the performance of our model architecture and to obtain pertinent and invariant information about the input skin image, We perform two preprocessing methods on the input image, including CLAHE and the Dull-Razor algorithm.
3. On several medical datasets such as ISIC2016, ISIC2017, ISIC2018, and PH2, we tested the network, and we obtained more refined results. Additionally, to further highlight the effectiveness of the network, the relevant outcomes are illustrated.
4. We deploy our approach into a desktop application named SegSkin.

The rest of this paper is structured as follows: In the second section a description of skin cancer, The related work is introduced in Sect. 3. The datasets we used and our suggested approach are explained in Sect. 4. The fifth section provide the implementation details and experimental findings. Section 6 is a discussion and limitation about our model. Section 7 concludes the paper.

2 Skin Cancer

Sometimes can be frustrating to have moles or other marks on the skin, and it can be difficult to recall what to look for when checking moles or growths to see whether they might be cancerous. The ABCDE rule for skin cancer can help. The ABCD rule was the first dermoscopy method developed to aid in distinguishing benign from malignant melanocytic lesions. This approach, as presented by Nachbar el al. [3], is based on a multivariate analysis of four criteria.

Table 1 demonstrates the indicators which are offered by the "ABCDE" memory aid from the American Academy of Dermatology [3] to determine if a lesion on the skin can be melanoma:

Table 1 Comparison between melanoma and normal lesion

Indicator	Melanoma	Normal
Asymmetry (A)	Asymmetrical	Symmetrical
Border (B)	Uneven	Even
Color (C)	Multiple colors	One color
Diameter (D)	Larger than $\frac{1}{4}$inch	Smaller than $\frac{1}{4}$inch
Evolving (E)	Changing in size, color, shape	Ordinary mole

Asymmetry : The two halves do not match exactly;
Border : Irregular, scalloped, or notched border;
Color : There could be various shades of tan, brown, and black. It's also possible to observe spots of white, gray, red, or blue. the color is mottled and irregular;
Diameter : The spot is larger than the eraser's tip (6.0 mm);
Evolving : Changes in size, shape, color, or symptoms over time.

Additionally, Fig. 2 illustrates the comparison of melanoma and non-melanoma skin lesions using the ABCDE rule.

3 Related Work

The recent research on skin lesion segmentation is presented in this section. It can be categorized into three groups: approaches based on deep learning, approaches based on U-Net architecture, and approaches using the attention mechanism.

A large part of the new works is principally founded on deep convolutional neural networks [1, 39] that cause a noticeable boost in the effectiveness of the results of semantic segmentation. In 2015, Ronneberger et al. [4] presented the U-Net network for segmenting medical images. The symmetric encoders and decoders of the U-Net neural network have demonstrated excellent performance in the area of medical imaging. The architecture comprises a contracting path to capture context and a symmetrically expanding path that permits exact localization. Yuan et al. [5] created a deep Fully Convolutional Networks (FCN) method for segmenting skin lesions by taking advantage of 19-layer CNNs. To improve segmentation performance even more, they created a new loss function based on the Jaccard distance to eliminate the need for sample re-weighting. Their technique was tested on two datasets: ISBI 2016 and PH2. Akyel et al. [6] proposed a novel FCN8 that contains 27 layers, the method for hair removal, and image segmentation in skin cancer. They added a new ResNet model known as ResNetC into FCN8. Finally, they evaluated their approach on both the ISIC 2018 and PH2 datasets.

Inspired by the U-Net architecture, Tanga et al. [9] proposed a skin lesion segmentation method according to the separable-U-Net combined with Stochastic Weight Averaging (SWA). This model in particular made use of the separable convolutional block and U-Net architectures, which are incredibly capable of cap-

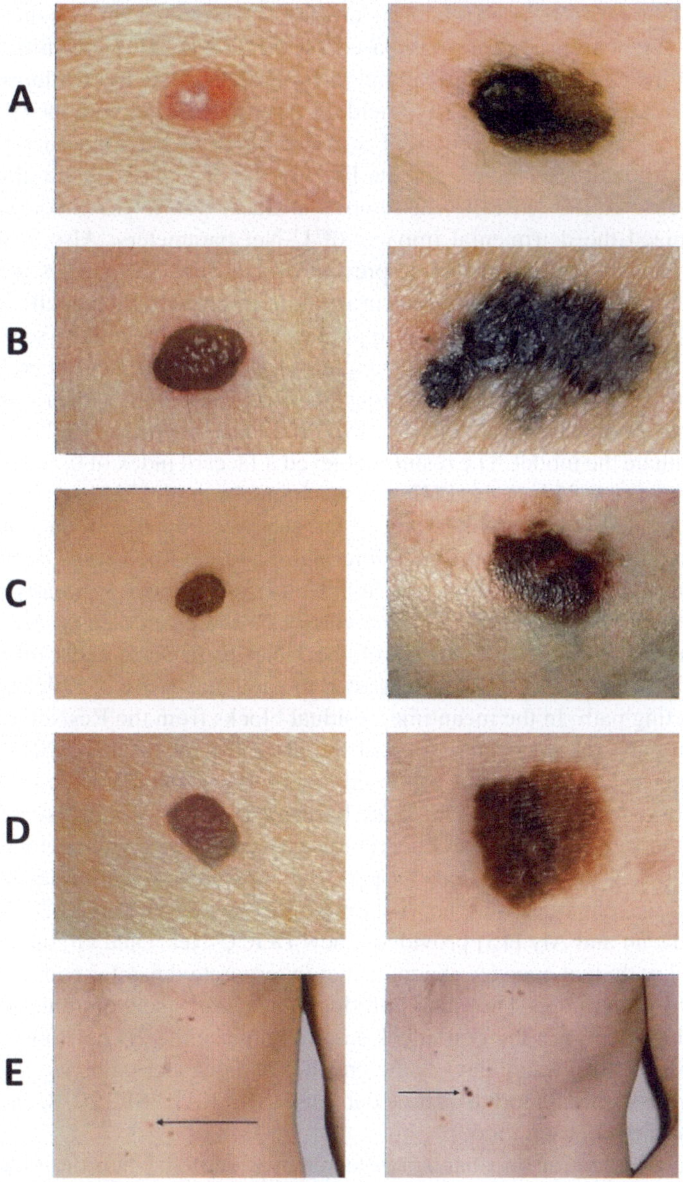

Fig. 2 Right: normal lesion. Left: melanoma lesion

turing context feature channel correlation and higher semantic feature information to improve pixel-level discrimination. Also, they used SWA to avoid the over-fitting problem. The suggested methodology's segmentation performance is evaluated on the ISBI 2016, ISBI 2017, and PH2 datasets, which reached an accuracy of 97.16,

94.31, and 96.69%, respectively. Liu et al. [27] provided an enhanced DCNN model for segmenting skin lesions based on the U-Net. The over-fitting issue is avoided by using the batch normalization layer. The dilated convolution layer is employed to increase the perceptive field all through training without affecting the resolution. Sanjar et al. [7] proposed to use a block of convolution layers and a bilinear interpolation technique for the FCN in the decoder stage combining with the Parametric ReLU (PReLU) to remove artifacts due to the theoretical issues and minimized the detrimental impacts of U-Net parameters. Also, a dropout is used after each convolution block to prevent over-fitting. The authors were able to segment skin lesions with a 94% accuracy and an 88.33% dice coefficient. Zafar et al. [10] proposed an automated approach for lesion boundary segmentation. This approach, known as Res-UNet, integrates the U-Net and ResNet architectures. In addition, they used image inpainting to remove the hair, which considerably improved the segmentation results. The ISIC 2017 test set and the PH2 datasets were used to evaluate the model. The results achieved a Jaccard index of 0.772 on the ISIC 2017 test set and 0.854 on the PH2 dataset. Iranpoor et al. [12] introduced a CNN with an upgraded U-Net architecture. In the suggested approach, the authors used a pre-trained architecture in the encoding phase and modified some of the pooling layers. After these modifications, the architecture's efficiency is greatly increased. The suggested method achieved 92% accuracy on the given dataset. Nguyen et al. [11] suggested an enhanced version of the UNet to perform tasks related to the segmentation of skin lesions. The suggested method makes use of EfficientNetB4 in the contracting path. In the meantime, residual blocks from the ResNet architecture are used to build the decoder portion of the proposed model. ISIC 2017 and 2018 datasets are used to evaluate the proposed model. Barın and Güraksın [8] suggested a novel hybrid deep learning architecture based on an FCN for skin lesion segmentation. The encoder part of this architecture uses deep learning architectures AlexNet and ResNet18. Whereas, the decoder part uses three deconvolution layers. Various preprocessing techniques were applied to two separate datasets ISIC 2017 and ISIC 2018. Ramadan and Aly [13] provided a new DGCU-Net (Dual Gradient-Color U-Net) model with dual encoder channels that incorporate the color and gradient data of the skin lesion image. They also introduced five atrous convolutional layers with various dilation rates in the bottleneck stage to replace the 2D convolutional layer. The proposed model interconnects the encoder and decoder paths via a spatial and channel-wise attention module. Three datasets, ISIC 2017, ISIC 2018, and PH2, are used to test the proposed model.

A wave of attention mechanism research was started when the Google Deep Mind team proposed the attention mechanism [32] in an image classification challenge. Woo et al. [33] developed Convolutional Block Attention Module (CBAM), a straightforward yet efficient attention module for feed-forward convolutional neural networks, using a feature map in between. Fengying et al. [34] proposed a new CNN architecture for skin lesion segmentation based on an attention mechanism. They have developed a high-resolution feature block with three branches, specifically, spatial attention, main, and channel-wise attention branches to maintain details throughout CNN. Chaitanya et al. [35] suggested a novel technique to incorporate attention within CNN using feature maps produced by different convolutional auto-encoder.

4 Materials and Methods

In this section, we provide more details about the used datasets as well as our proposed approach.

4.1 Dermoscopic Images

We used dermoscopic skin images from publicly available datasets acquired at the International Skin Imaging Collaboration (ISIC). These datasets contain dermoscopy images with ground truth masks that have been annotated by leading dermatologists. The dataset is designed to support the development and evaluation of computer-based algorithms for the diagnosis. It includes a diverse set of images representing different skin conditions, including melanomas, benign moles, and other skin diseases. Examples of images from these datasets are shown in Fig. 3.

4.1.1 ISIC 2016

We are using the dataset from the ISIC 2016 lesion segmentation task [19]. It consists of 900 dermoscopic training images and 379 testing images. In both the training and testing sets, there is a corresponding segmentation ground truth for every image.

4.1.2 ISIC 2017

The ISIC 2017 dataset [15] contains 2750 dermoscopy images from various healthcare organizations. 2000 images are used for training, 150 images are used for validation, and 600 images are used for testing, as the original challenge indicated. The ISIC 2017 dataset contains images with sizes varying from 540×722 to 4499×6748 pixels. A professional darmatologs carefully annotated each image with a skin lesion segmentation ground truth.

4.1.3 ISIC 2018

Dermoscopic images in the ISIC 2018 dataset [20, 21] are 8-bit RGB images with sizes ranging from 767×576 to 6682×4401. There are 2594 training images in the

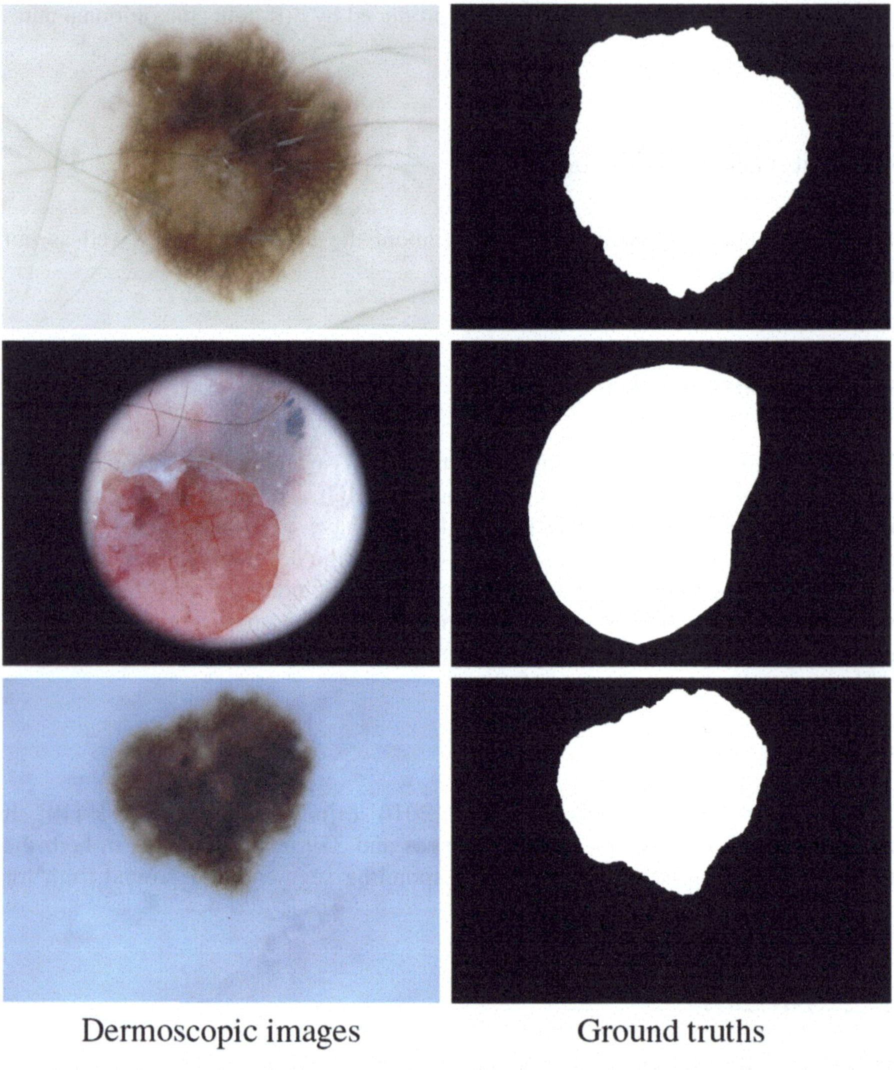

Fig. 3 Examples of skin lesion images from ISIC and PH2 datasets

dataset. Each image was assigned a skin lesion segmentation ground truth manually annotated by the professional darmatologs.

4.1.4 PH2

The PH2 dataset represents a set of skin lesion images that have been collected at the Dermatology Service of Hospital Pedro Hispano in order to create and test computer-aided diagnostic algorithms for skin cancer. The dataset is composed of 200 dermoscopic images. The dimensions of each image are around 768 × 560 pixels.

4.2 Proposed Approach

Creating our fully automatic segmentation model of skin lesions involves several crucial steps. First, we gather data from publicly available datasets acquired at ISIC. Additionally, one of the most crucial steps in deep learning is data preprocessing. It is a process of cleaning and scaling the data. In this step, we employed various preprocessing techniques such as image resizing, contrast enhancement, and also hair removal using Dull-Razor. After preprocessing the data, we created a model based on two architectures: VGG-19 and U-Net, as well as the attention mechanism that improves the efficiency of the architecture. At this step, the model's hyperparameters are adjusted, and its performance is evaluated. Once the model has been trained and evaluated, we deployed it into a desktop application to help the dermatologist segment the skin lesion for further diagnosis. Figure 4 illustrates all the steps of our approach.

4.2.1 Image Preprocessing

Image preprocessing refers to a series of operations performed on an image in order to enhance the quality of the image. Preprocessing improved segmentation performance, according to earlier approaches [22]. Consequently, we utilized various preprocessing techniques such as image resizing, contrast enhancement, hair removal, and normalization, before being provided to our model as input.

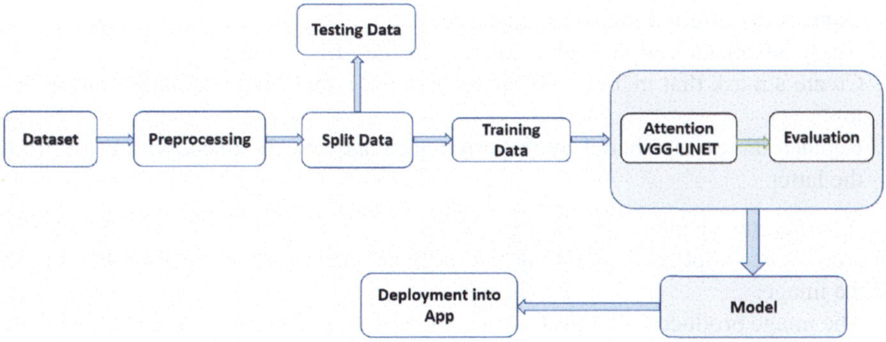

Fig. 4 Flowchart of our proposed approach

Image Resizing is a crucial step in the computer vision preprocessing process. Deep learning models are typically faster to train on small images. The neural network must learn from four times as many pixels in a larger input image, which lengthens the architecture's training period. Dermoscopic images come in various sizes. Therefore to account for these individual variations, images, and their corresponding ground truths were resized to 256×256 resolution.

Image Augmentation is a method for generating new images from old ones. To accomplish that, this included making small adjustments to the data, such as shifting the image either vertically or horizontally or rotating the image. Data augmentation can help our approach perform better and produce better results, by giving the model more data to train with and also improving the model's ability to recognize new patterns in the training data.

Contrast Enhancement CLAHE is a useful technique to improve the contrast which successfully increases the contrast of the images. The ideas of Adaptive Histogram Equalization (AHE) were used to develop the CLAHE approach [24]. AHE is an excellent contrast-enhancing algorithm for medical imaging. The adaptive approach varies from conventional histogram equalization in that it improves local contrast. The image is divided into different blocks, and each section's histogram equalization is computed. As a result, AHE generates numerous histograms, each of which represents a different element of the image. It improves the local contrast and edge definition in all clearly defined areas of the image. In relatively homogeneous areas of an image, AHE overamplifies the noise. To prevent this problem, we used CLAHE as depicted in Fig. 5.

Hair Removal Dermoscopy images encounter many skin lesion artifact types, such as hair. It might present some problems while segmenting skin lesions and introduce wrong information about their characteristics. To resolve these problems, a preprocessing method called Dull-Razor [23] is used to find and remove hairs. This entails applying several morphological procedures to the image to produce a mask that includes the hairs. The following steps present the Dull-Razor algorithm:

1. Convert the original image to grayscale;
2. Apply advanced morphological operations (i.e., Black-hat);
3. Create a mask that includes all the hairs in the image, and use binary thresholding;
4. Replace the pixels shared by the original image and the mask with those from the latter.

A structural element with a cross shape of 17×17 is described. Black-Hat filtering is accomplished by taking the original image and subtracting the closing of the image.

The image produced after performing the closing technique on a grayscale image is removed from the original image to produce hair-like structures. Then, we applied a threshold value of "10" to the image produced by the Black Hat filter resulting in the creation of a binary mask of the hair elements.

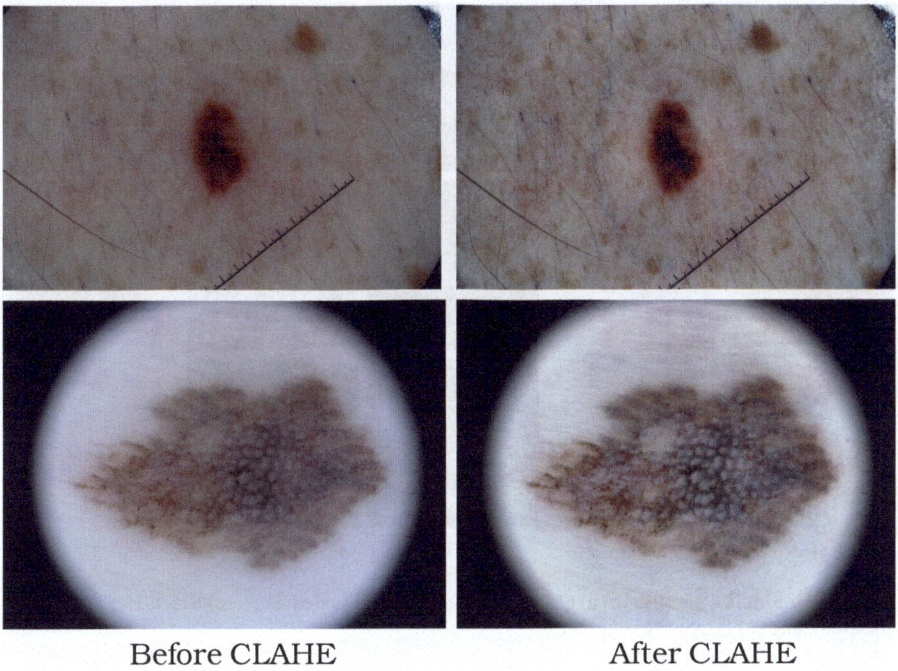

Fig. 5 CLAHE algorithm

The hair removal algorithm restores the original image by swapping out the hair structures with the surrounding pixels. This method is frequently used to recover outdated or noisy images. The mask created after thresholding was applied to the image to be inpainted, and the desired result was attained by inpainting the hairy regions that had been retrieved using the neighboring pixels as shown in Fig. 6.

Image Normalization Image normalization is the process of adjusting the intensity levels of an image so that it has a standard mean and standard deviation, to scale the input data so that it is centered on zero in all dimensions by altering the range of pixel values between 0 and 1. In order to normalize an image, its mean value is subtracted from the image, which is then divided by the image's standard deviation.

4.2.2 Network Structure

The VGG-19 network's architecture [2], as its name suggests, consists of 19 CNN layers and three fully connected layers. Basically, this architecture consists of three different types of layers:

- Convolution layers to extract the feature from the image using a variety of filter types and numbers;

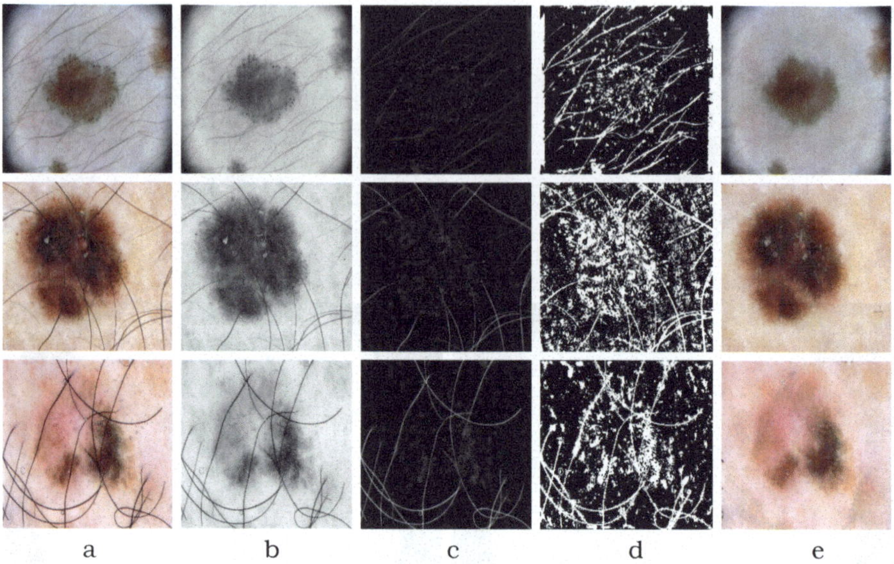

Fig. 6 Hair removal algorithm. (**a**) Original image, (**b**) Grayscale image, (**c**) Black-Hat, (**d**) Binary threshold, and (**e**) Image without hair

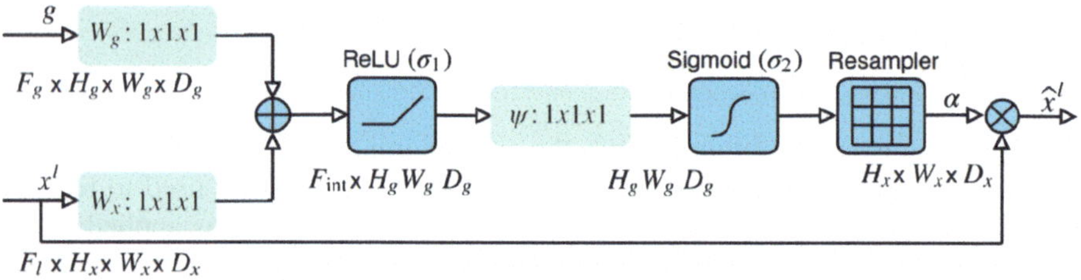

Fig. 7 Attention gate

- Max-pooling layers to reduce image size and extract the feature from the feature map created from these filters contained in the convolution layer;
- Flatten layers to generate a 1D tensor from the batches of feature maps;
- Fully-connected layers are the last layers in the convolutional neural network. The VGG-19 consists of three fully connected layers. The first ones contain dense units, while the last one contains the softmax layer.

The Attention Gate (AG) was initially proposed by Oktay et al. [26] in the U-Net architecture. In medical images, the AG attention module automatically and adaptively learns to focus on the various sizes and forms of the target structures. The model under the AG strain implicitly learns to highlight important features that are beneficial for a specific task while omitting superfluous regions from an input image. AG schematic is shown in Fig. 7.

The attention mechanism works as follows:

- There are two inputs to the attention gate, vectors x and g;
- g gating signal comes from the next lowest layer of the network;
- x comes from skip connections;
- The two vectors are added, element by element. This process results in aligned weights getting larger while unaligned weights get relatively smaller;
- The resulting vector passes through a Rectified Linear Unit (ReLU) activation layer and a 1×1 convolution that reduces the dimensions;
- This vector passes through a sigmoid layer that scales it between [0, 1], generating the attention coefficients (weights), where coefficients nearer 1 indicate more pertinent features;
- The attention coefficients are upsampled to the original dimensions of the x vector using trilinear interpolation. The attention coefficients are multiplied element-wise to the original x vector; this scales the vector based on relevance.

The U-Net architecture is one of the most frequently employed techniques for semantic segmentation. Encoding and decoding are the two main parts of this network. In this paper, the structure of the network includes two parts. In the first section, context is captured by employing four blocks of downsampling based on the VGG-19 network. The second section is based on the U-Net, which is composed of four up-sampling blocks and uses a symmetric expanding path to provide exact localization. In this path, we use the batch normalization layers to prevent the overfitting problem and also add an AG to precisely emphasize specific areas of the image while suppressing others. This can enhance the segmentation model's overall performance by allowing it to concentrate on the elements that are most crucial for the task being performed. The summary of our VGG-UNet architecture is illustrated in Fig. 8.

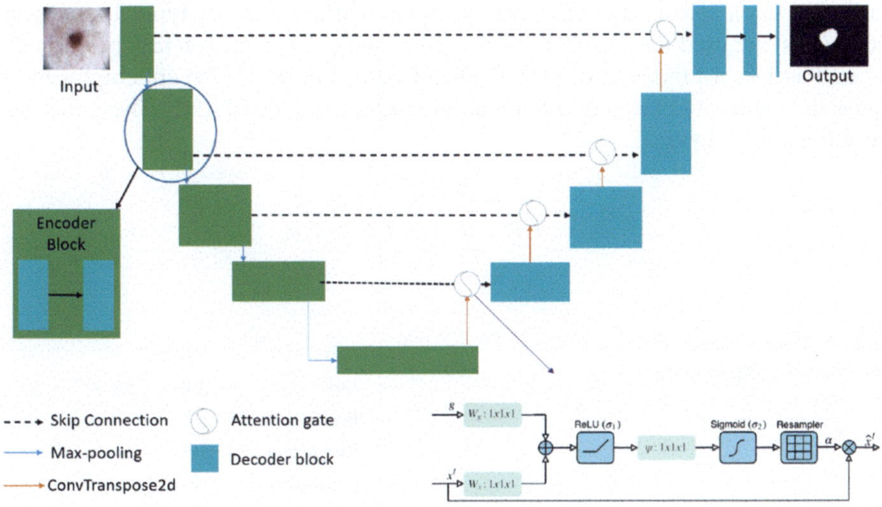

Fig. 8 Our network architecture VGG-UNet

5 Experiments and Results

5.1 Network Training

We carry out many different experiments to match the appropriate settings for the hyperparameter values. The important training parameters in our model, include learning rate, batch size, optimizer type, and the number of epochs.

We use the early stopping to prevent over-fitting, and we train our model around 100 epochs. The learning rate is decreased if, after 10 epochs, the model loss does not reduce. After nearly 40 epochs, our model came to an end. The hyperparameters used to train our model are presented in Table 2.

5.2 Implementation Details

In Google Colab, we built our network using TensorFlow and Python on GPUs T4 and P100 with 25 GB RAM. All training and testing phases were performed in the same environment, utilizing the TensorFlow 2.5.0 deep learning framework and Python 3.5 as the programming language.

5.3 Segmentation Metrics

In this paper, we use five metrics to evaluate the network performance, such as accuracy (Acc), sensitivity (SE), and specificity (SP), which are typical statistical metrics that are used for evaluating how well a binary segmentation task performed. As well as Jaccard index (JS)[28] and Dice Coefficient (DC) [29] are employed to assess the similarity between segmentation results and ground truth. These metrics are defined as follows:

$$AC = \frac{TP + TN}{TP + TN + FP + FN} \tag{1}$$

Table 2 Hyperparameters maintained during training

Parameter	Value
Input size	$256 \times 256 \times 3$
Batch size	32
Learning rate	10^{-4}
Optimizer	Adam
Epochs	100
Loss function	Binary crossentropy

$$JS = \frac{TP}{TP + FN + FP} \tag{2}$$

$$DC = \frac{2 \times TP}{2 \times (TP + FN + FP)} \tag{3}$$

$$SE = \frac{TP}{TP + FN} \tag{4}$$

$$SP = \frac{TN}{TN + FP} \tag{5}$$

5.4 Comparative Experiments

5.4.1 Comparison on the ISIC 2016 Dataset

Table 3 demonstrates that our suggested approach yields the best results on the ACC, SE, and SP compared against those of the current deep learning approaches. The ACC, SE, and SP are increased by 2.86, 0.92, and 2.89%, respectively, when compared to the Attention U-Net technique. which shows that the proposed approach has a highest ability to segment the skin lesion with high precision.

Also, Fig. 9 illustrates the results of visualizing the suggested network. The outcomes also demonstrated the highest performance of our suggested network VGG-UNet.

5.4.2 Comparison on the ISIC 2017 Dataset

Table 4 depicts that our method performs better than other existing state-of-the-art algorithms. When compared to the Separable-UNet method, the proposed method increases AC by roughly 3.21%, SE by 1.75%, and also SP by 1.47%.

Figure 10 shows the visualization of the segmentation results on the ISIC 2017 dataset. The outcomes also demonstrated the highest performance of our suggested network, VGG-UNet.

Table 3 Model performance on the ISIC 2016

Methods	AC(%)	JS(%)	DC(%)	SE(%)	SP(%)
U-Net[4]	94.3	81.2	89.5	90.7	96.2
Recurrent U-Net [25]	93.7	79.3	88.4	89.6	96.5
Attention U-Net [26]	94.4	81.1	89.0	90.8	96.3
Our VGG-UNet	**97.26**	**84.34**	**93.04**	**91.72**	**99.39**

Bold values are higher than the other values

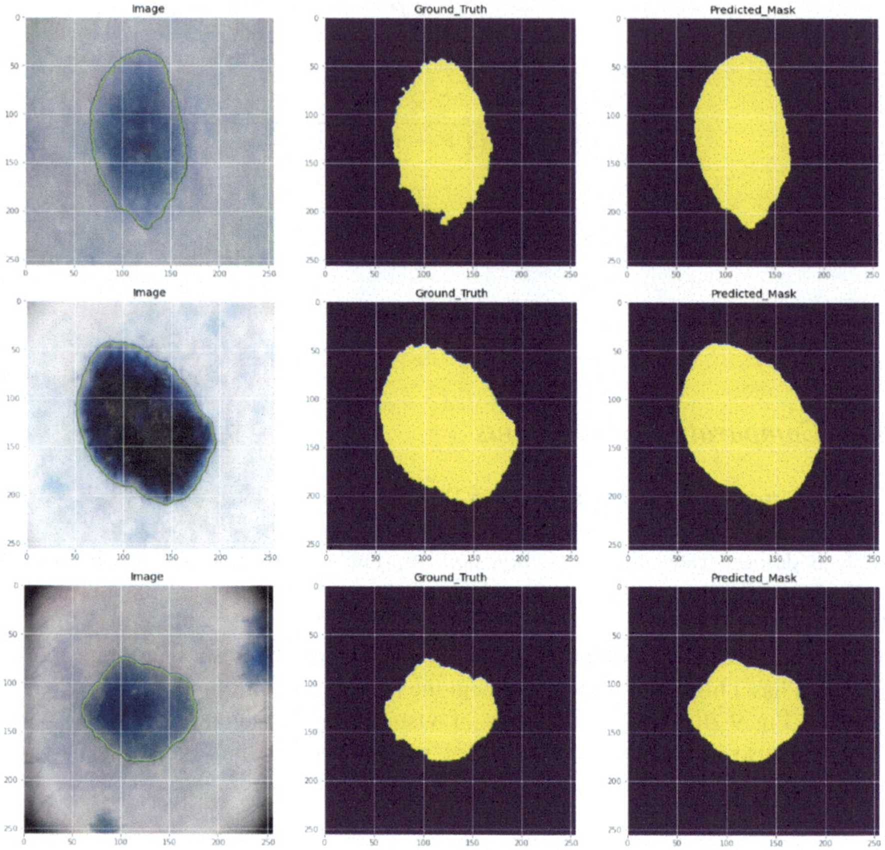

Fig. 9 Segmentation results of our model on ISIC 2016 dataset

Table 4 Model performance on the ISIC 2017

Methods	AC(%)	JS(%)	DC(%)	SE(%)	SP(%)
U-Net[4]	92.2	74.4	82.1	79.8	97.5
Recurrent U-Net[25]	90.5	64.3	78.2	81.6	95.3
Attention U-Net[26]	91.3	69.2	88.9	76.5	97.6
Separable-UNet[9]	94.31	79.26	86.93	89.53	96.32
Our VGG-UNet	**97.52**	75.79	**89.76**	**91.28**	**99.07**

Bold values are higher than the other values

5.4.3 Comparison on the ISIC 2018 Dataset

We assessed the model once more using the ISIC 2018 dataset, and we compared our segmentation findings with the most advanced methodologies to determine how robust our suggested model was. The results are shown in Table 5 below. We can

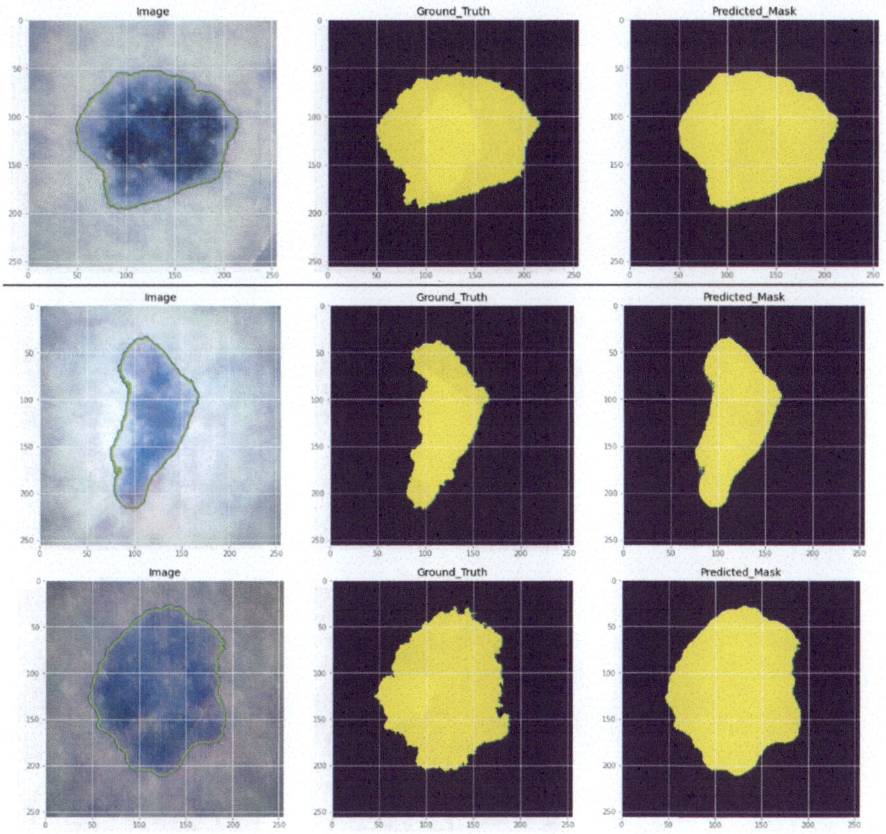

Fig. 10 Segmentation results of our model on ISIC 2017 dataset

Table 5 Model performance on the ISIC 2018

Methods	AC(%)	JS(%)	DC(%)	SE(%)	SP(%)
U-Net[4]	89.0	54.9	64.7	70.8	96.4
Recurrent U-Net[25]	88.0	58.1	67.9	79.2	92.8
Attention U-Net[26]	89.7	56.6	66.5	71.7	96.7
FCN-ResAlexNet[8]	94.65	84.17	91.40	95.85	87.86
Our VGG-UNet	**98.19**	80.94	**93.14**	95.38	**98.95**

Bold values are higher than the other values

remark that our approach produced important outcomes, especially for AC, DC, and SP.

Figure 11 provides a visual representation of our suggested network's segmentation of skin lesions. Experimental renderings can also be used to see how well the approach works when comparing the predicted mask with the ground truth.

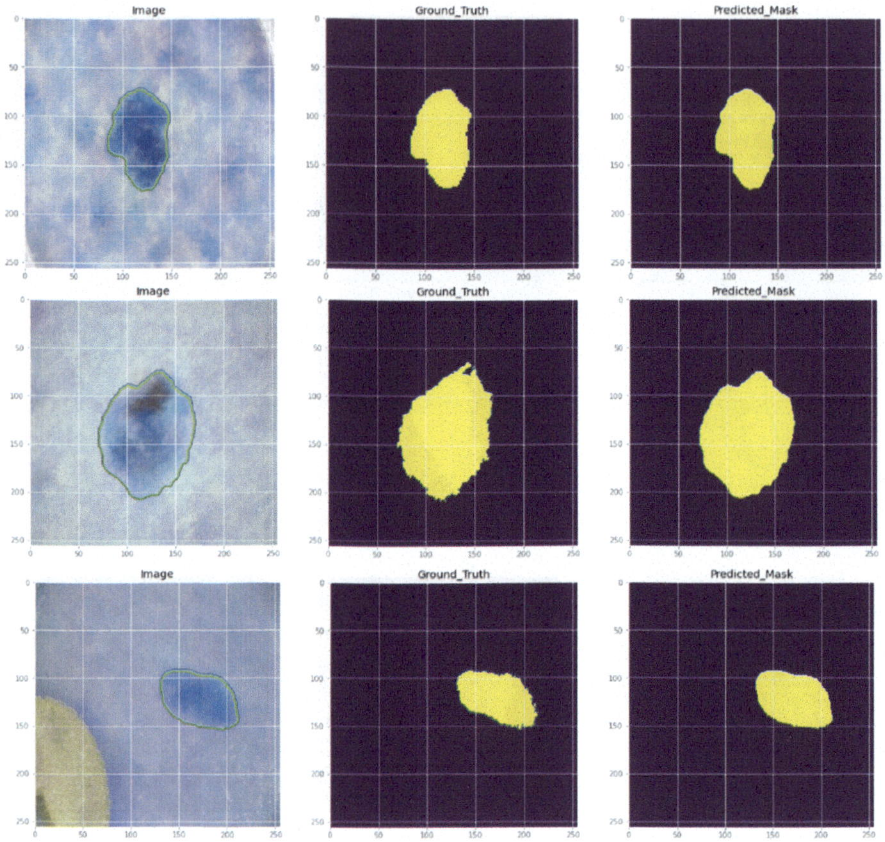

Fig. 11 Segmentation results of our model on ISIC 2018 dataset

5.4.4 Comparison on the PH2 Dataset

We further evaluated the architecture using the PH2 dataset Which one offers higher label quality with a smaller data size and compared our segmentations results with the current state-of-the-art approach in order to assess the robustness of our proposed model. In the PH2 we use data augementation to improve the representativeness, size, and diversity of the dataset. Additionally, to helps achieve a more accurate and robust model. The results are shown in Table 6 below. Our approach produced encouraging outcomes. We achieved an AC value of 99.09% and a DC of 97.58%. Whereas Fengying et al. [34] reached an AC of 94.9% and DC of 91.9%. Another architecture, MobileNetV3-UNet [36] obtained an AC of

Table 6 Model performance on the PH2

Methods	AC(%)	JS(%)	DC(%)	SE(%)	SP(%)
Fengying[34]	94.9	85.7	91.9	96.3	94.2
W-net[37]	97.23	–	93.82	96.43	97.71
MobileNetV3-UNet[36]	98.70	91.08	95.18	98.92	97.89
Our VGG-UNet	**99.09**	**93.63**	**97.58**	98.67	**99.28**

Bold values are higher than the other values

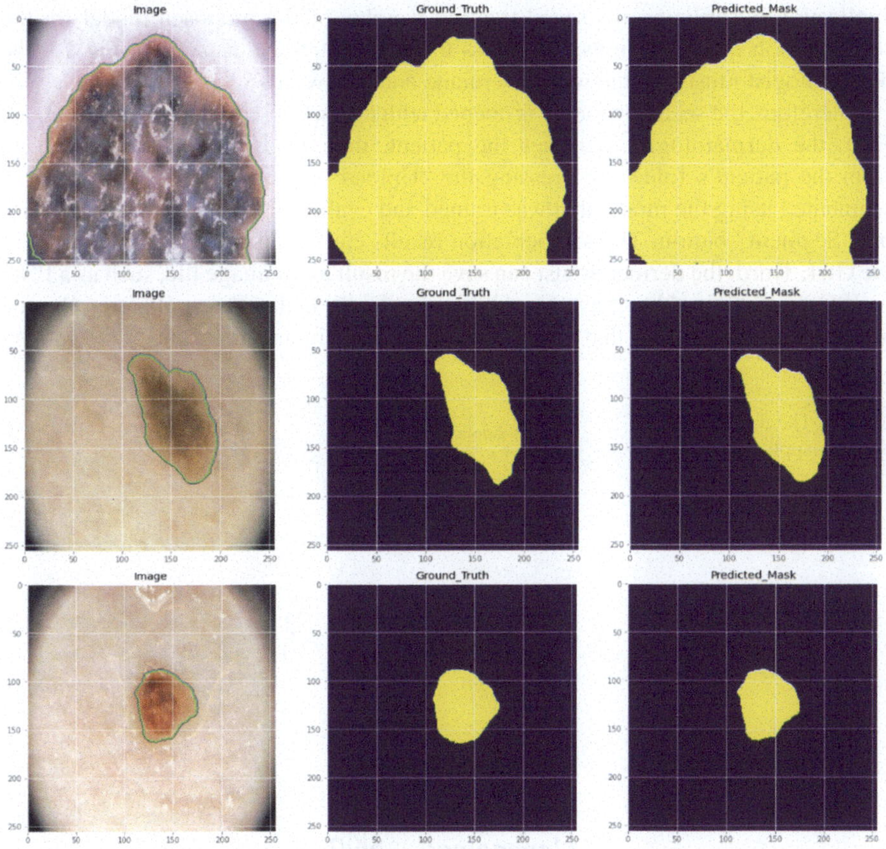

Fig. 12 Segmentation results of our model on PH2 dataset

98.70% and a DC of 95.18%. These results showed that our model outperformed the existing techniques used in the same field of study.

Figure 12 gives an illustration of our proposed method for segmenting skin lesions. The experimental renderings can also be used to see how well the method works.

5.5 Deployment of SegSkin Application

The proposed application, named "SegSkin", helps the dermatologist segment the skin lesion, as illustrated in Fig. 14. The SegSkin application was implemented with the Graphical User Interface (GUI) framework Tkinter. Tkinter is a built-in Python library that provides a set of tools and widgets that allow developers to create windows, menus, buttons, text boxes, and other GUI elements. The SegSkin application uses the power of deep learning to segment images. We created this application by utilizing the saved training weights of the proposed model for the segmentation of skin lesions. To access the main interface, as seen in Fig. 13, the dermatologist must first recover a username and password.

Therefore, the second window is opened with a simple GUI as depicted in Fig. 14. First, the dermatologist identifies the patient, then loads a dermoscopic image from the patient's folder by pressing the "Upload" button. Second, the image is segmented using the model that was trained and evaluated in the above phases with the "Segment" button. The segmentation results can be displayed on the screen in the GUI. Third, the dermatologist can save the result as an image file, such as a PNG or JPG, by pressing the "Save Mask" button. Additionally, the application has the ability to generate a PDF that contains the segmented image, the name of the patient,

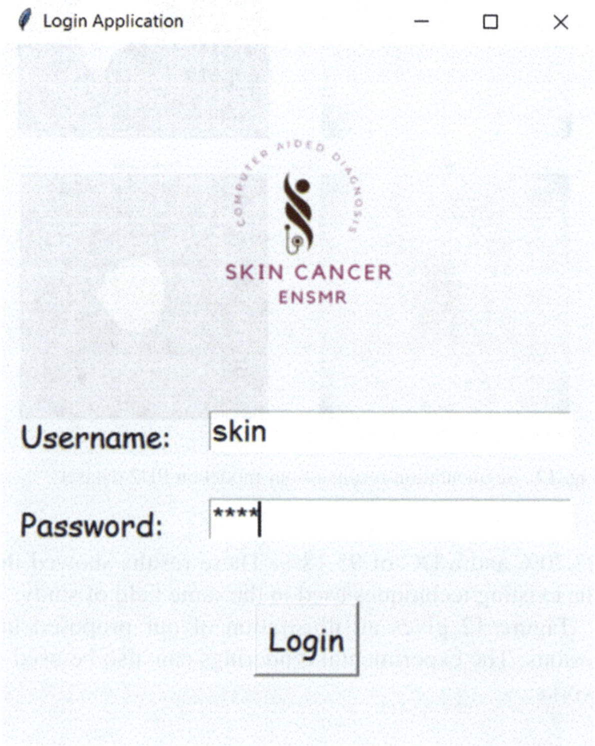

Fig. 13 The first window of SegSkin application: logging

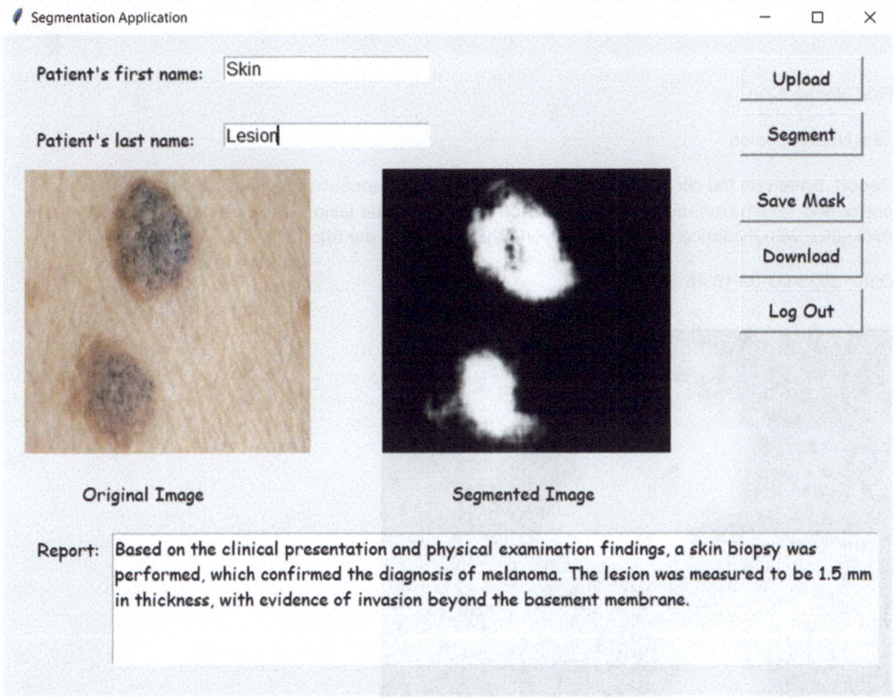

Fig. 14 The second window of SegSkin application: segment

the date the segmentation was done, and the medical report of the dermatologist (Fig. 15). The PDF document is created by the FPDF Python library. It is a pure Python library and does not require any external dependencies. FPDF generates PDF files dynamically by adding text, images, and other graphical elements to the document. The PDF can be stored locally for future use by pressing the "Download" button. Once dermatologists decide to complete the medical consultation, they can press the "Log Out" button to initialize the second window for further new consultations.

6 Discussion and Limitations

For computer-aided medical imaging analysis and diagnosis, it is crucial to develop an accurate and efficient automatic segmentation approach. In this paper, we developed a model for automatically segmenting skin lesions in dermoscopy images, which may aid in the early detection and treatment of skin lesions. The suggested VGG-UNet combines the characteristics of U-Net and VGG-19 and also we added the attention gate, which improves the performance of the basic version

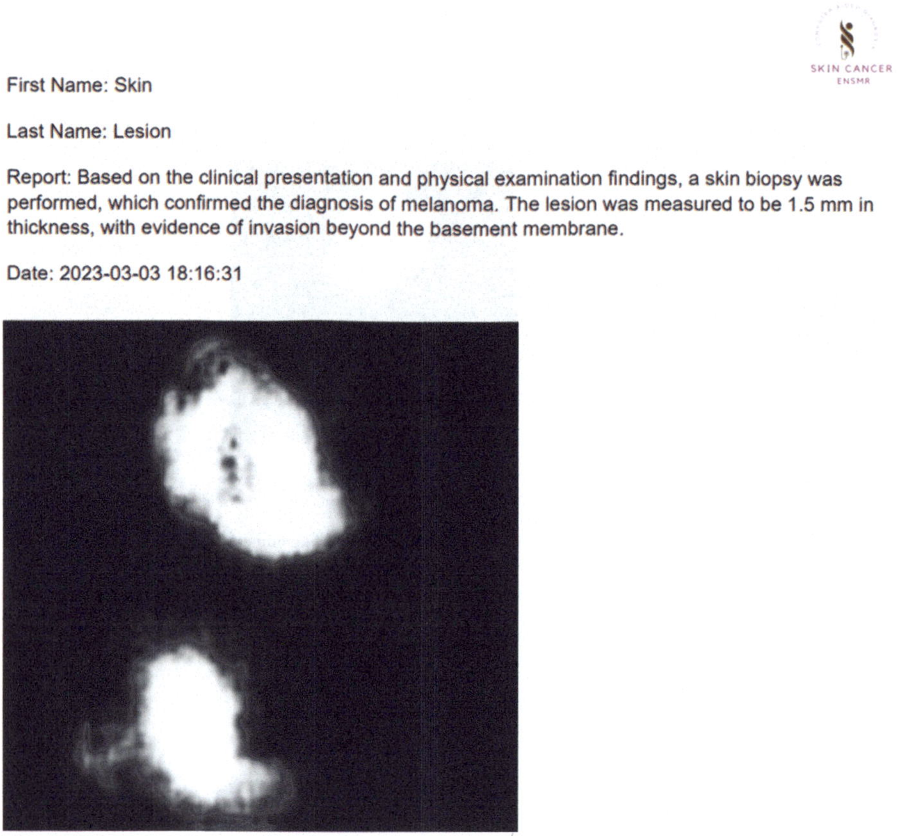
SKIN CANCER
ENSMR

First Name: Skin

Last Name: Lesion

Report: Based on the clinical presentation and physical examination findings, a skin biopsy was performed, which confirmed the diagnosis of melanoma. The lesion was measured to be 1.5 mm in thickness, with evidence of invasion beyond the basement membrane.

Date: 2023-03-03 18:16:31

Fig. 15 Structure of the medical report generated by SegSkin

of the U-Net. Moreover, to enhance the quality of dermoscopic images, we used the CLAHE approach and Dull-Razor algorithm. In particular, while methods based on deep learning necessitate an important amount of data to achieve effective segmentation, our model was trained with four datasets and used various image processing approaches for lesion segmentation in skin images. The results showed that the proposed approach provided beneficial results when compared to different methods based on deep learning. Regarding the experimental findings, VGG-UNet surpassed the five state-of-the-art models in the majority of metrics, and had the highest AC (97.26%), JS (84.34%), DC (93.04%), SE (91.72%) and SP (99.39%) in ISIC 2016, The best performing AC (97.52%), DC (89.76%), SE (91.28%) and SP (99.07%) in ISIC2017, the best AC (98.19%), DC (93.14%), and SP (98.95%) in ISIC2018, Furthermore the best AC (99.09%), JS (93.63%), DC (97.58%) and SP (99.28%) in PH2. Additionally, some illustrations of comparison outcomes are shown in Figs. 9, 10, 11, and 12 demonstrating the reliability of VGG-UNet in skin lesion segmentation.

The strength of the deep learning algorithm combined with the preprocessing technique is the primary benefit of the proposed approach. We also include batch normalization layers to improve the efficiency of our model by preventing overfitting. Moreover, the attention mechanism is used to focus on the most relevant inputs which could enhance the network's efficiency and accuracy.

Our model performs better on four skin lesion datasets that are publicly available. However, there is still space for improvement in the generalization capabilities of our suggested model, as demonstrated by the visual representation of datasets in Sect. 5.4. The inability of the convolution operation in the encoder to capture long-range dependencies, which is key to improving the generalization capabilities of the model, maybe the root cause of this issue. Additionally, the inference time in a single image still needs to be improved in our model. Obviously, the segmentation performance of the model must be ensured while the inference time is minimized. In order to balance model performance, inference time, and computational complexity, we will investigate a lightweight hybrid network architecture integrating CNNs and Transformers [41] for the segmentation of medical images in our upcoming study. In particular, we will combine the strengths of Transformers and CNNs to create an efficient network of encoder and decoder, that can be used the global and local information in order to enhance medical image segmentation.

7 Conclusion and Perspectives

Automatic lesion segmentation is a crucial step in computer-aided diagnosis and image-based medical analysis. Thanks to its great accuracy and speed as compared to manual analysis. Recently, deep neural networks have produced the best results for evaluating medical images. In this paper, we proposed a combination of the U-Net and VGG-19 architectures with an attention mechanism for enhancing the architectures. The approach used contrast-enhancing with CLAHE and a powerful hair removal algorithm as preprocessing steps. In the experiments, We used four publicly available benchmark datasets to validate the proposed approach. The results indicated that the model achieved significant improvements in the segmentation task and The results showed that the model surpassed both the initial U-Net network and its subsequent modified versions by generating more accurate segmentation results.

In further works, we will use Vision Transformers and CNNs for skin lesion segmentation and extend our SegSkin application.

References

1. Attia, M., Hossny, M., Nahavandi, S. & Yazdabadi, A. Skin melanoma segmentation using recurrent and convolutional neural networks. *2017 IEEE 14th International Symposium On Biomedical Imaging (ISBI 2017)*. pp. 292–296 (2017)
2. Simonyan, K. & Zisserman, A. Very deep convolutional networks for large-scale image recognition. *ArXiv Preprint ArXiv:1409.1556*. (2014)

3. Nachbar, F., Stolz, W., Merkle, T., Cognetta, A., Vogt, T., Landthaler, M., Bilek, P., Braun-Falco, O. & Plewig, G. The ABCD rule of dermatoscopy: high prospective value in the diagnosis of doubtful melanocytic skin lesions. *Journal Of The American Academy Of Dermatology*. **30**, 551–559 (1994)
4. Ronneberger, O., Fischer, P. & Brox, T. U-net: Convolutional networks for biomedical image segmentation. *International Conference On Medical Image Computing And Computer-assisted Intervention*. pp. 234–241 (2015)
5. Yuan, Y., Chao, M. & Lo, Y. Automatic skin lesion segmentation using deep fully convolutional networks with jaccard distance. *IEEE Transactions On Medical Imaging*. **36**, 1876–1886 (2017)
6. Akyel, C. & ARICI, N. Hair Removal and Lesion Segmentation with FCN8-ResNetC and Image Processing in Images of Skin Cancer. *Bilişim Teknolojileri Dergisi*. **15**, 231–238 (2022)
7. Sanjar, K., Bekhzod, O., Kim, J., Kim, J., Paul, A. & Kim, J. Improved U-net: fully convolutional network model for skin-lesion segmentation. *Applied Sciences*. **10**, 3658 (2020)
8. Barın, S. & Güraksın, G. An automatic skin lesion segmentation system with hybrid FCN-ResAlexNet. *Engineering Science And Technology, An International Journal*. pp. 101174 (2022)
9. Tang, P., Liang, Q., Yan, X., Xiang, S., Sun, W., Zhang, D. & Coppola, G. Efficient skin lesion segmentation using separable-Unet with stochastic weight averaging. *Computer Methods And Programs In Biomedicine*. **178** pp. 289–301 (2019)
10. Zafar, K., Gilani, S., Waris, A., Ahmed, A., Jamil, M., Khan, M. & Sohail Kashif, A. Skin lesion segmentation from dermoscopic images using convolutional neural network. *Sensors*. **20**, 1601 (2020)
11. Nguyen, D., Tran, T., Nguyen, C. & Pham, V. Skin lesion segmentation based on integrating efficientnet and residual block into U-Net neural network. *2020 5th International Conference On Green Technology And Sustainable Development (GTSD)*. pp. 366–371 (2020)
12. Iranpoor, R., Mahboob, A., Shahbandegan, S. & Baniasadi, N. Skin lesion segmentation using convolutional neural networks with improved U-Net architecture. *2020 6th Iranian Conference On Signal Processing And Intelligent Systems (ICSPIS)*. pp. 1–5 (2020)
13. Ramadan, R. & Aly, S. DGCU–Net: A new dual gradient-color deep convolutional neural network for efficient skin lesion segmentation. *Biomedical Signal Processing And Control*. **77** pp. 103829 (2022)
14. Miller, K., Ortiz, A., Pinheiro, P., Bandi, P., Minihan, A., Fuchs, H., Martinez Tyson, D., Tortolero-Luna, G., Fedewa, S., Jemal, A. & Others Cancer statistics for the US Hispanic/Latino population, 2021. *CA: A Cancer Journal For Clinicians*. **71**, 466–487 (2021)
15. Esteva, A., Kuprel, B., Novoa, R., Ko, J., Swetter, S., Blau, H. & Thrun, S. Dermatologist-level classification of skin cancer with deep neural networks. *Nature*. **542**, 115–118 (2017)
16. Binder, M., Schwarz, M., Winkler, A., Steiner, A., Kaider, A., Wolff, K. & Pehamberger, H. Epiluminescence microscopy: a useful tool for the diagnosis of pigmented skin lesions for formally trained dermatologists. *Archives Of Dermatology*. **131**, 286–291 (1995)
17. Vestergaard, M., Macaskill, P., Holt, P. & Menzies, S. Dermoscopy compared with naked eye examination for the diagnosis of primary melanoma: a meta-analysis of studies performed in a clinical setting. *British Journal Of Dermatology*. **159**, 669–676 (2008)
18. Litjens, G., Kooi, T., Bejnordi, B., Setio, A., Ciompi, F., Ghafoorian, M., Van Der Laak, J., Van Ginneken, B. & Sánchez, C. A survey on deep learning in medical image analysis. *Medical Image Analysis*. **42** pp. 60–88 (2017)
19. Gutman, D., Codella, N., Celebi, E., Helba, B., Marchetti, M., Mishra, N. & Halpern, A. Skin lesion analysis toward melanoma detection: A challenge at the international symposium on biomedical imaging (ISBI) 2016, hosted by the international skin imaging collaboration (ISIC). *ArXiv Preprint ArXiv:1605.01397*. (2016)
20. Codella, N., Rotemberg, V., Tschandl, P., Celebi, M., Dusza, S., Gutman, D., Helba, B., Kalloo, A., Liopyris, K., Marchetti, M. & Others Skin lesion analysis toward melanoma detection 2018: A challenge hosted by the international skin imaging collaboration (isic). *ArXiv Preprint ArXiv:1902.03368*. (2019)

21. Tschandl, P., Rosendah, C. & Kittler, H. Data descriptor: the HAM10000 dataset, a large collection of multi-source dermatoscopic images of common pigmented skin lesions. (2018)
22. De Raad, K., Garderen, K., Smits, M., Voort, S., Incekara, F., Oei, E., Hirvasniemi, J., Klein, S. & Starmans, M. The effect of preprocessing on convolutional neural networks for medical image segmentation. *2021 IEEE 18th International Symposium On Biomedical Imaging (ISBI)*. pp. 655–658 (2021)
23. Lee, T., Ng, V., Gallagher, R., Coldman, A. & McLean, D. Dullrazor®: A software approach to hair removal from images. *Computers In Biology And Medicine*. **27**, 533–543 (1997)
24. Pizer, S., Amburn, E., Austin, J., Cromartie, R., Geselowitz, A., Greer, T., Haar Romeny, B., Zimmerman, J. & Zuiderveld, K. Adaptive histogram equalization and its variations. *Computer Vision, Graphics, And Image Processing*. **39**, 355–368 (1987)
25. Alom, M., Hasan, M., Yakopcic, C., Taha, T. & Asari, V. Recurrent residual convolutional neural network based on u-net (r2u-net) for medical image segmentation. *ArXiv Preprint ArXiv:1802.06955*. (2018)
26. Oktay, O., Schlemper, J., Folgoc, L., Lee, M., Heinrich, M., Misawa, K., Mori, K., McDonagh, S., Hammerla, N., Kainz, B. & Others Attention u-net: Learning where to look for the pancreas. *ArXiv Preprint ArXiv:1804.03999*. (2018)
27. Liu, L., Mou, L., Zhu, X. & Mandal, M. Skin Lesion Segmentation based on improved U-net. *2019 IEEE Canadian Conference Of Electrical And Computer Engineering (CCECE)*. pp. 1–4 (2019)
28. Powers, D. Evaluation: from precision, recall and F-measure to ROC, informedness, markedness and correlation. *ArXiv Preprint ArXiv:2010.16061*. (2020)
29. Pereira, S., Pinto, A., Alves, V. & Silva, C. Brain tumor segmentation using convolutional neural networks in MRI images. *IEEE Transactions On Medical Imaging*. **35**, 1240–1251 (2016)
30. Doi, K. Computer-aided diagnosis in medical imaging: historical review, current status and future potential. *Computerized Medical Imaging And Graphics*. **31**, 198–211 (2007)
31. Korotkov, K. & Garcia, R. Computerized analysis of pigmented skin lesions: a review. *Artificial Intelligence In Medicine*. **56**, 69–90 (2012)
32. Mnih, V., Heess, N., Graves, A. & Others Recurrent models of visual attention. *Advances In Neural Information Processing Systems*. **27** (2014)
33. Woo, S., Park, J., Lee, J. & Kweon, I. Cbam: Convolutional block attention module. *Proceedings Of The European Conference On Computer Vision (ECCV)*. pp. 3–19 (2018)
34. Xie, F., Yang, J., Liu, J., Jiang, Z., Zheng, Y. & Wang, Y. Skin lesion segmentation using high-resolution convolutional neural network. *Computer Methods And Programs In Biomedicine*. **186** pp. 105241 (2020)
35. Kaul, C., Manandhar, S. & Pears, N. Focusnet: An attention-based fully convolutional network for medical image segmentation. *2019 IEEE 16th International Symposium On Biomedical Imaging (ISBI 2019)*. pp. 455–458 (2019)
36. Wibowo, A., Purnama, S., Wirawan, P. & Rasyidi, H. Lightweight encoder-decoder model for automatic skin lesion segmentation. *Informatics In Medicine Unlocked*. **25** pp. 100640 (2021)
37. Khouloud, S., Ahlem, M., Fadel, T. & Amel, S. W-net and inception residual network for skin lesion segmentation and classification. *Applied Intelligence*. pp. 1–19 (2022)
38. Jimi, A., Abouche, H., Zrira, N. & Benmiloud, I. Automated Skin Lesion Segmentation using VGG-UNet. *2022 IEEE/ACM International Conference On Advances In Social Networks Analysis And Mining (ASONAM)*. pp. 370–377 (2022)
39. Jimi., A., Abouche., H., Zrira., N. & Benmiloud., I. Skin Lesion Segmentation Using Attention-Based DenseUNet. *Proceedings Of The 16th International Joint Conference On Biomedical Engineering Systems And Technologies - BIOINFORMATICS,*. pp. 91–100 (2023)
40. Abouche, H., Jimi, A., Zrira, N. & Benmiloud, I. Segmentation and Classification of Dermoscopic Skin Cancer on Green Channel. *2022 IEEE/ACM International Conference On Advances In Social Networks Analysis And Mining (ASONAM)*. pp. 347–354 (2022)
41. Khan, S., Naseer, M., Hayat, M., Zamir, S., Khan, F. & Shah, M. Transformers in vision: A survey. *ACM Computing Surveys (CSUR)*. **54**, 1–41 (2022)

42. Moussaid, A., Zrira, N., Benmiloud, I., Farahat, Z., Karmoun, Y., Benzidia, Y., Mouline, S., El Abdi, B., Bourkadi, J. & Ngote, N. On the Implementation of a Post-Pandemic Deep Learning Algorithm Based on a Hybrid CT-Scan/X-Ray Images Classification Applied to Pneumonia Categories. *Healthcare*. **11**, 662 (2023).
43. Farahat, Z., Zrira, N., Souissi, N., Benamar, S., Belmekki, M., Ngote, M. & Megdiche, K. Application of Deep Learning Methods in a Moroccan Ophthalmic Center: Analysis and Discussion. *Diagnostics*. **13**, 1694 (2023).
44. Belharar, F. & Zrira, N. DeepRetino: Ophthalmic Disease Classification from Retinal Images using Deep Learning. *2022 IEEE 9th International Conference On Sciences Of Electronics, Technologies Of Information And Telecommunications (SETIT)*. pp. 392–399 (2022).

Segmentation and Classification of Dermoscopic Skin Images Using U-Net and Handcrafted Features

Hind Abouche, Anwar Jimi, Nabila Zrira, and Ibtissam Benmiloud

Abstract The most common type of cancer is skin cancer, which accounts for more than half of all cancer diagnoses. Melanoma is the rarest type of skin cancer, but it is the deadliest, with a high risk of spreading and death. On the other hand, melanoma is almost always treatable if detected early. In this regard, computer approaches for processing and analyzing skin lesion images have been investigated and developed. Our approach attempts to achieve this feat by developing a new method of melanoma segmentation and classification. The procedure begins with the preparation of dermoscopic images to remove hair using the Dull Razor algorithm, followed by image segmentation using a U-Net convolutional neural network to separate the skin lesion from the background. The segmented images obtained with the deep learning algorithm U-Net are then used to compute the Gray Level Co-occurrence Matrices (GLCM), followed by extracting Asymmetry, Border, Color, and Diameter (ABCD rule) features of the region of interest. Our approach achieves good results compared to the state-of-the-art.

Keywords Melanoma · U-Net · GLCM · ABCD · Dermoscopic images

1 Introduction

Skin cancer is one of the most popular and lethal cancers in the world, particularly as ozone levels decrease. Unprotected sunlight, which releases ultraviolet radiation, is the most common cause of skin cancer [25]. More of the sun's harmful ultraviolet rays meet the Earth's surface as the ozone layer's protective filtering function deteriorates. According to statistics, there are 300,000 non-melanoma cases and over 4000 melanoma cases for every 10% reduction in ozone levels. There are two

H. Abouche (✉) · A. Jimi · N. Zrira · I. Benmiloud
National Superior School of Mines, Rabat, Morocco
e-mail: hind.abouche@enim.ac.ma; anwar.jimi@enim.ac.ma; zrira@enim.ac.ma; benmiloud@enim.ac.ma

M. Kaya et al. (eds.), *Social Network Analysis and Mining Applications in Healthcare and Anomaly Detection*, Lecture Notes in Social Networks,
https://doi.org/10.1007/978-3-031-75204-9_9

types of skin cancer: malignant melanoma and benign non-melanoma. Each year, the World Health Organization estimates that two to three million non-melanoma cases and more than 130,000 melanoma cases occur worldwide. When a mole on the skin exhibits any non-cancerous growth, it is referred to as benign melanoma, as compared to malignant melanoma, which denotes a cancerous growth of the mole on the skin. Melanoma is the deadliest and most dangerous type of skin cancer, arising from the malignant growth of a pigmented skin lesion [23], and accounts for 75% of all skin cancer deaths. As reported by the World Cancer Research Fund International, malignant melanoma is the world's 17th most common cancer. Over 150,000 new cases of skin melanoma were diagnosed in 2020. It is the fifteenth most common cancer among women and the thirteenth most common cancer among men [33]. Malignant melanoma must be detected early by dermatologists. Unfortunately, evaluating visual features before identifying a malignant pigmented tumor can be difficult. Even skilled and experienced dermatologists can't tell the difference between melanoma and other skin tumors, such as nevus and more similar moles.

Skin cancer can be detected using two methods: computers or professional consultation. Lesions and wounds were discovered during a visual assessment of skin images. They analyze the scars to see if they are growing back and if the borders are growing unevenly [18]. Skin cancer can be identified immediately by processing the image from standard digital cameras or dermatoscopic exams.

Skin cancer diagnosis by hand is costly. As reported by the Skin Cancer Foundation, annual skin cancer treatment expenditures in the United States are estimated to be $8.1 billion, with $4.8 billion dedicated to non-melanoma cancer and $3.3 billion spent on melanoma.

In recent years, the use of advanced medical devices and the digitalization of medical services have resulted in massive volumes of medical images being generated. Deep learning (DL) has emerged as a potent tool across a wide range of imaging areas, including classification, prediction, detection, segmentation, diagnosis, interpretation, reconstruction, and so on. Deep neural networks were developed first in the computer vision sector, but they have quickly expanded to applications in medical imaging like lung diseases identification [30]. Diabetic retinopathy (DR) detection [32], eyes disease classification [31] and many more. This rising power of DL in illness diagnosis will empower clinicians and accelerate clinical decision making.

Computers today may be capable of identifying details, such as textural features, that the human eye cannot always detect. As a consequence, the use of computer vision and image processing techniques has played a role in enhancing dermoscopy to start producing equipment that is sufficiently effective for the correct diagnosis of lesions, seeking assistance to obtain precise data to assist experts [1, 4, 5, 24]. This improvement makes it easier to segment and classify various lesion types by identifying lesions, borders, and colors.

In this paper, we suggest a new method for computer-aided melanoma diagnosis. The automated diagnosis system is comprised of four major parts. The first part seeks to remove artifacts from the original images, such as hair, that may interfere with skin lesion detection using the Dull Razor algorithm. The second part is the segmentation algorithm U-Net which recognizes lesion boundaries based on the assumption that skin lesions are darker than healthy skin. The third part, which is inspired by the Haralick characteristics and the ABCD rule based on visual diagnosis, computes a collection of numerous parameters that allow melanoma and benign lesions to be distinguished. Finally, a classification technique is employed to obtain a diagnosis of the imaging lesion once these features that characterize each image are extracted.

In our work, we looked into the efficiency of the U-Net algorithm for skin cancer segmentation and feature extraction for lesion diagnosis. The following are the main contributions:

- Image segmentation using the deep learning U-Net algorithm;
- Haralick parameters such as Entropy; Energy, Contrast, Correlation, Homogeneity, Variance, Sum Of Average, Sum Of Variance, Sum Of Entropy, Difference Of Variance and Difference Of Entropy are recovered from the PH2 dataset;
- Asymmetry, border, color, and diameter characteristics are calculated based on the ABCD statistical features;
- As a result, Haralick, and ABCD features are used as consolidated features to evaluate performance with various GLCM offsets (i.e., 2, 4, 8, 12, 16, 20, 24, 28) and different orientations.

This paper is divided into four main sections, beginning with the introduction in Sect. 1. Section 2 outlines the proposed approach, which includes image pre-processing, image segmentation, feature extraction, and image classification. Section 3 presents the results of the experiments, and Sect. 4 concludes the paper.

2 Related Work

Sumithra et al. [17] employed three main features: texture, color, and RGB Histogram. The system's performance was evaluated using the author's dataset of 726 samples divided into five disease classes. Support Vector Machines (SVM) and K-Nearest Neighbor (KNN) classifiers produced 46.71% and 34% of the F-measure, respectively. When SVM and KNN were combined, F-measure was improved by 61%.

Almansour and Jaffar [8] presented a comparison of performance using accuracy between a different set of features to detect the skin lesion using the DermIs dataset and the SVM classifier, including GLCM (85%), Local Binary Patterns (LBP) (83%), color (87%), and the combination of LPB and GLCM (87%). They also combined LBP, GLCM, and color features, yielding an accuracy of 90.32%.

To extract shape features, Almaraz-Damian et al. [15] used texture, color, and the ABCD rule. For classification, they used the k-means algorithm. The approach was applied to DermQuest and the Dermatology Information System. The results achieved a performance of 75.1%.

As image features, Ashfaq et al. [16] used the ABCD rule and GLCM statistical parameters with a wide variety of offsets. Both dermIS and dermQuest were utilized as the datasets for this work. Melanoma and non-melanoma classification was separated into two experimental tests; the first used GLCM and color features and achieved an accuracy of 80%. While the second used only ABCD features and achieved an accuracy of 93%.

Moura et al. [10] proposed a feature extraction model based on the ABCD rule as well as a pre-trained Convolutional Neural Network (CNN). The model had an accuracy of 94.9%.

A classification approach was suggested by Majumder and Ullah [13] to predict the type of skin tumors based on eight characteristics of the ABCD rule on the PH2 dataset. The precision, specificity, and sensitivity of the results were calculated, resulting in 98%, 98%, and 97.5%, respectively.

Zaqout [14] used TDS (total dermoscopic score) and ABCD features on the PH2 dataset in another study. According to the results, this approach had a sensitivity rate of 85%, a specificity rate of 92%, and an accuracy rate of 90%.

Recently, Senan et al. [11] used a preprocessing method to remove hair and air bubbles. Following the segmentation phase, the segmented images were improved using a morphological method to extract the ABCD features. They put the proposed method to the test on the PH2 dataset. They achieved an 84% accuracy for the malignant and benign classes.

Tumpa et al. [12] suggested a method for classifying skin lesions into benign or malignant using an ABCD-based system combined with GLCM and LBP features. The images for the input are taken from the ISIC archive dataset and the PH2 dataset.

Sheha et al. [9] used the GLCM features as well as the Multilayer Perceptron classifier (MLP) to detect whether the lesion is Melanocytic Nevi or Malignant melanoma. In the training, the MLP achieved an accuracy of 100%, while in the testing the traditional MLP reached 92%.

Sheha et al. [9] used GLCM parameters as well as a Multilayer Perceptron Classifier (MLP) to determine whether a lesion was Melanocytic Nevi or Malignant Melanoma. The MLP achieved an accuracy of 92%.

Liu et al. [28] proposed a lesion segmentation approach that performed data augmentation on the ISIC 2017 dataset. Then, they compared the U-Net algorithm, which achieved an accuracy of 91.5%, SegNet, which reached an accuracy of 91.7%, and their proposed DCNN (deep convolution neural network), which attained an accuracy of 93%.

In another paper, Hasan et al. [29] used preprocessing techniques to improve the image quality of the ISIC 2018 dataset. Then, they applied the U-Net algorithm for segmentation with two different architectures. The first architecture of U-Net with 32 layers achieved 89% of the Jaccard coefficient, while the second architecture of U-Net with 46 layers achieved 93% for the same coefficient.

3 Methodology

Figure 1 depicts the proposed pipeline for distinguishing between malignant and benign skin cancer. The input dermoscopic dataset is gathered using the PH2 dataset. The procedure includes the following key steps: image pre-processing, ROI segmentation, handcrafted feature extraction, and classification.

Input images from PH2 datasets are used to provide data for training the model. The image is then processed with the Dull Razor algorithm to remove the artifacts. To segment the skin lesion in the image, the U-Net algorithm is used. All texture, shape, and color features of the skin lesions are extracted and fed into the network for further classification using the Haralick and ABCD techniques.

3.1 Dermoscopic Images

The gathering of relevant sets of input data is essential to the successful execution of the following steps as well as the resultant development of a coherent and powerful automated diagnostic system for skin lesions. The input dataset must include all possible lesion images. Dermoscopy images were taken from the PH2 dataset, which was developed as a result of collaborative research between the University of Porto and the Pedro Hispano Hospital's Dermatology Service in Portugal [7]. The dataset is freely available on the internet and can be used as a standard in any study. This dataset produced 200 melanocytic images, which we classified as 40 malignant lesions and 160 benign lesions, which include 80 common and 80 atypical nevus. These images were captured with the Tuebinger mole analyzer under

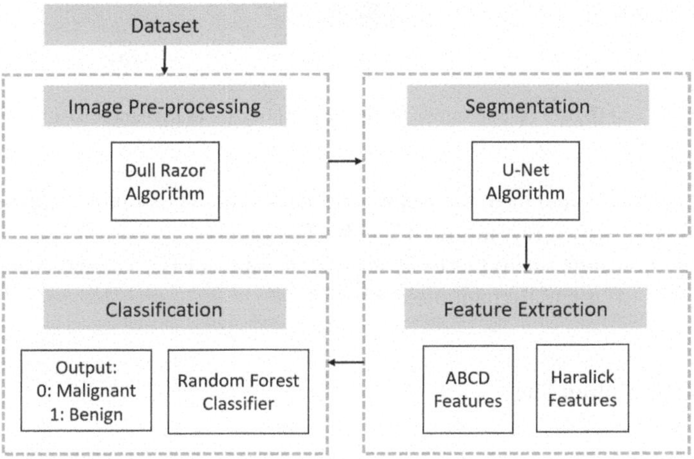

Fig. 1 The flowchart of our proposed approach

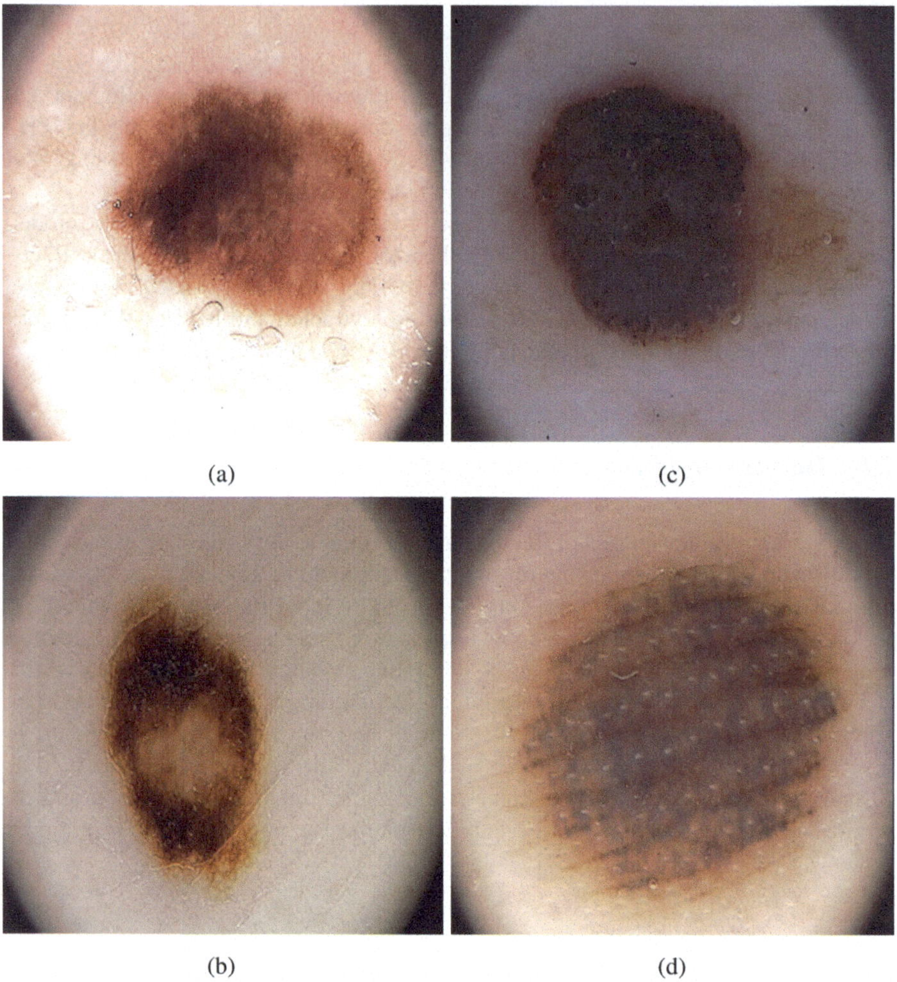

Fig. 2 Left: (**a**) and (**b**) are benign tumor, Right: (**c**) and (**d**) are malignant tumor

the same conditions and have the same properties. The RGB images are captured in the BMP format with a resolution of 764 by 574 pixels.

Figure 2 shows the two types of lesions from dataset PH2: (a) and (b) are benign nevus, (c) and (d) are malignant melanoma.

3.1.1 Image Enhancing

Due to high intra-class variation in melanoma images and low inter-class variation between melanoma and benign lesions, segmentation is one of the most difficult

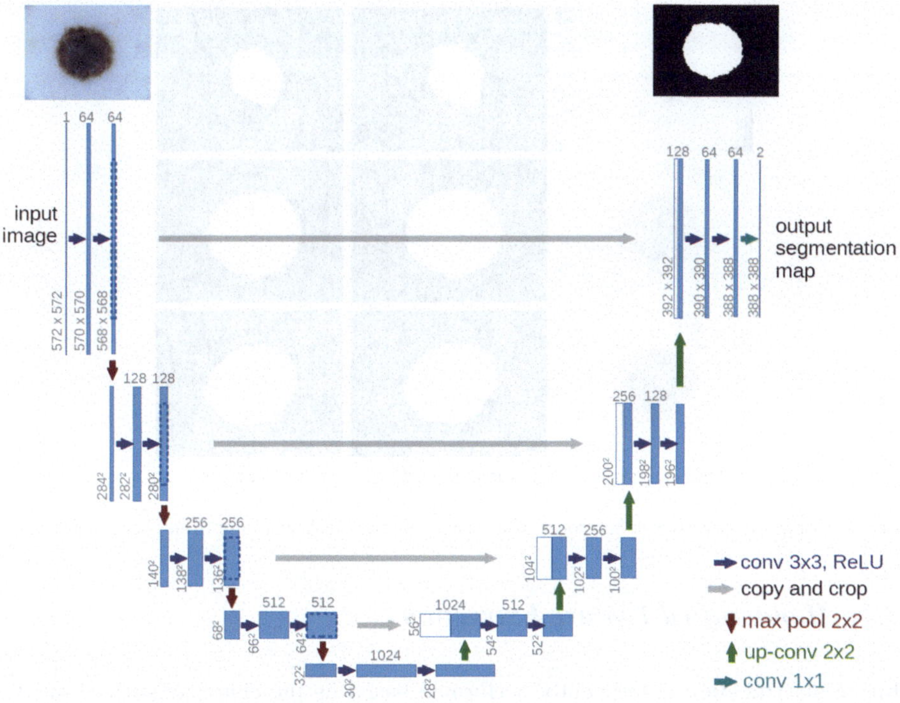

Fig. 3 U-Net algorithm architecture

steps. During the segmentation step of this work, the deep learning U-Net algorithm was used.

Olaf Ronneberger and his team created U-Net in 2015 for their work on biomedical images [20]. U-Net won the ISBI challenge by outperforming the sliding window technique by using fewer images and data augmentation to improve model performance. The name was inspired by the U-Net architecture. The "U-shaped" model is composed of convolutional layers and two networks. The encoder comes first, followed by the decoder, as shown in Fig. 3.

The U-Net is a convolutional network design for image segmentation with high accuracy. It has been demonstrated to attain excellent accuracy in a variety of segmentation tasks, most notably in medical image analysis. Its capacity to catch tiny details in images makes it ideal for applications requiring precise segmentation. It is also noted for its versatility in a variety of segmentation tasks. Its architecture is adaptable and extensible to handle various data kinds and requirements. Even with minimal training data sets, U-Net can perform well. This is useful in situations where gathering a large categorized dataset is difficult.

Figures 4 and 8 show a comparison between the output mask from lesion segmentation using U-Net and the ground truth masks.

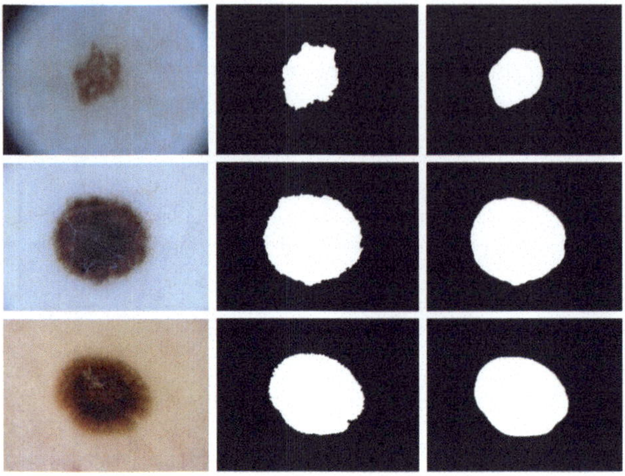

Fig. 4 Comparison between the ground truth mask and the mask resulting from U-Net algorithm

3.2 Handcrafted Feature Extraction

Image classification is frequently performed based on the characteristics of pixels within the segmented region of interest. As a result, extracting distinctive and significant features is a critical step in the classification process.

We were able to extract eleven Haralick features by tracking the gray-level co-occurrence probabilities based on the spatial relationships of pixels in various angular orientations. We computed the ABCD rule features, which include Asymmetry, Border, Diameter, and color features calculated using Mean, Skewness, Standard Deviation, and Variance for each channel in the RGB color space.

3.2.1 GLCM and Haralick's Statistical Texture Descriptors

The texture is a native attribute of skin that contains information about the structure or pattern arrangement of the skin. The texture feature depicts the relationship between spatial neighborhood pixels and image space gray values. The essential eleven values of the statistical texture measurements used by Haralick et al. [6] are Entropy, Energy, Contrast, Correlation, Homogeneity, Variance, Sum Of Average, Sum Of Variance, Sum Of Entropy, Difference Of Variance, and Difference Of Entropy, which were obtained from a GLCM matrix. The GLCM is a table that shows how often different pixel luminance value combinations appear in a specific pixel pair of an image. A two-dimensional gray-level co-occurrence matrix is commonly used in texture analysis to determine the locative dependency of gray-level values, assisting in the discovery of important details about nearby pixels in an image. Image texture can be evaluated using the Gray Level Co-occurrence Matrix (GLCM). The relationship between pixels with different gray levels is represented by GLCM. For this purpose, a separate matrix is generated for each set of pixel offset and orientation. Haralick proposed GLCM-based second-order statistical texture descriptors.

In this work, we calculated the average values of each pixel with offsets of 2, 4, 8, 12, 16, 20, 24, and 28 using four orientations: 0°, 45°, 90°, and 135°. The average values for each offset are then used to calculate the final Haralick features, allowing us to compare and select the offset value that provides the best accuracy.

The Haralick features are calculated as follows:

Contrast determines the textural roughness of a pixel's surrounding pixels across the entire image. As shown in Eq. 1, the contrast of a set of pixels is defined as the difference between their highest and lowest values.

$$Contrast = \sum_{i=1}^{Ng} \sum_{j=1}^{Ng} (i - j)^2 P(i, j) \tag{1}$$

Energy is equal to the sum of the squared components in the GLCM matrix (Eq. 2). Because it quantifies the level of texture disturbance or uniformity, it is also known as the non-homogeneity or angular second moment.

$$Energy = \sum_{i=1}^{Ng} \sum_{j=1}^{Ng} P(i, j)^2 \tag{2}$$

Homogeneity (or Inverse Difference Moment) refers to the effect of a pixel's surroundings on the overall image, it is a measure of how close the GLCM item distribution is to its diagonal. Homogeneity is maximized when all of the components are the same.

$$Homogeneity = \sum_{i=1}^{Ng} \sum_{j=1}^{Ng} \frac{P(i, j)}{1 + (i - j)^2} \tag{3}$$

Correlation is a measurement of the degree to which a pixel is connected to its neighbors across the entire image. It was graded between 1 and 0.

$$Correlation = \frac{[\sum_{i=1}^{Ng} \sum_{j=1}^{Ng} (ij) P(i, j)] - \mu_x \mu_y}{\sigma_x \sigma_y} \tag{4}$$

Entropy is a measure of randomness of the intensity image. Equation 5 calculates the entropy as follows:

$$Entropy = -\sum_{i=1}^{Ng}\sum_{j=1}^{Ng} P(i, j)ln(P(i, j) \tag{5}$$

Variance or the sum of squares, gives relatively high weights to elements that differ from the matrix's value.

$$Variance = \sum_{i=1}^{Ng}\sum_{j=1}^{Ng}(i - \mu)^2 * P(i, j) \tag{6}$$

Sum Of Average computes the average of all gray levels.

$$SAV = \sum_{i=2}^{2Ng} i P_{x+y}(i) \tag{7}$$

Sum Of Variance is a measure of heterogeneity that is strongly correlated with first-order statistical variables such as standard deviation. When the gray level values deviate from their mean, the variance increases.

$$SVA = \sum_{i=2}^{2Ng}(i - SEN)^2 P_{x+y}(i) \tag{8}$$

Sum Of Entropy is a measure of the proportion of non-consistency in the picture or the intricacy of the texture.

$$SEN = -\sum_{i=2}^{2Ng} P_{x+y}(i)ln(P_{x+y}(i)) \tag{9}$$

Difference Of Variance is defined as the variance of p_{xy} in a manner similar to its sum counterpart. The distinction change measure is characterized as the fluctuation of p_{xy}, in a way like its total partner

$$DVA = Variance(P_{x-y}) \tag{10}$$

Difference Of Entropy is a measure of the randomness or lack of structure or order in the variance of an image.

$$DEN = -\sum_{i=0}^{Ng} P_{x-y}(i)ln(P_{x-y}(i)) \tag{11}$$

Equations 1–11 depict eleven Haralick properties, namely: Entropy, Energy, Contrast, Correlation, Homogeneity, Variance, Sum Of Average, Sum Of Variance, Sum Of Entropy, Difference Of Variance, and Difference Of Entropy, where Ng is the number of gray levels found in the input image, $P(i, j)$ is the normalized entry in row i and column j of the GLCM, and I is the intensity of one pixel while j is that of the next pixel, constituting the pair for the GLCM.

3.2.2 ABCD Rule-Based Features

This rule defines and investigates a set of resilient criteria based on the ABCD (asymmetry, border irregularity, color, and diameter) rule to efficiently distinguish between melanoma and benign lesions. Concerning asymmetry, which is a clinical trait suggestive of malignancy, a set of strategies for detecting asymmetry is examined, and a new method for quantifying asymmetry is offered. In addition, we provide a new approach for measuring border irregularity. To quantify the border, it employs a hybrid approach that involves producing a circle whose form is indicative of pixel distribution within the lesion. Another goal of this research is to detect the color information in the lesion, which is thought to be a significant trait utilized to diagnose skin malignancies. For this part, texture properties are used to obtain color information. The diameter is the final factor we assess because melanomas typically begin with a diameter greater than 6–7 mm.

These are the characteristics that dermatologists frequently employ. The significance of these characteristics is that they help a dermatologist determine whether or not a skin lesion is a melanoma. The doctors' ABCD rule has been mathematically modeled and implemented in this paper. The following are the specifics of these features.

The ABCD rule is the second dermoscopy method introduced by Friedman et al. [2]. The ABCD rule has a high level of consistency in clinical diagnosis. Isasi et al. [3] proposed a system supported by traditional or clinical ABCD rules and dermatological protocols for pattern recognition. To reduce or eliminate system response time, quantitative features (inner patterns) from images are calculated using a simple operation algorithm, and the system achieves over 85% accuracy. Table 2 summarizes the ABCD rules, including conditions, descriptions, scoring, and factors.

3.2.3 Asymmetry

Asymmetry is one of the most essential parameters of melanoma; it defines the axis of symmetry [26]. Generally, the asymmetry value is calculated by dividing the lesion's segmented region into two sub-regions by an axis of symmetry and then determining the non-overlapping region across the axis. If the two sub-regions are very similar, the lesion is considered symmetric; otherwise, it is assumed to be

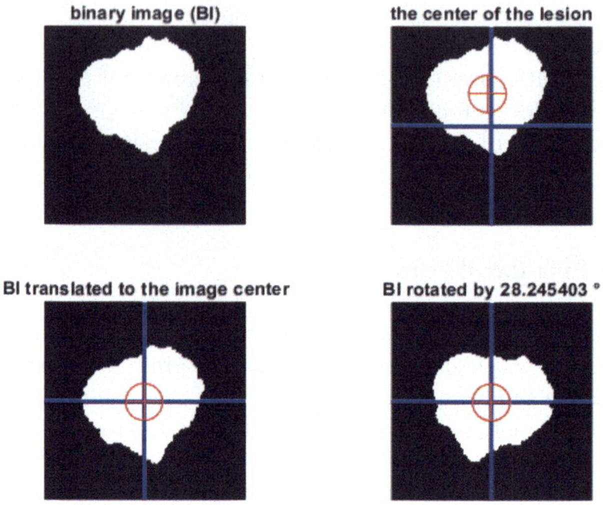

Fig. 5 Steps for aligning a binary image

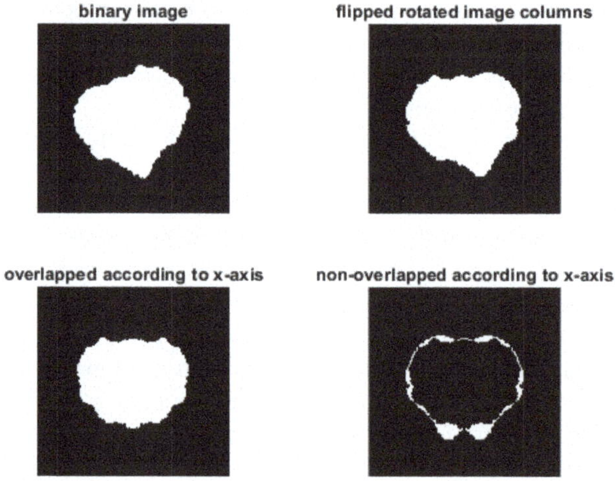

Fig. 6 The steps for computing Asymmetry A_1

unsymmetrical. Benign tumors have symmetric shapes, whereas malignant lesions have highly asymmetric shapes [13].

To determine the asymmetry feature, we had to align the segmented image with the image coordinate system. That was accomplished by translating its centroid into the coordinate system's origin and then rotating the image by its orientation angle to fit the image's major axis onto the x-axis as shown in Fig. 5. Figure 6 depicts a sample-aligned segmented image that has been flipped along the x-axis, and the non-overlapping region ($\delta\ L_x$) between the lesion image (L) and the flipped image

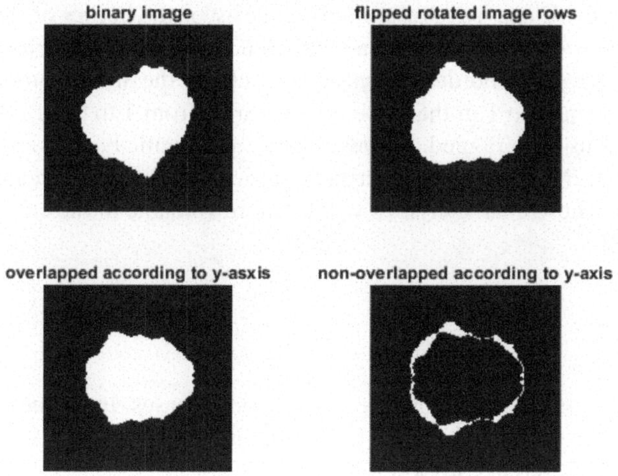

Fig. 7 The steps for computing Asymmetry A_2

(L_x) has been computed. Figure 7 shows the same sample-aligned segmented image flipped along the y-axis, with the non-overlapping region $(\delta\ L_y)$ computed between the lesion image (L) and the flipped image (L_y). The asymmetry score across the x-axis (A_1) and the y-axis (A_2) is calculated by the following equations:

$$\Delta L_{x'} = L \oplus L_x,\ A_1 = \frac{Area\ \ of\ \ L_x}{Area\ \ of\ \ L} \tag{12}$$

$$\Delta L_{y'} = L \oplus L_x,\ A_2 = \frac{Area\ \ of\ \ L_y}{Area\ \ of\ \ L} \tag{13}$$

3.2.4 Border Irregularity

To reveal the smoothness of the lesion boundary, the irregularity of the border is utilized as well to provide an overview of the various edge types that can be found. The irregularity parameter in a lesion is critical when evaluating a malignant lesion. Several measures can be used to calculate border irregularity, including the compactness index. The compact index was calculated using the following method in this paper.

$$B_1 = 4\pi A/P^2 \tag{14}$$

$$B_2 = A/P \tag{15}$$

$$B_3 = A \times P \tag{16}$$

Equations 14, 15, and 16 assess the irregularity of the border of the lesion [26]. A benign lesion is defined as having a regular and even border, whereas a malignant lesion has an irregular border. Because a circle is the most compact structure, compactness is equal to 1 in that case, and it varies from 1 to 0 for all other forms. Melanoma lesions have ragged, uneven, blurry, and erratic borders, so the B_1 value tends to be zero. B_2 is the Area to Perimeter ratio, and B_3 is the Area and Perimeter multiplication. These characteristics will be more valuable in the case of malignant melanoma [27].

3.2.5 Color

Color is an important feature for diagnosing skin diseases. In dermoscopic images, the first indicator that can be used to distinguish between benign and malignant melanoma is the difference in skin tone.

Color refers to how an item appears when exposed to light. Studying the three primary colors, red, green, and blue, assisted us in grasping the concept of color space. The exhibited colors of the segmented lesion areas must be identified using the color feature approach. While most other approaches used the ABCD rule to count the color score, which indicates how many colors the lesion contains, we chose to go further and deeper by calculating the mean, standard deviation, variance, and skewness of the segmented lesion region.

The four properties mentioned above are computed across each channel, yielding 12 color features (four features in RGB color space for each channel), which were retrieved as follows:

Mean is the average value obtained by adding all of the observed outcomes from the sample and dividing by the total number of events.

$$M = \frac{1}{x}\sum_{i=1}^{x} P \tag{17}$$

Standard deviation is the difference in distance between data values and the mean.

$$STD = \sqrt{\frac{1}{x}\sum_{i=1}^{x}(P_j - M)^2} \tag{18}$$

Skewness: the degree of asymmetry in the distribution, calculated by:

$$Skewness = \sqrt[3]{\frac{1}{x}\sum_{i=1}^{x}(P_j - M)^3} \tag{19}$$

Variance refers to the variation in color distribution.

$$S = \frac{1}{x}\sum_{i=1}^{x}(P_j - M)^2 \tag{20}$$

P_j denotes the jth pixel of a color channel P in the color space of an image I with x pixels.

3.2.6 Diameter

The diameter is the most important feature that is frequently overlooked. The distance between the capturing device and the lesion influences the diameter. To ensure a fair comparison, the distance between the camera and the lesion should be consistent across all images in a dataset [16]. If the diameter is greater than 6 mm and continues to grow over the next month, it is malignant melanoma [22]. The major axis length of the best-fitted ellipse [26] or the biggest distance between any two points on the lesion's border determines the diameter [21]. A melanoma-affected mole grows bigger than a normal mole, which is one of the most important criteria. A malignant lesion has a diameter greater than 6 mm. $D1$ denotes the average diameter of the lesion.

$$D1 = \frac{D1' + D''}{2} \tag{21}$$

Where D1'=$\sqrt{4A/\pi}$ and D''=(D+d)/2

$$D2 = D - d \tag{22}$$

$D2$ is the difference between the two principal axes' lengths. The major axis is D, and the minor axis is d. $D1$ and $D2$ will have a higher value in malignant melanoma than in benign melanoma [12].

3.3 *Classification*

Following feature extraction, the next procedure involves developing a model using the retrieved features from the PH2 dataset's 200 dermoscopic images. Because our final dataset contains two types of skin cancer lesions (i.e., melanoma and benign), the skin lesion identification function in this work is a standard binary categorization problem. The goal is to label each skin lesion in the dermoscopic images provided with an appropriate class label.

In this work, we used the random forest algorithm, which is a machine-learning technique used to solve regression and classification problems. It employs ensemble learning, a technique that combines many classifiers to provide solutions to complex problems. A random forest algorithm overcomes the limitations of the decision tree algorithm. It reduces dataset overfitting and improves precision. It generates predictions without requiring many package configurations [19].

In this scenario, there are 30 inputs in total, 11 from Haralick features and 19 from ABCD rule features. The label of the target is either 1 or 0, with 0 indicating malignancy and 1 indicating benignity.

4 Experimental Results

In this section, we present both segmentation and classification results for skin lesions.

4.1 Segmentation Results

Pixels in an image are divided into distinct groups. Segmentation is used in the detection of skin cancer to extract the lesion boundary that separates it from the surrounding non-cancerous tissue. The segmentation generates a binary mask at the location of the lesion. To assess the performance the performance of the U-Net algorithm during the segmentation phase, we employed the following measures:

Accuracy (ACC) of the model indicates how often it was correct overall:

$$ACC = \frac{TP + TN}{TP + FP + TN + FN} \tag{23}$$

Dice Coefficient (DC) measures the similarity between predicted and defined ground truths. A DC value can range from 0 to 1, with 0 representing no spatial overlap and 1 representing total overlap. And it was computed as follows:

$$DC = \frac{2 \times TP}{2 \times (TP + FN + FP)} \tag{24}$$

Jaccard Coefficient (JC) is a union over the intersection of segmented lesions and ground truth masks. The Jaccard coefficient can take values ranging from 0 to 1, with 0 representing no overlap and 1 representing the total overlap between the sets. And it is determined by:

$$JC = \frac{TP}{TP + FN + FP} \tag{25}$$

Sensitivity (SE) represents the percentage of successfully identified skin lesion pixels. And it is calculated by:

$$SE = \frac{TP}{TP + FN} \tag{26}$$

Specificity (SP) is the percentage of pixels classified as non-skin lesions. And it is computed by:

$$SP = \frac{TN}{TN + FP} \tag{27}$$

Where:

- **TP (True Positive)**: It is an abbreviation for malignant lesions that have been accurately diagnosed as malignant;
- **TN (True Negative)**: It assesses if benign lesions have been appropriately diagnosed as benign;
- **FN (False Negative)**: It stands for malignant tumors that were mistakenly recognized as benign;
- **FP (False Positive)**: It stands for benign lesions that were mistakenly diagnosed as malignant.

Since the deep learning U-Net model requires a large dataset to perform well, we proposed feeding the model with two datasets: the ISIC 2017 for training and validating the model and the PH2 for testing. Table 1 presents the hyper-parameters used while training the model.

Table 2 shows our segmentation results compared to some other papers that used the U-Net algorithm on different ISIC datasets. Liu et al. [28] used a data augmentation technique on the ISIC 2017 data set, as a data input, they combined the 3 RGB channels with 3 HSV channels, they compared three deep learning algorithms SegNet, U-Net, and DCNN, they achieved an accuracy of 91%, 91%, and 74% successively. In another paper, in the pre-processing step, Hasan et al. [29] implement Image Enhancement, Linear Filtering, and Image Restoration techniques. Also, the authors proposed two U-Net algorithms with different architectures (U-Net 32, and U-Net 46), The highest achieved accuracy value was 93%. Following the pre-processing stage for Dull Razor hair removal in

Table 1 U-Net training parameters

Parameter	Value
Input size	$256 \times 256 \times 3$
Batch size	32
Learning rate	SegNetne
Optimizer	Adam
Epochs	100
Loss function	Binary Crossentrop

Table 2 Comparison of segmentation results with the state-of-the-art

Approach	Methodology	JC	DC	ACC	SE	SP
Liu et al. [28]	SegNet	70%	79.7%	91.7%	81.5%	97.4%
	U-Net	68.6%	78.7%	91.5%	75.5%	96.9%
	DCNN	74%	83%	92.6%	82.8%	96.5%
Hasan et al. [29]	U-Net 32 layers	89%	–	–	–	97%
	U-Net 46 layers	93%	85%	93%	91%	97%
Our approach	U-Net	74.4%	**85.6%**	**95%**	83.5%	**98.7%**

our suggested method, we extracted Haralick and ABCD features to train our model using the ISIC 2017 dataset and test it using the PH2 dataset. Our model worked effectively and was able to reach a very high segmentation accuracy value of up to 95%.

Also, Fig. 8 shows qualitative results between the output mask from lesion segmentation using U-Net and the ground truth masks.

4.2 Classification Results

Image-based classification analysis was performed on 160 benign and 40 malignant lesion images. The data split for training versus test data is 70:30. Virtually all benign and malignant lesion images were classified correctly using the proposed method. It did, however, leave out a few. The model's effectiveness is evaluated using five criteria: Confusion matrix, accuracy, recall, f1-score, precision.

Confusion matrix summarizes the classification problem prediction outcomes. The number of correct and incorrect predictions is counted and divided by class.

Recall value indicates how many times the model identified the benign or malignant category:

$$Recall = \frac{TP}{TP + FN} \tag{28}$$

Precision quantifies how well a model predicts the skin lesion category

$$Precision = \frac{TP}{TP + FP} \tag{29}$$

F1-score which summarizes the predictive efficiency of a model by combining two seemingly opposing criteria: Precision and Recall.

$$F1 - Score = 2 \times \frac{Precision \times Recall}{Precision + Recall} \tag{30}$$

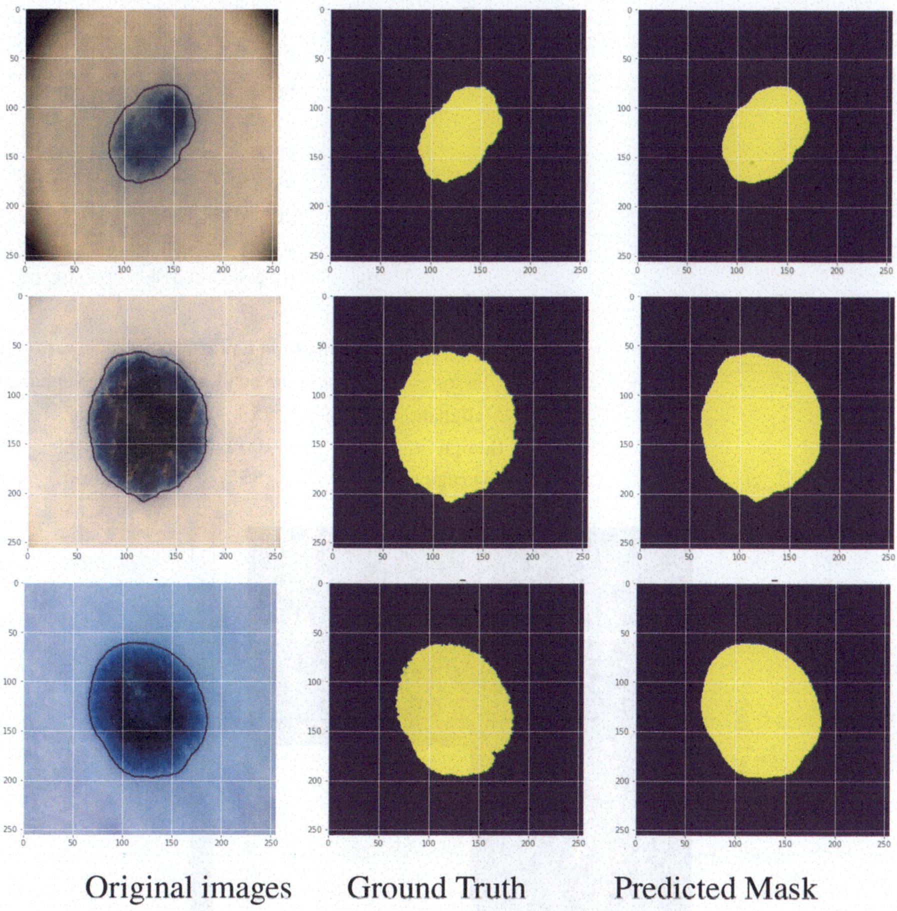

Fig. 8 Lesion segmentation results

We were capable of getting the optimal parameters of our model using the hyper-parameters tuning method Grid Search:

- N_Estimators=200
- Max_Depth=30
- Min_Samples_Split=3
- Min_Samples_Leaf=2
- Max_Features='sqrt'

The Random Forest model was used to generate results from Haralick parameters with various offsets in the range of 2–28, and the offset that produced the best results was chosen. All of the ABCD features were used to assess the RF's performance. As shown in Table 3, offset 4 produced the best results. As an outcome, the system has achieved a 95% overall accuracy in classification.

Table 3 Classification results with respect to the offset value

Offset	Accuracy	Precision	Recall
2	92%	92%	97%
4	**95%**	**95%**	**86%**
8	92%	92%	85.4%
12	93.3%	93.3%	86.4%
16	95%	95%	87.5%
20	90%	90%	84.3%
24	93.3%	93.3%	86.4%
28	91%	91%	85.4%

Table 4 The classification report of our proposed approach

	Classification report			
Classes	Precision	Recall	F1-score	Support
Malignant	100 %	75%	86%	12
Benign	94%	100%	97%	48
Average	**95%**	**95%**	**95%**	60

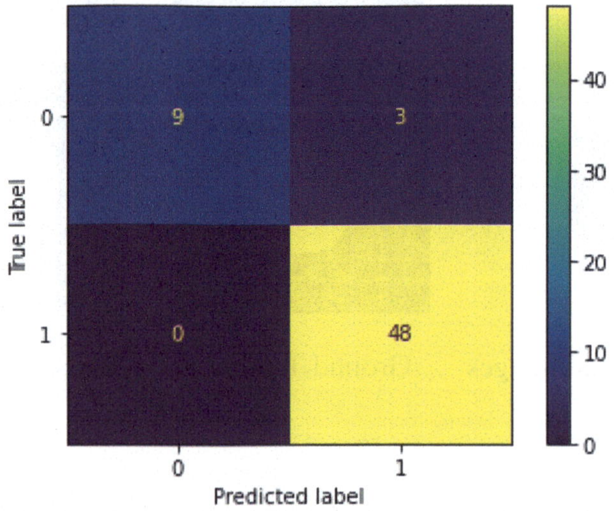

Fig. 9 Confusion matrix of our proposed approach

Our model made extremely precise predictions. According to the classification report shown in Table 4, the model correctly predicted that 94% of the skin cancer cases were benign. And all of the skin cancer cases predicted by the algorithm to be malignant were, in fact, malignant.

As illustrated by the confusion matrix in Fig. 9, which shows that our model only predicted three cases to be benign but turned out to be malignant; otherwise, the model was extremely accurate.

Table 5 Comparison of classification results with the state-of-the-art

Approach	Methodology	Accuracy
Zaqout [14]	Contrast Enhancing Segmentation thresholding ABCD features	90%
Senan et al. [11]	Gaussian filter Segmentation Morphological ABCD features TDS method	84%
Our approach	Dull Razor U-Net segmentation GLCM and ABCD features Random Forest	**95%**

In Table 5, we compared the results of the proposed approach to those of other techniques on the PH2 dataset. Senan et al. [11] used pre-processing methods to reduce noise, hair, and air bubbles. Following the segmentation step, the segmented images were improved using a morphological technique to get the ABCD attributes. Their system has an 84% accuracy. Zaqout et al. [14], on the other hand, used TDS and the ABCD features with the PH2 data set. The results showed that this approach had a 90% accuracy rate, whereas our system had a 95% accuracy rate.

5 Conclusion and Future Work

An efficient skin lesion diagnosis strategy was proposed in this work, beginning with the Dull Razor algorithm to locate and eliminate hair pixels in the image, followed by the U-Net algorithm for image segmentation, and various characteristics of the lesion are extracted using the Haralick and ABCD feature extraction methods. We concluded that combining these features improved the accuracy of the classification results.

In this paper, the handcrafted features are extracted. However, in the future, a large amount of data will be explored to enhance training and classification accuracy, and a deep learning algorithm could be used for melanoma classification.

References

1. Jimi, A., Abouche, H., Zrira, N. & Benmiloud, I. Automated Skin Lesion Segmentation using VGG-UNet. *2022 IEEE/ACM International Conference On Advances In Social Networks Analysis And Mining (ASONAM)*. pp. 370–377 (2022)
2. Friedman, R., Rigel, D. & Kopf, A. Early detection of malignant melanoma: the role of physician examination and self-examination of the skin.. *CA: A Cancer Journal For Clinicians*. **35**, 130–151 (1985)
3. Isasi, A., Zapirain, B. & Zorrilla, A. Melanomas non-invasive diagnosis application based on the ABCD rule and pattern recognition image processing algorithms. *Computers In Biology And Medicine*. **41**, 742–755 (2011)

4. Abouche, H., Jimi, A., Zrira, N. & Benmiloud, I. Segmentation and Classification of Dermoscopic Skin Cancer on Green Channel. *2022 IEEE/ACM International Conference On Advances In Social Networks Analysis And Mining (ASONAM)* (2022)
5. Jimi, A., Abouche, H., Zrira, N. & Benmiloud, I. Skin Lesion Segmentation Using Attention-Based DenseUNet. *Proceedings Of The 16th International Joint Conference On Biomedical Engineering Systems And Technologies - BIOINFORMATICS,*. pp. 91–100 (2023)
6. Haralick, R., Shanmugam, K. & Dinstein, I. Textural features for image classification. *IEEE Transactions On Systems, Man, And Cybernetics*, 610–621 (1973)
7. Mendonça, T., Celebi, M., Mendonca, T. & Marques, J. Ph2: A public database for the analysis of dermoscopic images. *Dermoscopy Image Analysis*. (2015)
8. Almansour, E. & Jaffar, M. Classification of Dermoscopic skin cancer images using color and hybrid texture features. *IJCSNS Int J Comput Sci Netw Secur*. **16**, 135–139 (2016)
9. Sheha, M., Mabrouk, M., Sharawy, A. & Others Automatic detection of melanoma skin cancer using texture analysis. *International Journal Of Computer Applications*. **42**, 22–26 (2012)
10. Moura, N., Veras, R., Aires, K., Machado, V., Silva, R., Araújo, F. & Claro, M. ABCD rule and pre-trained CNNs for melanoma diagnosis. *Multimedia Tools And Applications*. **78**, 6869–6888 (2019)
11. Senan, E. & Jadhav, M. Analysis of dermoscopy images by using ABCD rule for early detection of skin cancer. *Global Transitions Proceedings*. **2**, 1–7 (2021)
12. Tumpa, P. & Kabir, M. An artificial neural network based detection and classification of melanoma skin cancer using hybrid texture features. *Sensors International*. **2** pp. 100128 (2021)
13. Majumder, S. & Ullah, M. Feature extraction from dermoscopy images for melanoma diagnosis. *SN Applied Sciences*. **1**, 1–11 (2019)
14. Zaqout, I. Diagnosis of skin lesions based on dermoscopic images using image processing techniques. *Pattern Recognition-Selected Methods And Applications*. (2019)
15. Almaraz-Damian, J., Ponomaryov, V. & Rendon-Gonzalez, E. Melanoma CADe based on ABCD rule and haralick texture features. *2016 9th International Kharkiv Symposium On Physics And Engineering Of Microwaves, Millimeter And Submillimeter Waves (MSMW)*. pp. 1–4 (2016)
16. Ashfaq, M., Minallah, N., Ullah, Z., Ahmad, A., Saeed, A. & Hafeez, A. Performance analysis of low-level and high-level intuitive features for melanoma detection. *Electronics*. **8**, 672 (2019)
17. Sumithra, R., Suhil, M. & Guru, D. Segmentation and classification of skin lesions for disease diagnosis. *Procedia Computer Science*. **45** pp. 76–85 (2015)
18. Lacy, K. & Alwan, W. Skin cancer. *Medicine*. **41**, 402–405 (2013)
19. Breiman, L. Random forests. *Machine Learning*. **45** pp. 5–32 (2001)
20. Ronneberger, O., Fischer, P. & Brox, T. U-net: Convolutional networks for biomedical image segmentation. *Medical Image Computing And Computer-Assisted Intervention–MICCAI 2015: 18th International Conference, Munich, Germany, October 5–9, 2015, Proceedings, Part III 18*. pp. 234–241 (2015)
21. Alasadi, A. & AL-Safy, B. Early detection and classification of melanoma skin cancer. (LAP LAMBERT Academic Publishing, 2016)
22. Shaw, H., Rigel, D., Friedman, R., Mccarthy, W. & Kopf, A. Early diagnosis of cutaneous melanoma: revisiting the ABCD criteria. *Jama*. **292**, 2771–2776 (2004)
23. Zagrouba, E. & Barhoumi, W. A prelimary approach for the automated recognition of malignant melanoma. *Image Analysis & Stereology*. **23**, 121–135 (2004)
24. Codella, N., Cai, J., Abedini, M., Garnavi, R., Halpern, A. & Smith, J. Deep learning, sparse coding, and SVM for melanoma recognition in dermoscopy images. *International Workshop On Machine Learning In Medical Imaging*. pp. 118–126 (2015)
25. Javed, R., Rahim, M., Saba, T. & Rehman, A. A comparative study of features selection for skin lesion detection from dermoscopic images. *Network Modeling Analysis In Health Informatics And Bioinformatics*. **9**, 1–13 (2020)

26. She, Z., Liu, Y. & Damatoa, A. Combination of features from skin pattern and ABCD analysis for lesion classification. *Skin Research And Technology*. **13**, 25–33 (2007)
27. Clawson, K., Morrow, P., Scotney, B., McKenna, J. & Dolan, O. Analysis of pigmented skin lesion border irregularity using the harmonic wavelet transform. *2009 13th International Machine Vision And Image Processing Conference*. pp. 18–23 (2009)
28. Liu, L., Mou, L., Zhu, X. & Mandal, M. Skin Lesion Segmentation based on improved U-net. *2019 IEEE Canadian Conference Of Electrical And Computer Engineering (CCECE)*. pp. 1–4 (2019)
29. Hasan, S., Gezer, M., Azeez, R. & Gülseçen, S. Skin lesion segmentation by using deep learning techniques. *2019 Medical Technologies Congress (TIPTEKNO)*. pp. 1–4 (2019)
30. Moussaid, A., Zrira, N., Benmiloud, I., Farahat, Z., Karmoun, Y., Benzidia, Y., Mouline, S., El Abdi, B., Bourkadi, J. & Ngote, N. On the Implementation of a Post-Pandemic Deep Learning Algorithm Based on a Hybrid CT-Scan/X-Ray Images Classification Applied to Pneumonia Categories. *Healthcare*. **11**, 662 (2023)
31. Farahat, Z., Zrira, N., Souissi, N., Benamar, S., Belmekki, M., Ngote, M. & Megdiche, K. Application of Deep Learning Methods in a Moroccan Ophthalmic Center: Analysis and Discussion. *Diagnostics*. **13**, 1694 (2023)
32. Belharar, F. & Zrira, N. DeepRetino: Ophthalmic Disease Classification from Retinal Images using Deep Learning. *2022 IEEE 9th International Conference On Sciences Of Electronics, Technologies Of Information And Telecommunications (SETIT)*. pp. 392–399 (2022)
33. Jimi, A., Abouche, H., Zrira, N. & Benmiloud, I. Skin Lesion Segmentation Using Attention-Based DenseUNet. *BIOINFORMATICS*. pp. 91–100 (2023)

Global Prevalence Patterns of Anti-Asian Prejudice on Twitter During the COVID-19 Pandemic

Brittany Wheeler, Monika Purohit, Patrick Furman, Seong Jung, Deborah L. Hall, Maria Camila N. Barioni, and Yasin N. Silva

Abstract Anti-Asian prejudice increased during the COVID-19 pandemic, evidenced by a rise in physical attacks on individuals of Asian descent. Concurrently, as many governments enacted stay-at-home mandates, the spread of anti-Asian content increased in online spaces, including social media platforms such as Twitter. In the present study, we investigated temporal and geographic patterns in the prevalence of social media content relevant to anti-Asian prejudice within the U.S. and worldwide. Specifically, we used the Twitter Data Collection API to query over 13 million tweets posted during the first 15 months of the pandemic (i.e., from January 30, 2020 to April 30, 2021), for both negative (e.g., #kungflu) and positive (e.g., #stopAAPIhate) hashtags and keywords related to anti-Asian prejudice. Results of a range of exploratory and descriptive analyses offer novel insights. For instance, in the U.S., results from a burst analysis indicated that the prevalence of negative (anti-Asian) and positive (counter-hate) messages fluctuated over time in patterns that largely mirrored salient events relevant to COVID-19 (e.g., political tweets, highly-visible hate crimes targeting Asians). Other representative findings include geographic differences in the frequency of negative and positive keywords that shed light on the regions within the U.S. and the countries worldwide in which negative and positive messages were most frequent. Additional analyses revealed informative patterns in the prevalence of original tweets versus retweets, the co-occurrence of negative and positive content within a tweet, and fluctuations in content in relation to the number of new COVID-19 cases and reported COVID-related deaths. Together,

B. Wheeler · S. Jung · D. L. Hall (✉)
Arizona State University, Glendale, AZ, USA
e-mail: bmwheel5@asu.edu; shjung3@asu.edu; d.hall@asu.edu

M. Purohit · P. Furman · Y. N. Silva
Loyola University Chicago, Chicago, IL, USA
e-mail: mpurohit@luc.edu; pfurman@luc.edu; ysilva1@luc.edu

M. C. N. Barioni
Federal University of Uberlândia, Uberlândia, Brazil
e-mail: camila.barioni@ufu.br

M. Kaya et al. (eds.), *Social Network Analysis and Mining Applications in Healthcare and Anomaly Detection*, Lecture Notes in Social Networks,
https://doi.org/10.1007/978-3-031-75204-9_10

these findings underscore the value of research examining trends in social media messages of hate and counter-hate during the COVID-19 pandemic.

Keywords Anti-Asian prejudice · COVID-19 pandemic · Twitter · Counter-hate

1 Introduction

The World Health Organization (WHO) reported on January 4, 2020, that it was monitoring an outbreak of a new virus in the Wuhan, Hubei Province of China [1]. At this time, knowledge of and concern about the virus from the public was limited. Less than one month later, however, on January 30, the WHO declared the spread of the virus, termed COVID-19, a public health emergency, bringing global attention to this widespread health concern [1, 2]. The name 'coronavirus' was developed according to WHO's "Best Practices for the Naming of New Human Infectious Diseases," which recommends avoiding cultural, social, regional, or ethnic associations when naming a disease [3]. Despite these recommendations, because of the origins of the virus, COVID-19 was frequently referred to in the media as the "Chinese virus," the "Wuhan virus," and the "Asian virus" [4–7]. To illustrate, a widely-shared image revealed that President Trump had crossed out the word "corona" in "coronavirus" from his notes and replaced it with the word "Chinese" [8].

While some have argued that this terminology is not inherently racist, given the virus' origin, anti-Asian prejudice notably increased in prevalence and salience during this time [9–14]. For example, police reports in the U.S. involving anti-Asian hate and physical violence against Asian Americans and Pacific Islanders (AAPI) increased 145% in 2020 compared to previous years [11] and Stop AAPI Hate—a non-profit organization dedicated to reducing anti-Asian prejudice—reported 2583 incidents of anti-Asian prejudice between March 18, 2020 and August 5, 2020 [15]. This number of incidents may, in fact, be higher given that these only represent reported instances and do not account for unreported acts of hate or harassment [16].

Online anti-Asian hate speech, defined as any online message that includes "profanity, offensive language, or toxicity" directed at Asian individuals [18], also increased during this time. The Anti-Defamation League, for instance, reported an 85% increase in anti-Asian discrimination online [19]. To illustrate, during the first months of the pandemic, 72,000 posts on Instagram contained the hashtag #WuhanVirus, while another 10,000 contained the hashtag #KungFlu [20]. Notably, social media posts (i.e., tweets) generated by President Trump and other political leaders used the phrase "Chinese Virus" [9]. The role of these tweets in promoting the continued use of the term is perhaps reflected by the finding that 18% of tweets using anti-Asian hashtags referred to Trump in some capacity [9, 21]. In fact, recent research by Kim and Kesari [22] identified marked increases in anti-Asian terminology after President Trump first started using similar language.

Whereas some have argued that the use of this language is benign, others have found its deliberate and continued use signals support for anti-Asian attitudes and contributes to the proliferation and wider dissemination of hateful messages [9, 23]. The increased prevalence of hate in online spaces is also particularly concerning, given that it has paralleled increases in real-life (i.e., offline) hate crimes [17, 24]. Indeed, the use of these terms is one of the most frequently cited reasons for the increase in anti-Asian hate crimes, according to individuals of Asian descent [10, 11].

Research has demonstrated that, despite its widespread nature, hateful content on Twitter tends to be produced by a small number of users—an alarming finding given the amount of content produced [25]. Interestingly, counter-hate content (i.e., positive language intended to combat hateful messages) that drew connections between anti-Asian terminology and xenophobia and prejudice also increased during this time [22]. Producers of counter-hate content were more likely to be women, younger adults, and—perhaps not surprisingly in light of the profound impact on their lives—Asian-American reporters, professors, and politicians [26].

Although a number of studies on anti-Asian sentiment during the COVID-19 pandemic have been conducted within the United States, comparatively fewer studies have taken a global perspective on this issue. Yet, it is important to recognize that violent attacks and hate speech online are not limited to one particular geographic location. Reports from the United Kingdom, for instance, have shown that Asian individuals were also subjected to physical assaults and exclusion from various social settings [27–29].

In order to better understand national-level cultural differences related to anti-Asian sentiment, Hofstede's cultural dimensions [30, 31] have been used in previous research. Hofstede's framework suggests that there are several key factors associated with evaluating cultural differences, including individualism (i.e., the extent to which individuals are integrated within the community), masculinity (i.e., the extent to which emotional roles are distributed evenly across genders), uncertainty avoidance (i.e., the extent to which individuals within a culture can feel comfortable in uncertain situations), and power distance (i.e., the extent to which power is distributed equally across members of the community).

Building on this, Ng [31] found that cultures high in individualism, power distance, and uncertainty avoidance, such as the United Kingdom, India, and Ghana, exhibited higher levels of negative, anti-Asian sentiment during the pandemic. This phenomenon can be attributed to various factors that are unique to each cultural dimension. In societies that value individualism, individuals tend to prioritize their personal opinions and express their emotions more openly [31]. Consequently, there was a greater tendency to direct blame and anger toward Asian individuals during the pandemic, resulting in a higher level of negative sentiments [31]. Cultures with high power distance tend to exhibit greater inequality, which perpetuates social hierarchies and fuels xenophobic sentiments toward individuals perceived to have a lower status. Thus, high power distance predicted a heightened level of negative sentiment directed toward Asian individuals, who were deemed unworthy of respect due to their perceived lower status [31]. Cultures with high uncertainty avoidance tend to label others based on a variety of stigmas that reinforce negative stereotypes and perpetuate a lack of tolerance toward certain groups of people [31]. In the case of the COVID-19 pandemic, this construct was also associated with increased negative sentiment directed toward Asian individuals [31].

In addition to research that adopts a global perspective, studies that build on and speak to the relationship between online hate and real-world outcomes [17, 24] may be particularly beneficial. By the middle of 2021, the COVID-19 pandemic had caused the loss of over four million lives globally, with more than 188 million individuals contracting the virus [32]. One important consideration is how the prevalence of online anti-Asian content may have varied in relation to COVID-19 milestones and transmission rates, such as the number of new COVID-19 cases and COVID-19-related deaths.

Finally, it is worth noting that prejudicial attitudes have also been observed during other infectious disease outbreaks [33–36]. In the U.S., the 2009 H1N1 outbreak originating in Mexico led to a surge in stigma against Mexicans and people of Hispanic descent [34, 36]. Similarly, after the 2003 Severe Acute Respiratory Syndrome (SARS) outbreak, which was linked to China, Asian Americans were targeted with disease-related stigma [33]. A crucial difference between these prior outbreaks and the COVID-19 pandemic, however, is the pervasiveness of social media in the daily lives of individuals on a global scale. Thus, understanding temporal and geographic patterns in anti-Asian content online during the COVID-19 pandemic—especially in the context of influential events and pandemic-related milestones—can provide unique insights about the spread of online hate, more generally, during global public health crises.

In this paper, we present the results of a range of exploratory and descriptive analyses to shed light on anti-Asian prejudice—as well as messages to counter this hate—on Twitter during a 15-month span of the COVID-19 pandemic. We begin by reviewing findings originally discussed in our previous work [37] that offer insights on temporal and geographic patterns in the frequency of anti-Asian and counter-hate content. Crucially, however, we extend our previous work in several important ways. For instance, one concern with the frequent use of anti-Asian rhetoric on social media has been the potential for the re-circulation of this content. On Twitter, re-circulation can occur through replies (i.e., a tweet directed at the original poster by utilizing the ‘reply’ button) and retweets (i.e., a pure echoing of content created by another user) [38]. Retweeting hateful anti-Asian content is particularly harmful, as it allows the content to be amplified and reach new and wider audiences, signals support from a listening audience, and validates the original poster’s ideas [39]. While limited research has evaluated this re-circulation with a focus on anti-Asian messages, research by Lindgren [38] examining other online movements found that increased retweets can be viewed as micro-acts of support. This is further illustrated by the work of Solovev and Prollochs [40], who found that tweets initially containing more negative sentiment are more likely to contain higher levels of hate speech within replies.

In our previous work [37], we sought to contribute to the body of research regarding anti-Asian prejudice by covering a significantly longer time frame, considering both anti-Asian and positive keywords, and employing a relatively under-utilized method (i.e., burst analysis) to understand trends in keyword use associated with anti-Asian prejudice. In the present paper, we seek to expand on these findings by taking a more fine-grained approach to evaluating anti-Asian and counter-hate content on Twitter. Specifically, in our previous work, we covered broad trends in the use of specific hateful and counter-hate terminology—which, although beneficial, does not account for the differences in how users can engage with this content (i.e., reply, retweet, post original content). Additionally, given that previous research has indicated that most hateful content is produced by a relatively limited number of users [25], we seek to evaluate trends in anti-Asian and counter-hate messages within the top 10% of producers of relevant content. That is, understanding the trends associated with the most "influential" users can provide valuable insights, given their centrality within online discussions. Also, while global trends were touched upon within our previous paper, we dis-aggregate this content to better understand negative and positive content trends from the top three countries producing this content. Drawing on Hofstede's work on cultural dimensions [30], we aim to develop an understanding of why certain countries generated more anti-Asian and counter-hate content. Furthermore, new additions to this work include an evaluation of the co-occurrence of anti-Asian and counter-hate keywords at the level of individual tweets and a descriptive analysis of reply conversion (i.e., when replies to a message change sentiment). These analyses can provide a better understanding of the interplay of anti-Asian and counter-hate messages within tweets and the subsequent online interactions they elicit. Lastly, we re-generated several of the figures presented in our previous work which only considered U.S. data with a broader focus on global trends and integrated data on new COVID-19 cases and COVID-related deaths with temporal trends in anti-Asian and counter-hate tweets.

The remainder of the paper is organized as follows: In Sect. 2, we discuss in greater detail the procedures we employed to collect and clean two complementary sets of Twitter data. In Sect. 3, we present the results of a set of diverse analyses examining temporal and geographic patterns in the data, as well as exploratory findings that shed light on more nuanced aspects of anti-Asian and counter-hate content. Finally, in Sect. 4, we discuss implications, limitations, and crucial directions for future research.

2 Methods

2.1 Data

All data were collected according to Twitter data collection guidelines and using the proper API access provided to researchers [41, 42]. In the following sections, we refer to anti-Asian content as "negative" and counter-hate content as "positive."

Archive Dataset Using the Twitter Data Collection API [43], we queried tweets containing negative and positive hashtags and keywords related to anti-Asian prejudice from January 30, 2020 to April 30, 2021. This time frame was selected to correspond with the date on which the World Health Organization indicated the spread of COVID-19 was a global health issue and the start of AAPI Heritage Month the following year (when positive AAPI messages might increase independent of COVID-19). We used 12 specific negative hashtags/keywords as indicators of anti-Asian prejudice (#batsoup, #chinavirus, #gobacktochina, #chinesevirus, #chineseplague, #gook, #chinaliedpeopledied, #kungflu, #wuflu, #chingchong, #makechinapay, #ccpvirus) and 5 specific positive hashtags/keywords (#hateisavirus, #Iamnotavirus, #racismisavirus, #washthehate, #stopasianhate), which were chosen based on the relevant literature [44], news publications [45–47], and social media posts discussing anti-Asian attitudes during the beginning of the pandemic. The total sample consisted of 13,008,053 tweets from 3,298,940 distinct users.

1% Dataset The 1% sample stream dataset was generated from Twitter's sample stream endpoint [49] which provides access to a roughly 1% random sample of publicly available tweets in real-time. This dataset was compiled from the tweets gathered over the course of 24 hours (August 1–2, 2021) to estimate the amount of activity that 1% of the Twitter platform could generate in one day. 4,093,933 tweets were collected in this sample from 2,956,806 distinct users.

2.2 *Geographic Location Labeling*

During the collection of both datasets, a filter was applied to collect a list of users who had publicly available geolocation data through their location settings. To perform descriptive analyses based on geographic location, we devised a geolocation labeling strategy similar to Jiang et al. [48]. This strategy was necessary because less than 0.5% of the tweets in our dataset had available geo_place information. For our analysis, we considered the state granularity for the tweets originating in the U.S. and the country granularity for the tweets originating in other countries, based on self-reported user profile locations. Using a fuzzy text matching algorithm [50], pre-processed user-reported locations were matched against a set of predetermined locations inside and outside of the U.S. The similarity between user-reported locations and predetermined locations was computed using the edit distance metric. The score threshold to consider a matching pair of locations, which was set to 80%, was defined based on a validation analysis conducted by an external human annotator who manually verified a random sample of labeled locations considering country names and U.S. state names. Considering the precision validation measure (TP/(TP + FP)), the geolocation labeling strategy achieved a predictive positive value of 99.8% for the U.S. locations and varied from 89.8% to 100% for the other countries that, together with the U.S., account for 90% of the collected data. The set of predetermined locations inside the U.S. consisted of state names and state abbreviations. The set of predetermined locations outside the U.S. was built using the top 20 countries with the most Twitter users as of July 2020 [53] and their 5 most populous cities [54]. To avoid ambiguity, only the country abbreviations that didn't overlap with a U.S. state abbreviation were included. Additionally, we used an ambiguous locations list—built throughout the testing process—to adjust the geolocation labeling by removing ambiguous matches. (An example of an ambiguous match is the token 'valencia,' which can refer to a city in Spain and a town in California.)

2.3 Analytic Plan

Using the previously described datasets, a series of descriptive analyses were performed to investigate the overall prevalence of negative and positive keyword use, as well as trends over time and across locations. We then performed a burst analysis to examine whether there were significant increases in the frequency of negative and positive keywords and, if so, whether such bursts in activity followed similar trends associated with offline hate directed at individuals of Asian descent. (Additional information about the burst detection analysis is presented in the following section.)

3 Results

3.1 Descriptive Analyses

Overall Tweet Frequency As shown in Fig. 1a, the use of negative keywords before March 2020 was relatively low. However, within that month, there was a marked increase in the use of negative keywords, with the frequency of negative keywords reaching its peak later in that month. Although considerably less frequent throughout most portions of the timeline, the use of positive keywords, in contrast, culminated in major spikes in late February 2021. Similar trends are also apparent in Fig. 1b for the top 10% of users, as the frequency of these negative and positive keywords shows similar peaks in activity. The top 10% producers in our dataset generated 56.1% of tweets and the top 1% were responsible for 24.2%. Figure 1c displays the frequency of new COVID-19 cases and COVID-related deaths globally, based on data from the Centers for Disease Control [55]. Interestingly, there were two major spikes in the number of reported COVID-related deaths—the first occurring between the months of March 2020 and May 2020, coinciding with the surge in positive keyword frequencies seen in Fig. 1a. The second spike occurred in early 2021, when the number of positive keywords, especially "stopasianhate," increased sharply again. These findings suggest a potential link between real-world outcomes, such as the prevalence of COVID-19 cases and deaths, and the generation of counter-hate messages.

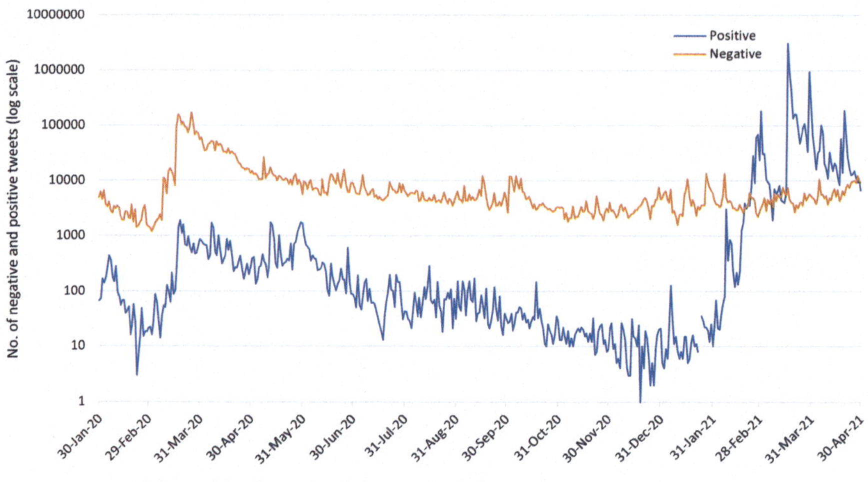

(a) Logarithmic scale of the number of negative and positive tweets.

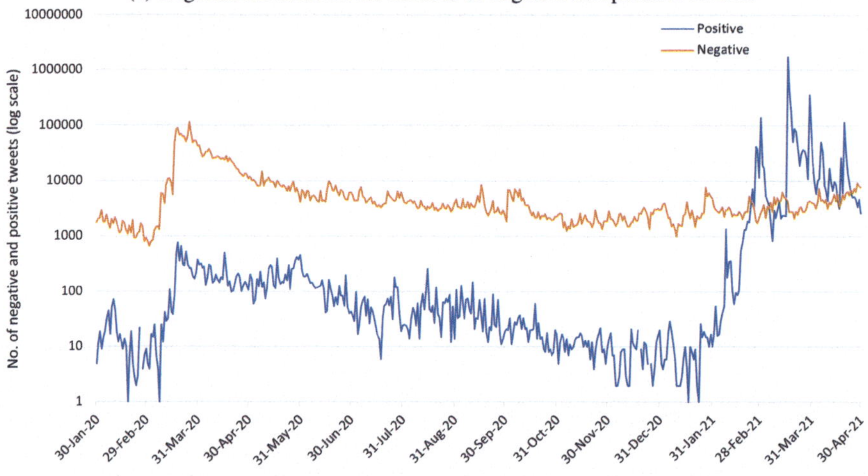

(b) Logarithmic scale of the number of negative and positive tweets for the top 10% of producers.

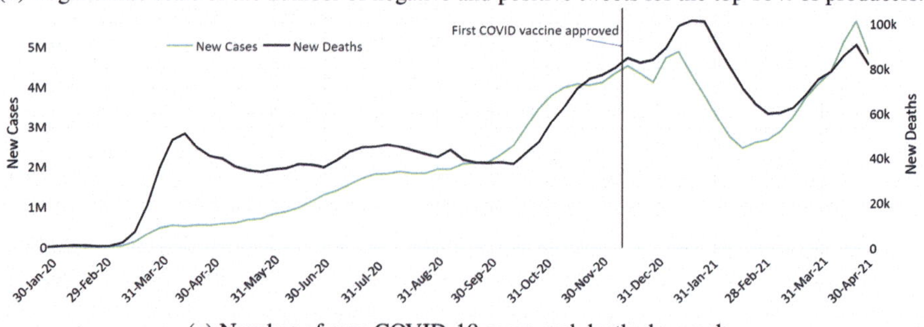

(c) Number of new COVID-19 cases and deaths by week.

Fig. 1 Global number of negative and positive tweets and the number of new COVID-19 cases and deaths between January 2020 and April 2021. (**a**) Logarithmic scale of the number of negative and positive tweets. (**b**) Logarithmic scale of the number of negative and positive tweets for the top 10% of producers. (**c**) Number of new COVID-19 cases and deaths by week

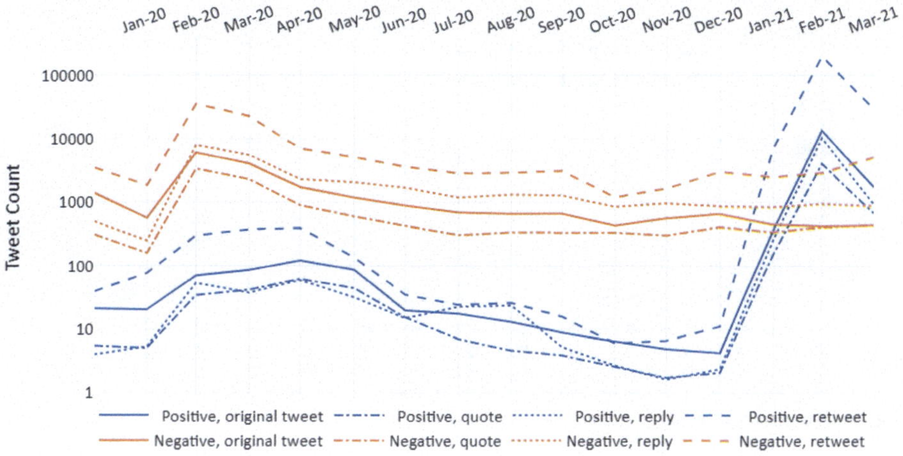

Fig. 2 Number of negative and positive tweets between January 2020 and April 2021 by type of tweet

Trends by Type of Tweet To analyze the relation between different types of tweets, we broke down the data presented in Fig. 1a to examine trends over time based on tweet type (i.e., original tweet, quote, reply, retweet). Retweets, in particular, may be useful for gauging agreement with an original tweet, as they do not alter its meaning. As depicted in Fig. 2, the vast majority of tweets (78.39%) were retweets, indicating that most tweets containing our selected keywords were not original content. Additionally, while 87.72% of positive tweets were retweets, only 62.99% of negative tweets were retweets, suggesting that tweets containing negative keywords may have been less popular to share overall. Quotes were the least common tweet type, accounting for only 3.75% of tweets. Similar to Fig. 1a, the dis-aggregated trends in Fig. 2 exhibited comparable patterns over time, with the ratio between the different tweet types remaining relatively constant, particularly for negative tweets. However, we noted a significant spike in the frequency of retweets containing positive keywords around December 2020, compared to subsequent months. This shift was remarkable given that, for several months prior to December, the number of positive retweets was not substantially greater than replies or original tweets. During these same months, negative retweets were far more prevalent than other types of negative tweets, but this dynamic abruptly reversed between December 2020 and February 2021. Replies, unlike retweets, were primarily negative, with 71.76% of them containing negative keywords, and they were also less common, accounting for only 9.73% of tweets in our dataset.

Sentiment Transitions Figure 3 displays daily counts of the number of replies where the original tweet contained a positive keyword and the reply contained a negative keyword or vice versa. We refer to a negative response to a positive tweet as a "positive to negative transition" in the figure. Across all tweets in our data, we only observed 454 transitions of any kind, which amounts to less than 0.04% of

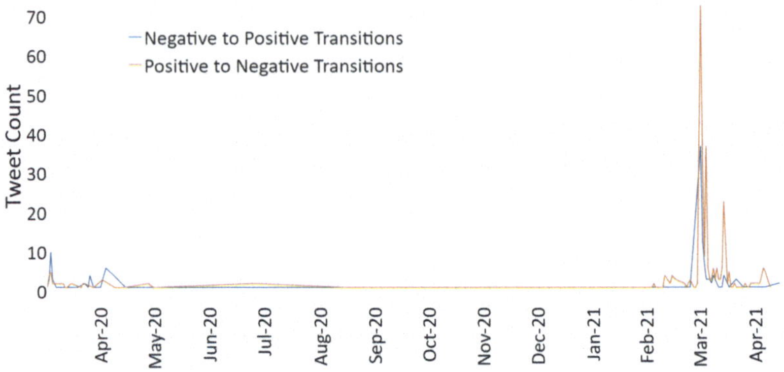

Fig. 3 Frequency of reply conversions

the total number of replies—in short, transitions were a particularly rare occurrence. The vast majority of these transitions occurred between February and April of 2021, the same period in which the "stopasianhate" keyword peaked in frequency. Most of these transitions were positive to negative transitions, suggesting a strong response by users of negative keywords to the sudden surge in positive keyword frequency, which was not observed in other time periods.

Trends by Type of Keyword Figure 4 depicts trends in negative and positive keyword use for the whole dataset over time. As shown, sharp spikes in negative activity occurred following President Trump's first use of the term "Chinese Virus" in March 2020 [4]. Additionally, although there were more tweets containing positive keywords, overall, these tweets were mainly generated between February 2021 and April 2021. That is, they coincided with a prominent event that occurred in the U.S.—the Atlanta-area spa shootings that resulted in the deaths of multiple individuals of Asian-descent [51]. There was minimal use of these keywords during the early months of the pandemic. As shown in Fig. 4a, the most frequently used negative keyword was "ccpvirus," followed by "chinavirus" and "chinesevirus." The most frequently used positive keywords were "stopasianhate" and "hateisavirus."

Tweets Vs. Retweets for Individual Keywords Given the proportion of retweets within the data, we also evaluated the proportion of frequently used keywords within types of retweets, specifically (see Figs. 5, 6, and 7). Three of the four most frequently retweeted keywords were positive, implying that tweets containing negative keywords may have been less appealing to share (i.e., retweet). Furthermore, reflecting its popularity, 88.02% of tweets referencing the "stopasianhate" keyword were retweets. The only keyword with a higher proportion of retweets was "chineseplague," with 89.35% of tweets being retweets.

Co-occurrence Patterns Figure 8 displays the frequency of pairs of keywords used together in the same conversation (defined as an original tweet and all replies to

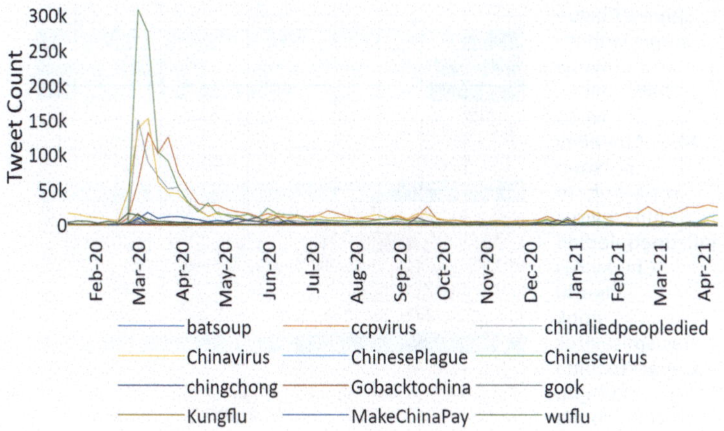

(a) Frequency of Negative Keyword Use on Twitter

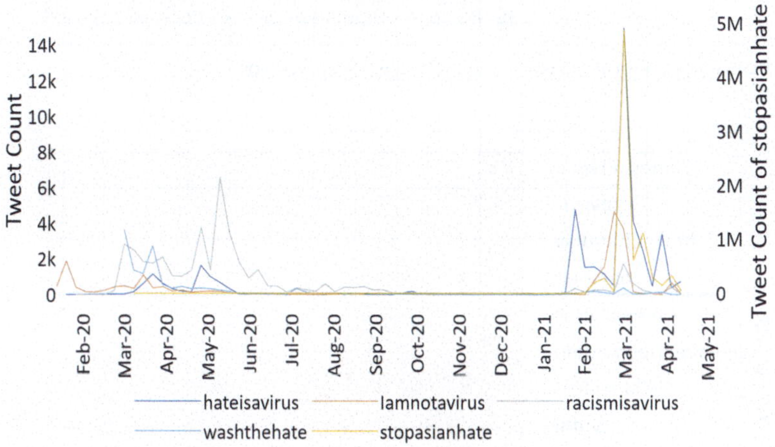

(b) Frequency of Positive Keyword Use on Twitter

Fig. 4 Frequency of negative and positive keywords on Twitter between January 2020 and April 2021. (**a**) Frequency of negative keyword use on Twitter. (**b**) Frequency of positive keyword use on Twitter

that tweet). We can observe that, except for "chineseplague," "hateisavirus," and "racismisavirus," when more than one keyword appeared in the same conversation, the subsequent keyword(s) tended to be the same (instead of a different) keyword. We did not find this pattern of mirroring, or repetition, for the positive keywords, perhaps because "stopasianhate" alone comprised more than 98% of all positive keyword use. That is, other positive keywords tended to appear alongside "stopasianhate." One possible explanation is that "iamnotavirus" and "washthehate" were either popular with different users from those who used "stopasianhate" or

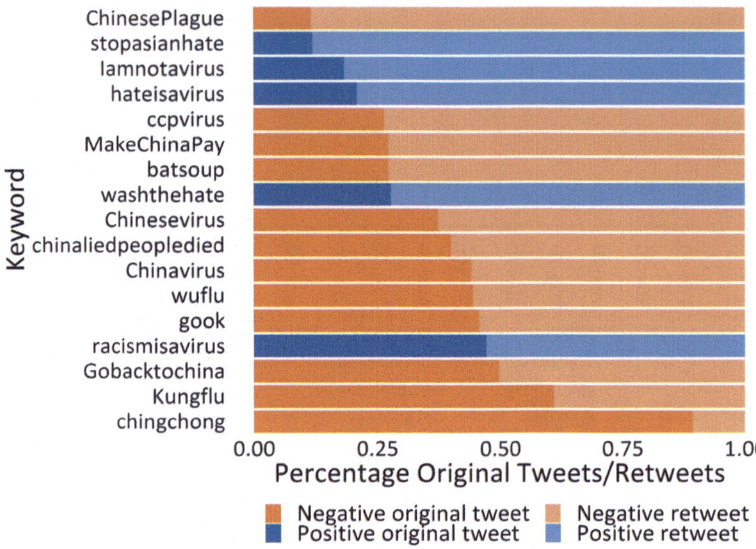

Fig. 5 Percentages of original tweets and retweets for all keywords

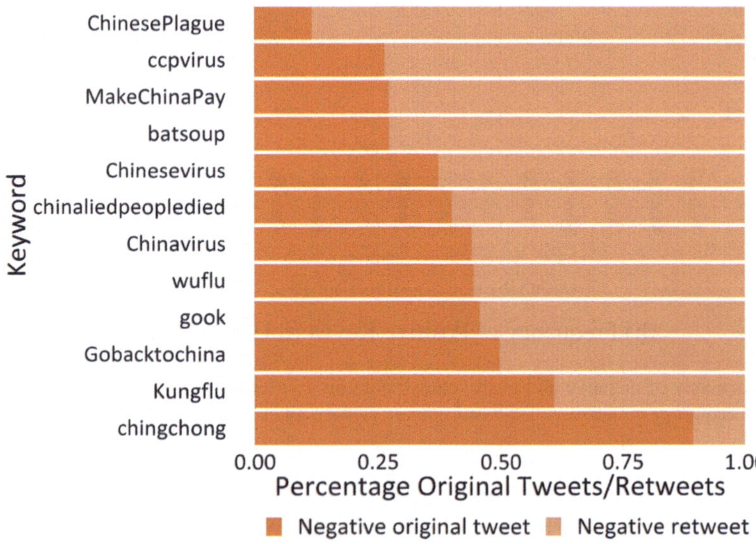

Fig. 6 Percentages of original tweets and retweets for negative keywords

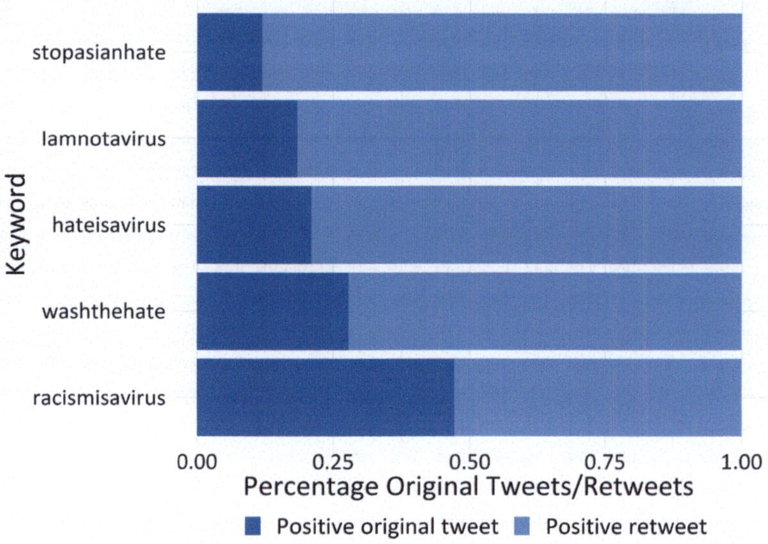

Fig. 7 Percentages of original tweets and retweets for positive keywords

	ccpvirus	batsoup	chinaliedpeopledied	chinavirus	chineseplague	chinesevirus	chingchong	gobacktochina	gook	hateisavirus	iamnotavirus	kungflu	makechinapay	racismisavirus	washthehate	wuflu	stopasianhate
ccpvirus	252331																
batsoup	103	33329															
chinaliedpeopledied	87092	157	364055														
chinavirus	110649	32711	160750	438155													
chineseplague	93	0	315	567	972												
chinesevirus	118472	32651	226883	317586	1525	962131											
chingchong	67	2	196	373	1	1437	1857										
gobacktochina	0	0	0	4	0	2	0	6									
gook	36	2	49	55	0	115	53	0	30935								
hateisavirus	10	0	11	26	0	141	0	0	2	70683							
iamnotavirus	12	1	10	31	0	184	0	0	2	1824	6164						
kungflu	2024	127	5917	11017	36	20106	63	0	34	39	35	24548					
makechinapay	30167	19	41315	27827	9	29439	13	0	9	0	0	129	91781				
racismisavirus	75	0	306	176	0	598	0	0	0	4690	2762	74	23	12379			
washthehate	0	0	53	27	0	120	0	0	0	3535	2398	32	11	4330	15376		
wuflu	4101	35	3119	21309	24	11109	16	0	11	2	0	3368	205	8	0	32959	
stopasianhate	25723	6	809	24480	0	5952	2645	0	3034	229277	3233	3235	6	46216	2212	243	501514264

Fig. 8 Frequency table of the number of times keywords co-occur in the same conversation

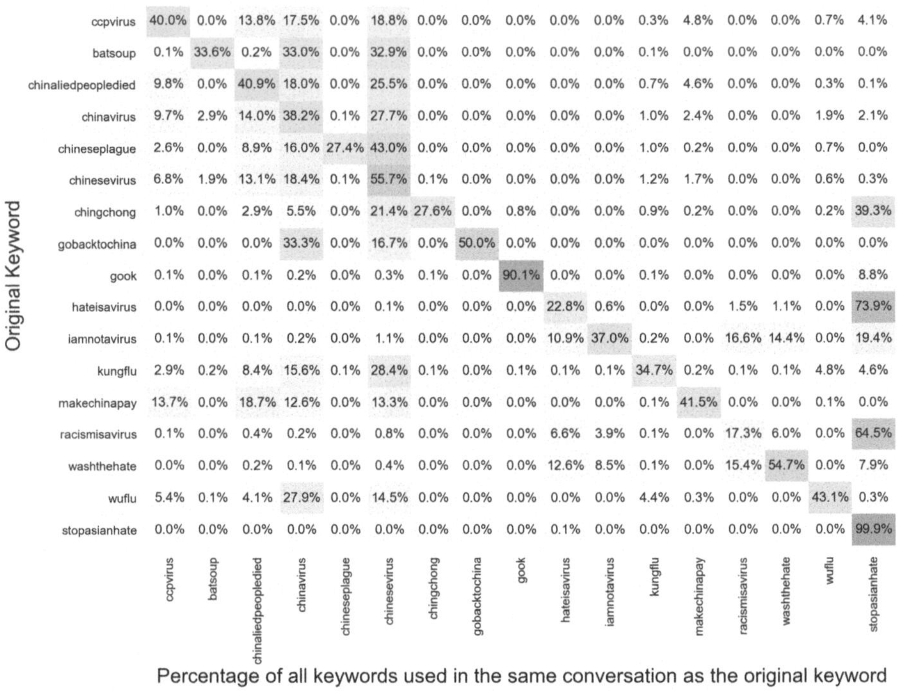

Fig. 9 Percentage of times keywords co-occur in the same conversation

were popular at different points in time. While some keywords, such as "gook," were almost never used together with other keywords in a conversation, most keywords showed some level of co-occurrence with other keywords. In cases of co-occurrence, positive keywords tended to be paired with other positive keywords, and negative keywords with other negative keywords.

Notably, the negative keywords "chinesevirus," "chinavirus," "chinaliedpeopledied," "batsoup," and "ccpvirus" frequently appeared together relative to their individual usage. This implies that these particular negative keywords might have either a similar meaning or a common group of supporters and users. Figure 9 provides a simplified comparison between keywords of varying frequencies. It is a scaled version of Fig. 8, where each entry represents the percentage of co-occurrences of the original keyword on the left with the corresponding keyword on the bottom, within the same conversation. This is based on the condition that the conversation contained at least two keywords. Although positive keywords rarely appeared with negative keywords and vice versa, "chingchong" was an exception. Specifically, given an initial tweet containing the keyword "chingchong," 39.3% of keywords that appeared in the same conversation were "stopasianhate." This may be partly explained by the overwhelmingly greater frequency of "stopasianhate" than "chingchong" and the finding that other negative keywords appeared alongside a

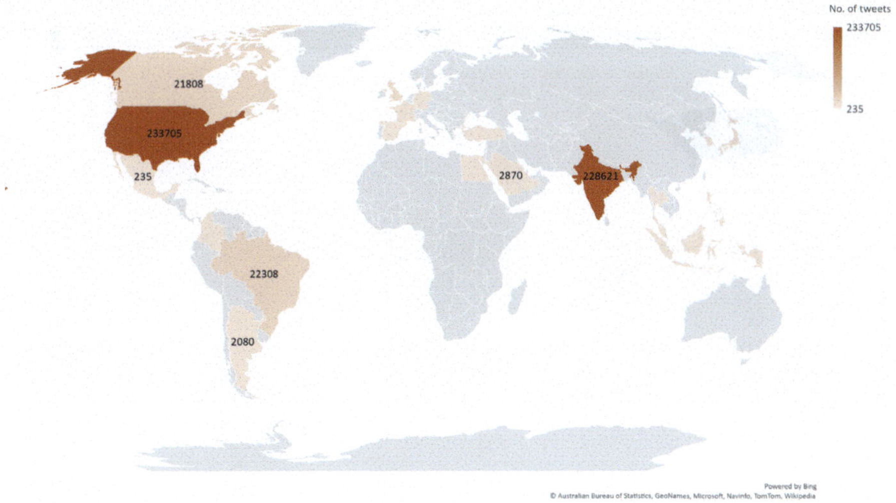

Fig. 10 Count of negative tweets per country

positive keyword less than 10% of the time. This suggests that "chingchong" was more likely than other negative keywords to spark discourse on Twitter between users of positive and negative keywords, although further analysis is needed to determine the exact nature of these interactions.

3.2 Regional Trends

Despite its global impact, the COVID-19 pandemic affected different parts of the world at differing rates. Whereas trends in various geographic regions share similarities with the aggregated global trends, exploration of regional differences in negative and positive tweets can yield novel insights.

Negative Keyword Use As shown in Figs. 10, 11, 12, and 13, globally, 4,521,457 distinct tweets contained at least one of the 12 negative keywords, with most of this content generated in the U.S. and India (USA = 233,705 tweets; IND = 228,621 tweets). Within the U.S., New York, California, and Florida were the largest producers of negative content (NY = 37,986 tweets; CA = 30,139 tweets; FL = 27,076).

Figure 14a shows that within the U.S., the country with the highest frequency of negative content, most negative keywords were used infrequently until February 2020, after which point, there was a gradual increase. The majority of negative keywords were used between February and March 2020; after this, there was a clear decline in negative keyword use. The term "Chinesevirus" was the most frequently used negative keyword in the U.S., peaking in March 2020 before declining. In March and April 2020, the most commonly used negative keywords were

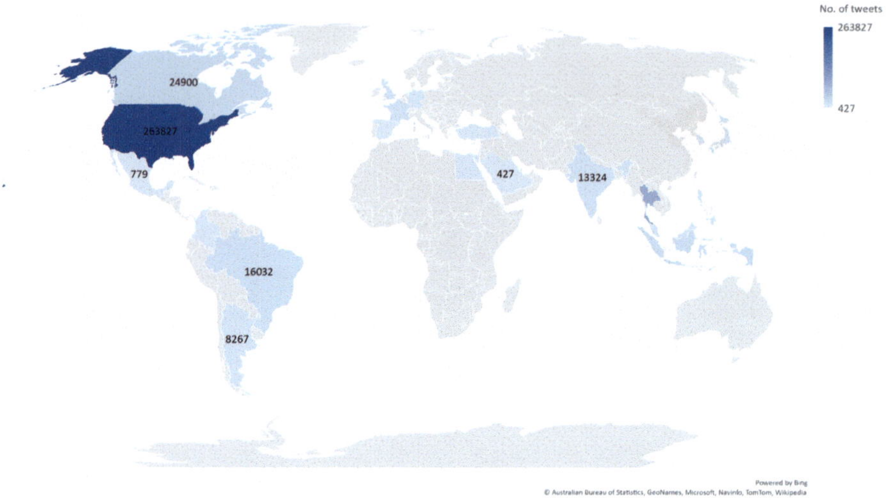

Fig. 11 Count of positive tweets per country

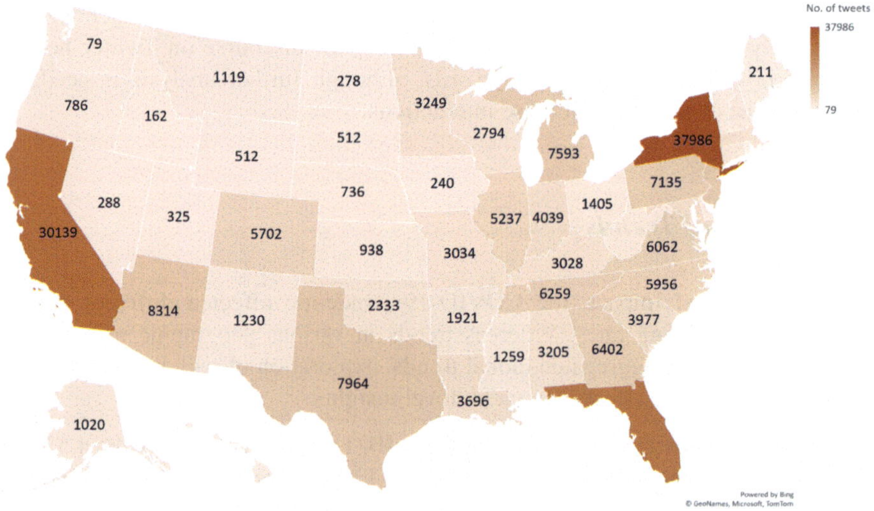

Fig. 12 Count of negative tweets in the U.S.

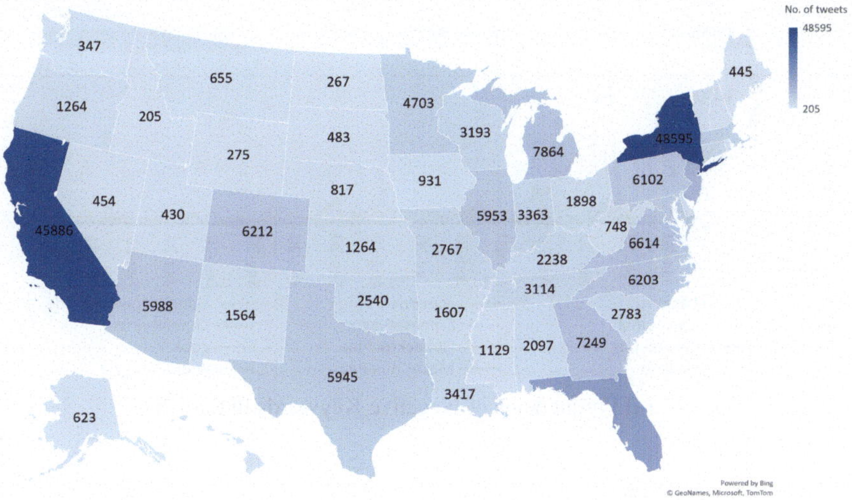

Fig. 13 Count of positive tweets in the U.S.

"Chinavirus," "ccpvirus," "wuflu," "kungflu," "makechinapay," and "Chinesevirus." Although negative keyword use declined after April 2020, small spikes in "kungflu" and "Chinavirus" were observed in June 2020.

As shown in Fig. 14b, India—the second-highest producer of negative content—showed similar trends. Negative keyword use in India began in February 2020, peaked between February and July 2020, and then gradually declined. "Chinavirus" was the most frequently used negative keyword in India, mainly in March, April, and July 2020. Other frequently used negative keywords in India were "Chinaliedpeopledied," "ccpvirus," and "MakeChinaPay." Figure 14c shows that in Brazil, the third-highest producer of negative content, negative keyword use did not begin until February 2020, at which point it began to rise. "Chinavirus" was the most frequently used negative keyword in Brazil, peaking in March 2020 before declining. After April 2020, the use of negative keywords in Brazil was minimal.

Positive Keyword Use The analysis of positive content in different regions revealed interesting trends across different countries (Figs. 10, 11, 12, and 13). 6,660,469 distinct tweets contained at least one of the 5 positive keywords, with most of the positive content also generated in the U.S., followed by Thailand (USA = 263,827 tweets; TH = 82,696 tweets). Notably, California and New York also produced the most content containing positive keywords (CA = 45,886; NY = 48,595). As depicted in Fig. 15a, in the U.S., the top producer of positive tweets, positive keyword use was low until February 2020, after which point it began to rise steadily. The most frequently used keyword was "stopasianhate," followed by "racismisvirus" and "hateisavirus," which reached their peaks in May 2020 and March 2021, respectively. "Washthehate" and "hateisavirus" showed surges in

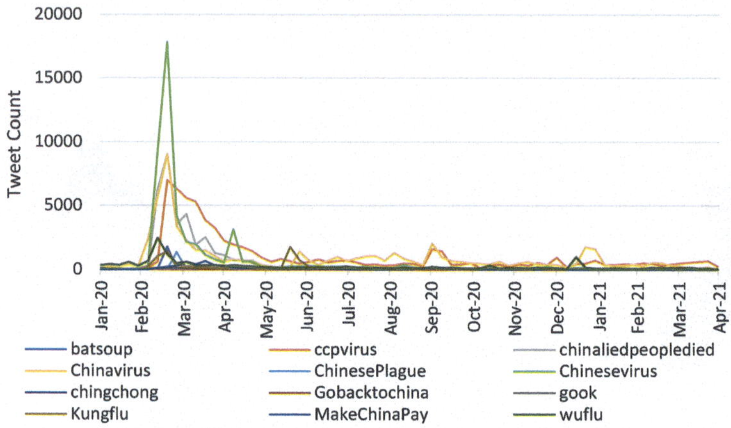

(a) Frequencies of Negative Keywords in the US

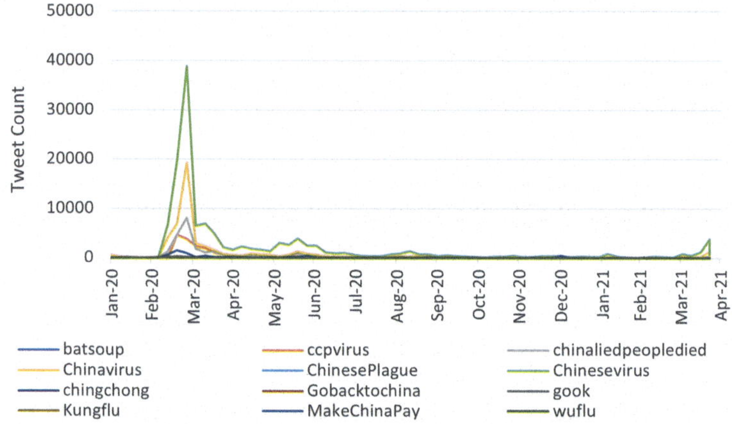

(b) Frequencies of Negative Keywords in India

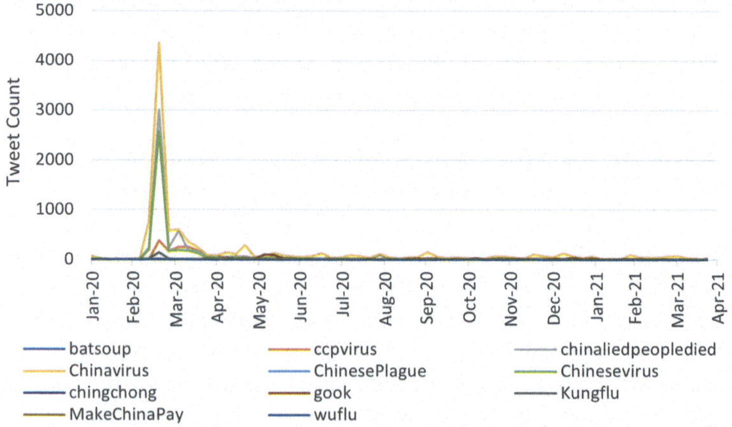

(c) Frequencies of Negative Keywords in Brazil

Fig. 14 Frequencies of each negative keyword over the data collection period created by the top three countries of production. (**a**) Frequencies of negative keywords in the US. (**b**) Frequencies of negative keywords in India. (**c**) Frequencies of negative keywords in Brazil

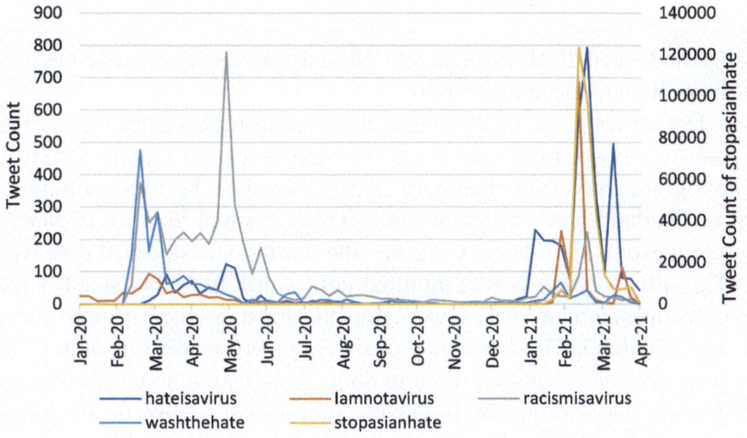

(a) Frequencies of Positive Keywords in the US

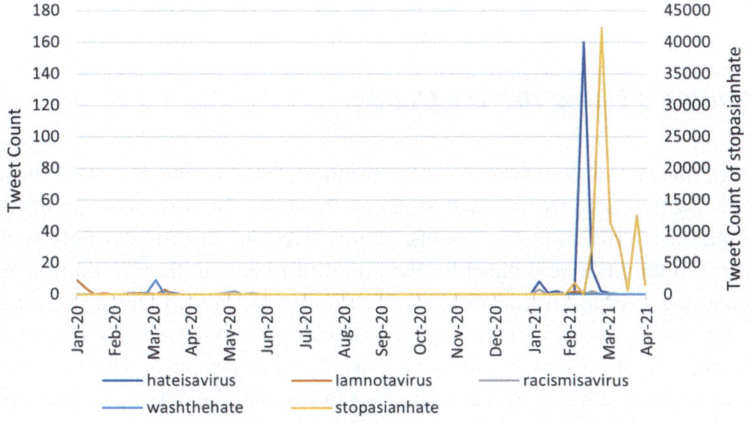

(b) Frequencies of Positive Keywords in Thailand

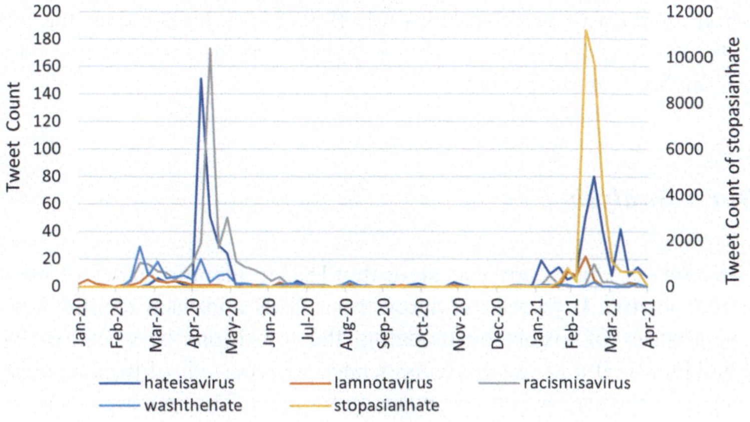

(c) Frequencies of Positive Keywords in Canada

Fig. 15 Frequencies of each positive keyword over the data collection period created by the top three countries of production. (**a**) Frequencies of positive keywords in the US. (**b**) Frequencies of positive keywords in Thailand. (**c**) Frequencies of positive keywords in Canada

March 2020 and April 2021, respectively. Notably, the use of positive keywords was minimal from June to December 2020.

Figure 15b shows that in Thailand, the second-highest producer of positive tweets, positive keyword use was almost non-existent until January 2021, but then picked up significantly from February 2021 onwards. The most commonly used keyword in Thailand was "stopasianhate," which reached its peak in March 2021. Lastly, as depicted in Fig. 15c, in Canada—the third top producer of positive tweets, the use of positive keywords was minimal until April 2020, but steadily increased thereafter. "Stopasianhate" was once again the most frequently used term, as in the U.S. and Thailand. The frequency of this keyword peaked in March 2021 and then began to decline. Together, these findings demonstrate that different countries showed distinct patterns in the frequency of positive keywords over time. The widespread use of "stopasianhate" across all three countries highlights the urgency of addressing anti-Asian sentiment globally.

3.3 Analyses Using the 1% Dataset

The goal of this task was to normalize the frequencies of tweets based on the amount of overall Twitter activity in each state of the U.S. To this end, an initial ratio was computed by dividing the counts of positive and negative tweets with valid geolocation in the archive dataset by the count of tweets in the 1% dataset for each state. Then, the average initial ratio was computed across all states (i.e., 4.277 for positive keywords and 3.786 for negative keywords). A new ratio was calculated for each state by dividing the initial ratio by the average ratio. The final ratios for negative and positive keywords are reported in Fig. 16. As depicted, Tennessee had the highest ratio of negative keywords (i.e., 201% higher than the average), followed by Alaska, which was 151% higher than the average. In contrast, Washington D.C. had the highest ratio of positive keywords (i.e., 211% higher than the average), followed by Washington state (i.e., 203% higher than the average) and New York (i.e., 148% higher than the average).

3.4 Burst Analysis

We used Kleinberg's burst analysis algorithm [52] to identify bursts of heightened negative and positive keyword use across time. This approach identifies bursts of activity in a series of events by modeling the transitions between two states—baseline and bursty. Bursty states are associated with periods of time when an event (e.g., negative or positive tweets) is unusually frequent. The approach uses two main parameters, s and *gamma*, which affect different aspects of the way the algorithm detects bursts.

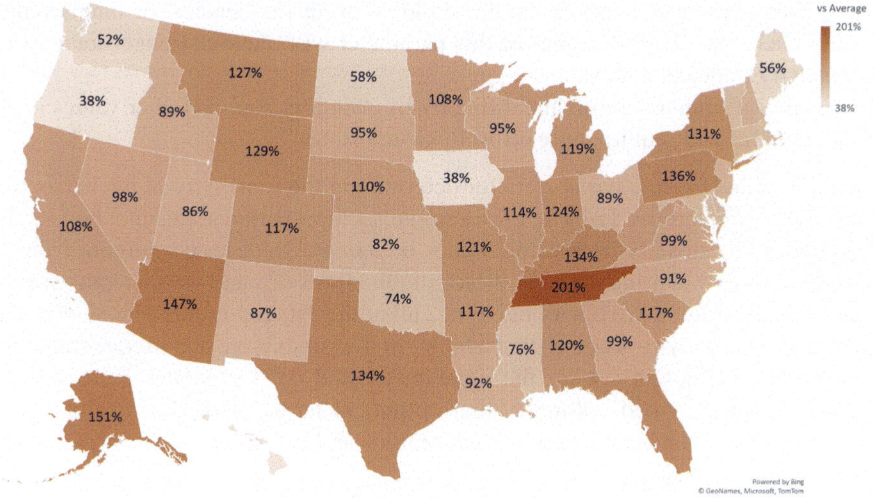

(a) Normalized Frequencies - Negative Keywords

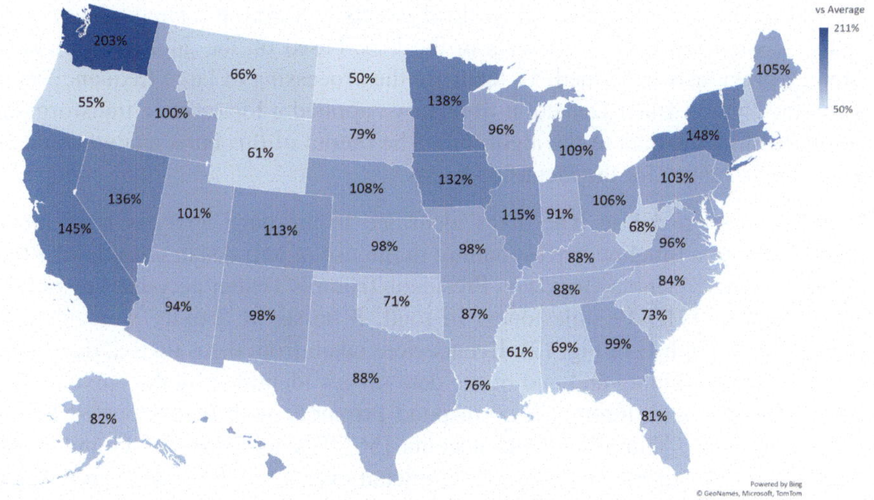

(b) Normalized Frequencies - Positive Keywords

Fig. 16 Normalized comparison of the frequencies of negative and positive keywords. The raw frequencies of the sample stream were first divided by the total number of tweets in the archive search produced in each state. Then, these ratios were averaged across all states. (**a**) Normalized frequencies—negative keywords. (**b**) Normalized frequencies—positive keywords

- *s*: This parameter controls the threshold of event frequencies, or intensiveness, for each state. Higher values of this parameter will require stronger increases of activity to detect a burst.
- *gamma*: Gamma controls the difficulty of changing states. Higher values of this parameter will require more effort to switch states.

Multiple *s* and *gamma* parameters for determining the sensitivity of the bursts were assessed in an iterative fashion. For example, as the *s* parameter cannot be less than or equal to 1, steadily decreasing values of *gamma* were tested ranging from the default of 1 to 0. During many of these combinations of *s* and *gamma* values, either the analysis resulted in a binary burst (i.e., all of the data represents a burst of activity or none of the activity is considered a burst) or the bursts were inconsequential. From this testing, values of 1.1 for the *s* parameter and 0.0 for *gamma* were selected. These values provided optimal visual output, in terms of producing the clearest separation between burst and non-burst regions and using multiple levels to capture burst intensity [52].

We performed separate burst analyses (with the same parameters) for the datasets with negative and positive keywords. Specifically, we used the burst detection algorithm to identify bursts in discrete bundles of events, where each bundle was defined as the set of negative or positive tweets received in a single day. For this analysis, we considered the tweets in the U.S. based on the geolocation labeling strategy previously described. To facilitate the processing of large frequency values using the Python Burst Detection library, we applied a logarithmic transformation before feeding the data to the algorithm. The output of this burst analysis step was a set of date ranges for the identified bursts.

Negative Keyword Use The dates identified in the burst analysis were labeled with events on a timeline corresponding to the use of anti-Asian terminology (e.g., “Chinese virus,” “China virus”) on President Trump’s Twitter account, key political events, and COVID-19 milestones. In total, 8 bursts of activity were identified (labeled A through H in Fig. 17). Events were taken from dates up to 2 days before and after the beginning and end of the date ranges identified by the burst analysis. Events for Bursts A through F correspond primarily with tweets posted by (and originating from) Trump’s Twitter account [56]. Events for Bursts G and H were taken from news media coverage of significant events [57, 58] that occurred at the time, as well as from the CDC’s COVID-19 pandemic timeline [59].

Positive Keyword Use Evaluating positive keyword use, 3 bursts of activity were identified, ranging from March 17, 2020 to June 16, 2020; June 19, 2020 to June 30, 2020; and February 2, 2021 to April 4, 2021 (Fig. 18). These bursts in positive keyword use immediately followed increases in physical violence and offline hate toward Asian Americans. For example, from March to June 2020, the Federal Bureau of Investigation reported increases in crimes directed toward Asian Americans [60]. Further, the burst of positive activity following February 2, 2021 culminates when there was a marked increase in physical violence against Asian individuals. For example, within this time frame, the highly-publicized Atlanta-area

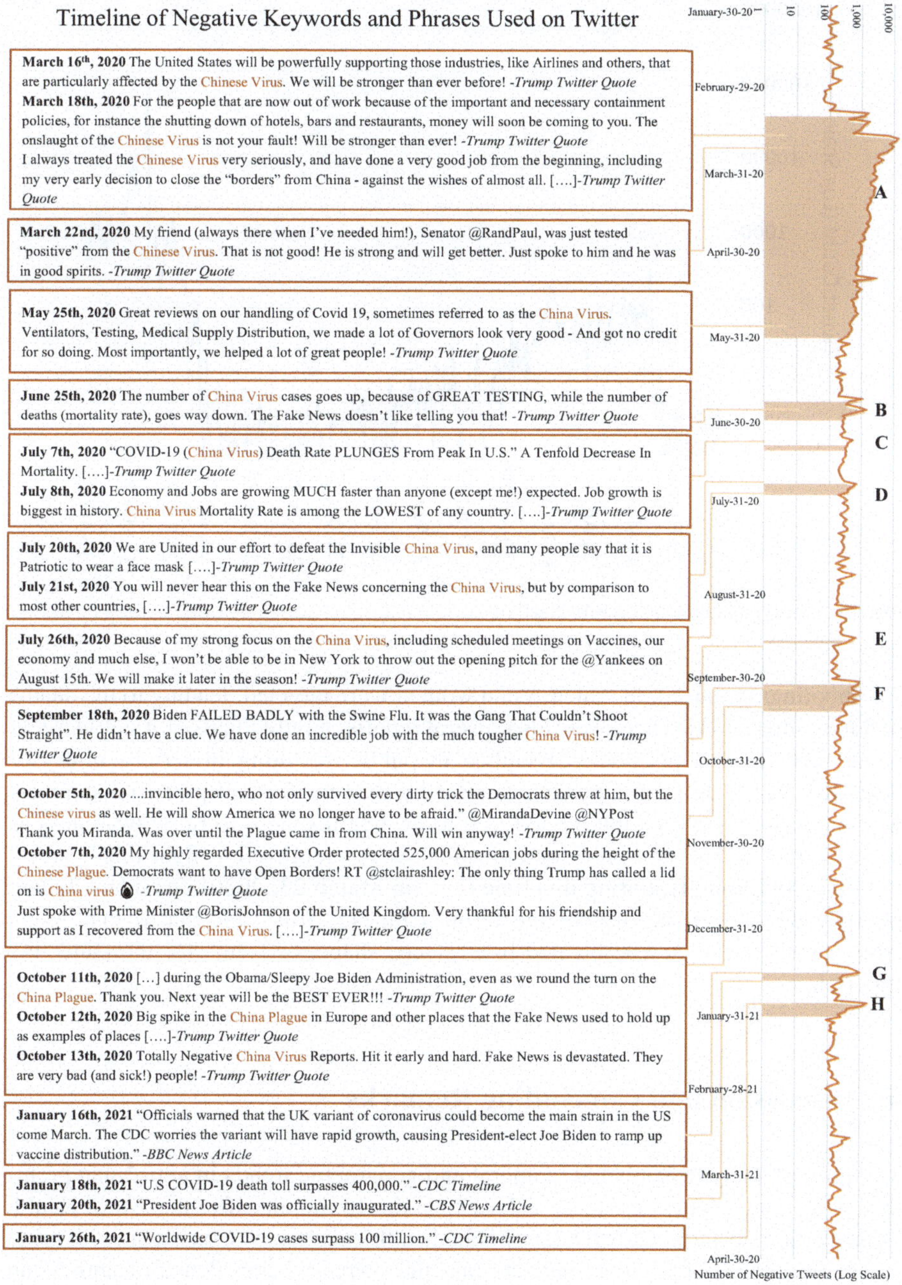

Fig. 17 Timeline of negative keywords and phrases with a subset of representative tweets occurring within bursts of heightened anti-Asian activity

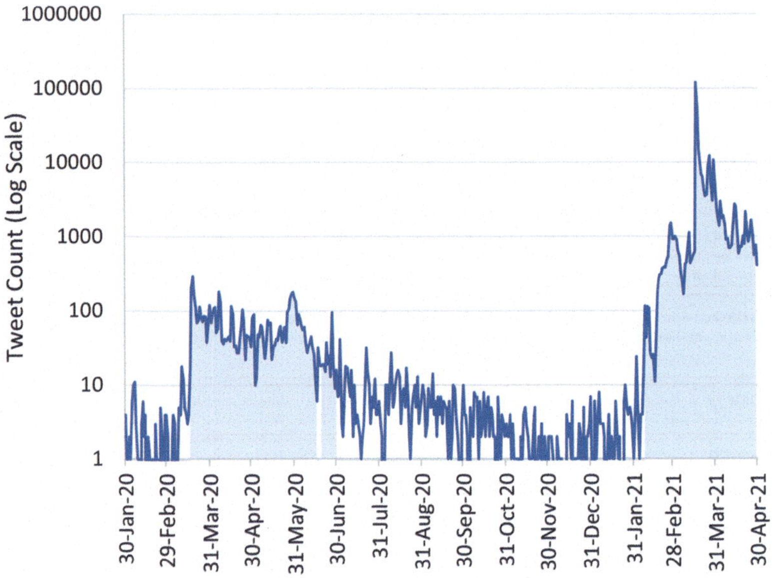

Fig. 18 Bursts of heightened positive activity

spa shootings occurred, in which Asian women were targeted, leading to the deaths of 8 individuals [51]. There were also several reports of individuals of Asian-descent being verbally and physically assaulted in public, resulting in serious injury or death [61, 62]. The burst in positive keyword use, in the form of prosocial, counter-hate messages, could be interpreted as a protective response to raise awareness as protests, rallies, and non-profit organizations were mobilized to fight this hostility [63–65]. Additionally, during this time (i.e., on March 23, 2020), President Trump publicly denounced his use of the term "Chinese virus" and stated that Asian Americans should "not be blamed in any way, shape, or form" for the pandemic [66, 67].

4 Discussion and Concluding Remarks

The present study investigated temporal and geographic trends in anti-Asian prejudice and counter-hate messages on Twitter in the 15 months after the World Health Organization declared COVID-19 a public health emergency. Consistent with other recent research, our findings indicate that the increased prevalence of anti-Asian prejudice during the early stages of the pandemic was a global phenomenon [68, 69]. Specifically, marked increases in anti-Asian hate on Twitter occurred during the months of February 2020 and March 2020. Strong similarities in the trends for the overall data and for the data from the top 10% of producers provide some evidence that a relatively small but influential number of users were contributing largely to anti-Asian and counter-hate discussions online. Further, dis-aggregation of the data by type of tweet (e.g., original tweet vs. retweet) provided a more nuanced look at how and the extent to which anti-Asian and counter-hate messages are shared. The finding that replies were more likely to contain negative content might be an indication of a call to discuss anti-Asian hate online, given the interactive nature of replying. In contrast, retweets were more likely to contain positive content. Because retweeting may reflect the motive to share, promote, or express agreement with an original tweet, this finding may be indicative of greater support for positive content compared to negative content on Twitter [39]. Although we did not have access to information regarding users' motives for retweeting, our interpretation is consistent with prior research finding that retweets are a good indicator of links between like-minded individuals [70] and that retweeting content is associated with increased trust in, interest in, and agreement with the original message [71].

Our analyses also revealed geographic differences in the frequency of negative (anti-Asian) and positive (counter-hate) content generated by Twitter users, both within the U.S. and on a global scale. Although we did not directly assess Hofstede's cultural dimensions [30], our findings are largely aligned with this theoretical framework. That is, Hofstede has indicated that the U.S. is high on individualism, India is high on power distance, and Brazil is high on uncertainty avoidance. This is particularly insightful, as it lends support to Ng's [31] findings that countries high on these factors might have a greater inclination to attribute blame to others in the face of uncertain events. The spread of positive keywords was more geographically focused in the U.S. Because individuals around the world increasingly view the U.S. as a source of influence [72], greater positivity (e.g., anti-racist messages) in online discourse within the U.S. may be beneficial for increasing positive online discourse on a global scale.

New York, California, and Florida were the largest producers of anti-Asian keywords within the U.S. in our archive dataset (based on our query of over 13 million tweets). However, a complementary analysis performed on a random sample of approximately 1% of publicly available tweets from a single date yielded additional insights. When considering the 1% of tweets on a given day, the states with the highest ratio of anti-Asian keywords to all Twitter content generated by users in the state were Tennessee and Alaska. In contrast, whereas California and New York were the largest producers of counter-hate keywords in our archive dataset, Washington D.C. had the highest ratio of counter-hate keywords in the 1% dataset, followed by Washington state and New York. The greater positive Twitter content generated by users in New York, in particular, is interesting in light of the relatively higher rate of crime targeting AAPI individuals in this state. That is, data from Stop AAPI Hate [73] indicates that out of 9081 reported incidents of anti-Asian hate (i.e., physical violence, online harassment, civil rights violations) in the U.S. from March 2020 to June 2021, roughly 15% occurred in New York. The dynamic ways in which prejudice manifests itself in face-to-face interactions and online spaces—and the role of social media in conveying messages of support and solidarity in response to acts of racial animosity—warrant further empirical attention.

Using burst analysis, we identified several significant surges (i.e., bursts) in the frequency of both anti-Asian and counter-hate keywords on Twitter. Examination of these bursts in relation to relevant content generated by President Trump on Twitter, political events, and key milestones in the COVID-19 timeline helps contextualize these temporal findings and underscores the extent to which social media can both reflect and potentially influence anti-Asian sentiment. Crucially, our results are largely consistent with previous research indicating that President Trump's use of politically incorrect terminology when discussing political events precipitated increases in White nationalist ideals and racism [74], broadly, and the finding that bursts of negative activity occurred after President Trump started using anti-Asian rhetoric in his tweets, speeches, and interviews during the pandemic [9]. Furthermore, the complexity of the prejudice fueled by and evident throughout the pandemic is perhaps illustrated by the political connotation of some of the anti-Asian keywords. For example, "ccpvirus"—in reference to the Chinese Communist Party—likely stemmed from news reports that this political party withheld information about COVID-19 during the early months of the pandemic [75]. A better understanding of the link between these bursts of activity and offline behavior may be particularly beneficial for social media platforms. For example, following a hate-speech triggering event (e.g., a violent attack or hate crime), social media companies might closely monitor hateful keywords and evaluate the use of mechanisms to amplify anti-hate messaging.

Finally, although there were more transitions from positive to negative (counter-hate to anti-Asian) than from negative to positive (anti-Asian to counter-hate) content within Twitter replies, bursts in the frequency of positive messages following violent attacks directed at Asian individuals highlight the protective nature of counter-hate messages online. This heightened positive activity can bring increased awareness of anti-Asian prejudice through "hashtag activism." It remains unclear, however, whether surges in the use of counter-hate keywords (e.g., #hateisavirus, #stopasianhate) led to a measurable reduction in verbal and physical attacks against AAPI individuals; notably, similar campaigns aimed at reducing violence have lost momentum over time [37].

4.1 Limitations and Future Directions

A few noteworthy limitations of this research stem from the data sample. For example, only tweets containing one of the English keywords or hashtags were collected and subsequently analyzed. Although over 1.4 billion individuals speak English globally [76] and about 53% of all tweets are in English [77], given that the COVID-19 pandemic and violence directed at individuals of Asian-descent occurred on a global scale (including in regions where English is not a commonly-spoken language), our exclusive reliance on tweets written in English limits the generalizability of our results. Future research using culturally-relevant anti-Asian and counter-hate keywords in other languages will contribute to a more complete understanding of the spread of anti-Asian hate online during this time.

Furthermore, we only utilized the top 20 countries with the most Twitter users (as of July 2020) along with their 5 most populous cities as locations within our geolocation strategy. Although we were able to classify roughly 10% of the collected data using this strategy, approximately 50% of our data did not contain a valid geolocation and approximately 40% did not contain any geolocation at all. This decreased the usable sample size for our analyses and leaves open questions about related phenomena in smaller countries and nations with limited access to Twitter. Although research focusing on Canadian [78] and U.K. [29] populations and findings from other global analyses (e.g., [31]) are largely consistent with our results, future research should evaluate these geographical trends across a wider range of countries.

Finally, it is important to note that the patterns of findings discussed in this research are correlational in nature. It is thus not possible to conclude that hateful messages directed toward Asian individuals caused or were caused by increases in offline violent attacks, salient events, statements by prominent figures, etc. It is also not possible to infer that rises in COVID-19 cases or deaths caused increases in anti-Asian or counter-hate messages. These relationships could also be impacted by a variety of confounding factors, such as individuals' political beliefs, access to and willingness to receive the COVID-19 vaccine, knowledge about the pandemic, and coverage of violent attacks against Asian individuals in the news media. Interestingly, however, we note that some research has supported the effectiveness of using Twitter activity as an indicator of the "wisdom of crowds." Specifically, Turiel et al. [79] found that the intensity of COVID-19-related tweets in different geographic regions during incipient stages of the pandemic predicted COVID-19 morbidity rates in these regions one month later.

This research aims to build initial awareness of patterns of hate and counter-hate on social media, with important questions remaining regarding the mechanisms underlying these observations. Our hope is that our efforts to expand on recent research in this area will contribute to a deeper understanding of how prejudice and hatred, as well as empathy and counter-hate, proliferate online during global crises.

Acknowledgments This work was supported by the National Science Foundation under awards #2036127 and #2227488. Additionally, the authors would like to thank Johnny Hudson (Arizona State University) for his contributions to an early version of the Twitter timeline.

References

1. World Health Organization, "Timeline: WHO's COVID-19 response", https://www.who.int/emergencies/diseases/novel-coronavirus-2019/interactive-timeline, 2021.
2. Google Trends, "Coronavirus search trends", https://trends.google.com/trends/story/US_cu_4Rjdh3ABAABMHM_en, 2021.

3. World Health Organization, "World health organization best practices for the naming of new human infectious diseases", https://apps.who.int/iris/bitstream/handle/10665/163636/WHO_HSE_FOS_15.1_eng.pdf, 2015.
4. S. Darling-Hammond, E. K. Michaels, A. M. Allen, D. H. Chae, M. D. Thomas, T. T. Nguyen, M. M. Mujahid, and R. C. Johnson, "After "the China virus" went viral: Racially charged coronavirus coverage and trends in bias against Asian Americans," *Health Education and Behavior*, vol. 47, ed. 6, pp. 870-879, https://doi.org/10.1177/1090198120957949, 2020.
5. A. R. Gover, S. B. Harper, and L. Langton, "Anti-Asian hate crime during the COVID-19 pandemic: Exploring the reproduction of inequality," *American Journal of Criminal Justice*, pp. 1–21, https://doi.org/10.1007/s12103-020-09545-1, 2020.
6. T. Levenson, "Stop trying to make "Wuhan virus" happen," https://www.theatlantic.com/ideas/archive/2020/03/stop-trying-make-wuhan-virus-happen/607786/, 2020.
7. World Health Organization, "A guide to preventing and addressing social stigma," https://www.who.int/docs/default-source/coronaviruse/covid19-stigma-guide.pdf, 2020.
8. A. Smith, "Photo of Trump remarks shows 'corona' crossed out and replaced with 'Chinese' virus", *NBC News*, 2020, https://www.nbcnews.com/politics/donald-trump/photo-trump-remarks-shows-corona-crossed-out-replaced-chinese-virus-n1164111
9. Y. Hswen, X. Xu, A. Hing, J. B. Hawkins, J. S. Brownstein, and G. C. Gee, "Association of #COVID19 versus #Chinesevirus with anti-Asian sentiments on Twitter: March 9–23, 2020," *American Journal of Public Health*, vol. 111, ed. 5, pp. 956–964, 2021.
10. N. G. Ruiz, K. Edwards, and M. H. Lopez, "One-third of Asian Americans fear threats, physical attacks and most say violence against them is rising," *Pew Research Center*, https://www.pewresearch.org/fact-tank/2021/04/21/one-third-of-asian-americans-fear-threats-physical-attacks-and-most-say-violence-against-them-is-rising/, 2021.
11. B. Levin, and A. Grisham, "Fact sheet: Anti-Asian prejudice March 2021," *Center for the Study of Hate and Extremism*, https://www.csusb.edu/sites/default/files/FACT%20SHEET-%20Anti-Asian%20Hate%202020%20rev%203.21.21.pdf, 2021.
12. M. Costello, L. Cheng, F. Luo, Ho. Hu, S. Liao, N. Vishwamitra, M. Li, and E. Okpala, "COVID-19: A pandemic of anti-Asian cyberhate", *Journal of Hate Studies*, vol. 17 ed. 1, pp. 108–118, https://doi.org/10.33972/jhs.198, 2020.
13. H. Tessler, M. Choi, and G. Kao, "The anxiety of being Asian American: Hate crimes and negative biases during the COVID-19 pandemic," *American Journal of Criminal Justice*, vol. 45, ed. 4, pp. 636-646, https://doi.org/10.1007/s12103-020-09541-5, 2020.
14. T. T. Nguyen, S. Criss, P. Dwivedi, D. Huang, J. Keralis, E. Hsu, L. Phan, L. H. Nguyen, I. Yardi, M. M. Glymour, A. M. Allen, D. H. Chae, G. C. Gee, and Q. C. Nguyen, "Exploring U.S. shifts in anti-Asian sentiment with the emergence of Covid" *International Journal of Environmental Research and Public Health*, vol. 17, ed. 19, https://doi.org/10.3390/ijerph171970323, 2022.
15. Stop AAPI Hate, "Stop AAPI hate national report 3.19.20 - 8.5.20," https://www.asianpacificpolicyandplanningcouncil.org/wp-content/uploads/STOP_AAPI_Hate_National_Report_3.19-8.5.2020.pdf 2020.
16. J. Cao, C. Lee, W. Sun, and J.C. De Gagne, "The #StopAsianHate movement on Twitter: A qualitative descriptive study", *International Journal of Environmental Research and Public Health*, vol. 19(7), 3757, https://doi.org/10.3390/ijerph19073757, 2022.
17. Harrison, R. and Hamilton, K., "Hate speech on Twitter predicts frequency of real-life hate crimes", *NYU*, https://www.nyu.edu/about/news-publications/news/2019/june/hate-speech-on-twitter-predicts-frequency-of-real-life-hate-crime.html, 2019.
18. A. Toliyat, S. I. Levitan, Z. Peng, and R. Etemadpour, "Asian hate speech detection on Twitter during COVID-19", *Frontiers in Artificial Intelligence*, vol. 5, https://doi.org/10.3389/frai.2022.932381, 2022.

19. Anti-Defamation League, "ADL report: Anti-Asian hostility spikes on Twitter after President Trump's COVID diagnosis", https://www.adl.org/news/press-releases/adl-report-anti-asian-hostility-spikes-on-twitter-after-president-trumps-covid 2020.
20. E. Mcguire, "Anti-Asian hate continues to spread online amid COVID-19 pandemic", https://www.aljazeera.com/news/2020/04/anti-asian-hate-continues-spread-online-covid-19-pandemic-200405063015286.html, 2020.
21. A. D. Dubey, "The resurgence of cyber racism during the COVID-19 pandemic and its after effects: Analysis of sentiments and emotions in Tweets," *JMIR Public Health and Surveillance*, vol. 6, ed. 4, https://doi.org/10.2196/19833, 2020.
22. J. Y. Kim, and A. Kesari, "Misinformation and hate speech: The case of anti-Asian hate speech during the COVID-19 pandemic", *Journal of Online Trust and Safety*, vol. 1, ed. 1, https://doi.org/10.54501/jots.v1i1.13, 2021.
23. F. Miro-Llinares, and J.J. Rodrigez-Sala, "Cyber hate speech on twitter: Analyzing disruptive events from social media to build a violent communication and hate speech taxonomy", *WIT Press*, vol. 11, pp. 406–415, https://doi.org/10.2495/DNE-V11-N3-406-415, 2016.
24. B. Kim, E. Cooks, and S.-K. Kim, "Exploring incivility and moral foundations toward Asians in English-speaking tweets in hate crime-reporting cities during the COVID-19 pandemic", *Internet Research*, vol. 32, ed. 1, pp. 362–378, https://doi.org/10.1108/INTR-11-2020-0678, 2020.
25. J. An, H. Kwak, C. S. Lee, B. Jun, Y-Y. Ahan, "Predicting anti-Asian hateful users on Twitter during COVID-19", *arXiv*, vol. 1, https://doi.org/10.48550/arXiv.2109.07296, 2021.
26. H. Lyu, Y. Fan, Z. Xiong, M. Komisarchik and J. Luo, "Understanding public opinion toward the #StopAsianHate movement and the relation with racially motivated hate crimes in the US", *IEEE Transactions on Computational Social Systems*, vol. 10, no. 1, pp. 335-346, doi: https://doi.org/10.1109/TCSS.2021.3136858, 2023.
27. S. O. Cheng, "Xenophobia due to the coronavirus outbreak – A Letter to the editor in response to "the socio-economic implications of the coronavirus pandemic (COVID-19): A review"", *Int J Surg*, vol. 79, pp. 13–14, https://doi.org/10.1016/j.ijsu.2020.05.017, 2020.
28. M. Coates, "Covid-19 and the rise of racism." *BMJ*, vol. 06, 369:m1384, 2020.
29. S. Schumann, and Y. Moore, "The COVID-19 outbreak as a trigger event for sinophobic hate crimes in the United Kingdom." *The British Journal of Criminology*, vol. 63, pp. 367–383, https://doi.org/10.1093/bjc/azac015, 2023.
30. Hofstede Insights, "Tool to compare countries", https://www.hofstede-insights.com/fi/product/compare-countries/, 2023.
31. R. Ng, "Anti-Asian sentiments during the COVID-19 pandemic across 20 countries: Analysis of a 12-billion-word news media database", *Journal of Medical Internet Research*, vol. 8, ed. 23, https://doi.org/10.2196/28305, 2021.
32. W. Sun, "Introduction to the Special Issue: "Media and communication during the COVID-19 (coronavirus) pandemic", *Howard Journal of Communications*, vol. 32, ed. 5, pp. 415–420, https://doi.org/10.1080/10646175.2021.1966857, 2021.
33. L. Y. Dhanani and B. Franz, "Unexpected public health consequences of the COVID-19 Pandemic: A national survey of anti-Asian attitudes in the USA" *Int J Public Health*, vol. 65, ed. 6, pp. 747–754, doi: https://doi.org/10.1007/s00038-020-01440-0, 2020.
34. R. Goodwin, S. Haque, F. Neto, and L. B. Myers, "Initial psychological responses to influenza A, H1N1 ("swine flu")". *BMC Infectious Diseases*, vol. 9, ed. 166, doi: https://doi.org/10.1186/1471-2334-9-166, 2009.
35. M. S. Khan, A. Osei-Kofi, A. Omar, H. Kirkbride, A. Kessel, A. Abbara, D. Heymannm, A. Zumla, and O. Dar, "Pathogens, prejudice, and politics: The role of the global health community in the European refugee crisis", *Lancet Infect Dis*, vol. 16, pp. e173–e177, doi: https://doi.org/10.1016/S1473-3099(16)30134-7, 2016.
36. M. McCauley, S. Minsky, and K. Viswanath, "The H1N1 pandemic: media frames, stigmatization and coping", *BMC Public Health*, vol. 13, pp. 1116, doi: https://doi.org/10.1186/1471-2458-13-1116, 2013.

37. B. Wheeler, S. Jung, M.C. Barioni, M. Purohit, D. Hall, and Y. Silva, "#WashTheHate: Understanding the prevalence of anti-Asian prejudice on Twitter during the COVID-19 pandemic", *Proceedings of the 2022 IEEE/ACM International Conference on Advances in Social Networks Analysis and Mining*, https://doi.org/10.1109/ASONAM55673.2022.10068578, 2022.
38. S. Lindgren, "Movement mobilization in the age of hashtag activism: Examining the challenge of noise, hate, and disengagement in the #MeToo campaign", *Policy & Internet*, vol. 11, ed. 4, pp. 418–438, https://doi.org/10.1002/poi3.212, 2019.
39. D. Boyd, S. Golder and G. Lotan, "Tweet, tweet, retweet: Conversational aspects of retweeting on twitter", *43rd Hawaii International Conference on System Sciences,* Honolulu, HI, USA, pp. 1–10, doi: https://doi.org/10.1109/HICSS.2010.412, 2010.
40. K. Solovev, N. Prollochs, "Hate speech in the political discourse on social media: Disparities across parties, gender, and ethnicity", *Association for Computing Machinery*, pp. 3656–3661, https://doi.org/10.1145/3485447.3512261, 2022.
41. C. Rivers, B. Lewis, and S. Marmagas. "A framework for ethical use of Twitter for public health research", vol. 11, 2013.
42. Twitter. "Developer terms: Developer policy", https://developer.twitter.com/en/developer-terms/policy, 2022.
43. Twitter, "Developer Twitter API," *Twitter Developer*, https://developer.twitter.com/en/docs/twitter-api, 2021.
44. B. He, C. Ziems, S. Soni, N. Ramakrishnan, D. Yang, and S. Kumar, "Racism is a virus: Anti-Asian hate and counterspeech in social media during the COVID-19 crisis", *Proceedings of the 2021 IEEE/ACM International Conference on Advances in Social Networks Analysis and Mining*, https://doi.org/10.1145/3487351.3488324, 2021.
45. A. Chiu, "Trump has no qualms about calling coronavirus the 'Chinese Virus.' That's a dangerous attitude, experts say", *Washington Post*, https://www.washingtonpost.com/nation/2020/03/20/coronavirus-trump-chinese-virus/, 2020.
46. E. Shim, "Asian Americans take campaign against 'Kung Flu' slur to the streets", *UPI*, https://www.upi.com/Top_News/US/2020/06/27/Asian-Americans-take-campaign-against-Kung-Flu-slur-to-the-streets/8321593296741/", 2020.
47. M. D. Cava, and K. Lam, "Coronavirus is spreading and so is anti-Chinese sentiment and xenophobia", *USA Today*, https://www.usatoday.com/story/news/nation/2020/01/31/coronavirus-chinese-xenophobia-racism-misinformation/2860391001/, 2020.
48. J. Jiang, E. Chen, S. Yan, K. Lerman, and E. Ferrara, "Political polarization drives online conversations about Covid-19 in the United States", *Human Behavior and Emerging Technologies*, vol. 2, ed. 3, pp. 200–211, https://doi.org/10.1002/hbe2, 2020.
49. Twitter, "Volume Streams," *Twitter Developer*, https://developer.twitter.com/en/docs/twitter-api, 2021.
50. A. Cohen. "Fuzzy string matching in Python", https://pypi.org/project/fuzzywuzzy/, 2022.
51. R. Fausset, N. Bogel-Burroughs, and M. Fazio. "8 dead in Atlanta spa shootings, with fears of anti-Asian bias", *New York Times*, https://www.nytimes.com/live/2021/03/17/us/shooting-atlanta-acworth, 2021.
52. J. Kleinberg, "Bursty and hierarchical structure in streams," *Data Mining and Knowledge Discovery*, vol. 7, ed. 4, pp. 373–397, https://doi.org/10.1023/A:1024940629314, 2003.
53. Statistica, "Number of Active Twitter Users in Selected Countries," *Statistica*, https://developer.twitter.com/en/docs/twitter-api, 2021.
54. World Population Review, "Largest Cities by Population," *World Population Review*, https://worldpopulationreview.com/world-cities, 2023.
55. World Health Organization, "WHO COVID-19 Dashboard," *World Health Organization*, https://covid19.who.int/data, 2023.
56. Trump Twitter Archive. "Trump twitter archive V2", https://www.thetrumparchive.com, 2021.
57. BBC US Canada. "Covid: UK variant could drive "rapid growth" in US cases, CDC warns", https://www.bbc.com/news/world-us-canada-55684878, 2021.

58. S. Becket, G. Segers, K. Watson, M. Quinn, and C. Linton, "President Biden takes office, moving quickly to implement agenda", https://www.cbsnews.com/live-updates/biden-inaugurated-46th-president-united-states/, 2021.
59. Centers for Disease Control and Prevention. "CDC museum Covid-19 timeline" https://www.cdc.gov/museum/timeline/covid19.html, 2021.
60. Federal Bureau of Investigation, "Hate Crime," *Crime Data Explorer*, https://crime-data-explorer.fr.cloud.gov/pages/explorer/crime/hate-crime, 2023.
61. K. Tran, "2 elderly Asian women punched in the head in separate attacks on NYC subway", *Yahoo News*, https://news.yahoo.com/2-elderly-asian-women-punched-235848778.html?soc_src=social-sh&soc_trk=ma, 2021.
62. W. G. Kantor, "Filipino American man recounts brutal attack with box cutter on N.Y.C. subway: 'nobody helped'.", *People, Meredith Corporation*, https://people.com/crime/filipino-american-man-recounts-brutal-attack-with-box-cutter-on-n-y-c-subway-nobody-helped/, 2021.
63. A. V. Lozano, "People across U.S. protest anti-Asian hate following deadly spa shootings", *NBC News*, https://www.nbcnews.com/news/us-news/people-across-u-s-protest-anti-asian-hate-following-deadly-n1261677, 2021.
64. A. Roginand, A. Nawaz, "We have been through this before. Why anti-Asian hate crimes are rising amid coronavirus", *PBS News Hour*, https://www.pbs.org/newshour/nation/we-have-been-through-this-before-why-anti-asian-hate-crimes-are-rising-amid-coronavirus, 2020.
65. Stop AAPI Hate, "About" https://stopaapihate.org/about/, 2022.
66. K. Leigh, "Trump says he'll stop using the term 'Chinese Virus'", *Bloomberg*, https://www.bloomberg.com/news/articles/2020-03-25/trump-says-he-ll-stop-using-chinese-virus-easing-blame-game, 2020.
67. B. Samuels, "Americans after repeatedly using term 'Chinese virus'", *THE HILL*, https://thehill.com/homenews/administration/489107-trump-expresses-support-for-asian-americans-after-repeatedly-using, 2020.
68. X. Tan, R. Lee, and L. Ruppanner, "Profiling racial prejudice during COVID-19: Who exhibits anti-Asian sentiment in Australia and the United States?", *Australian Journal of Social Issues*, vol. 6, ed. 5, https://doi.org/10.1002/ajs4.176. 2021.
69. R. Tekumalla, Z. Baig, M. Pan, L. A. R. Hernandez, M. Wang, and J. M. Banda, "Characterizing anti-Asian rhetoric during the COVID-19 pandemic: A sentiment analysis case study on Twitter", *Proceedings of the ICWSM Workshops*, https://doi.org/10.36190/2022.81, 2022.
70. B. Evkoski, A. Pelicon, I. Mozetič, N. Ljubešić, and P. Kralj Novak, "Retweet communities reveal the main sources of hate speech", *PloS One*, vol. 17 ed. 2, e0265602, 2022.
71. P. T. Metaxas, E. Mustafaraj, K. Wong, L. Zeng, M. O'Keefe, and S. Finn, "What do retweets indicate? Results from user survey and meta-review of research", *In Proceedings of The International AAAI Conference on Web and Social Media*, vol. 9, no. 1, pp. 658–661, 2015.
72. J. Gramlich and K. Devlin, "More people around the world see U.S. power and influence as a 'major threat' to their country". *United States of America* https://policycommons.net/artifacts/616940/more-people-around-the-world-see-us/1597687/, 2019.
73. A. J. Y. Horse, R. Jeung, R. Lim, B. Tang, M. Im, L. Higashiyama, ... and M. Chen, "Stop AAPI hate national report", https://stopaapihate.org/wp-content/uploads/2021/08/Stop-AAPI-Hate-Report-National-v2-210830.pdf, 2020.
74. J. G. Shafer, "Donald Trump's political incorrectness: Neoliberalism as frontstage racism on social media", *Social Media + Society*, https://doi.org/10.1177/2056305117733226, 2017.
75. C. Buckley and S. L. Myers, "As new coronavirus spread, China's old habits delayed fight" *New York Times*, https://www.nytimes.com/2020/02/01/world/asia/china-coronavirus.html, 2020.
76. Statistica, "The most spoken languages worldwide in 2023", https://www.statista.com/statistics/266808/the-most-spoken-languages-worldwide/, 2023.
77. Semiocast, "Semiocast – Top languages on Twitter-stats", https://semiocast.com/top-languages-on-twitter-stats/, 2023.

78. S. Chen, and C. Wu, "#StopAsianHate: Understanding the global rise of anti-Asian racism from a transcultural communication perspective", *Journal of Transcultural Communication*, vol.1, ed. 1, pp. 5–19. https://doi.org/10.1515/jtc-2021-2002, 2022.
79. J. Turiel, D. Fernandez-Reyes, and T. Aste, "Wisdom of crowds detects COVID-19 severity ahead of officially available data", *Scientific Reports*, vol. 11, 13678. https://doi.org/10.1038/s41598-021-93042-w, 2021.

Enhancing Fraud Detection in SWIFT Financial Systems Through Ontology-Based Knowledge Integration and Graph-Driven Analysis

Lylia Abrouk, Hamza Chergui, Hamid Ahaggach, and Nicolas Cabioch

Abstract Fraud detection within financial institutions presents a multifaceted challenge, necessitating robust tools for both the prevention and identification of fraudulent activities. In this article, we detail our methodology for detecting fraud within the SWIFT network, leveraging a domain-specific ontology. Our approach unfolds in two primary phases. Initially, we construct the OntoFiC ontology, tailored specifically for modeling SWIFT transactions and associated actors. This ontology is then populated with a real dataset. Following this foundational step, we employ rules-based reasoning, crafting SWRL (Semantic Web Rule Language) rules that correspond to various fraud scenarios. Subsequently, we construct a comprehensive graph representation to detect fraudulent customers and transactions, and we visualize the results of our fraud detection efforts. To assess the efficacy of our approach, we compare the performance of four anomaly graph detection algorithms (DOMINANT, GADNR, ONE and CoLA) with Isolation Forest algorithm. The results indicate that graph-based detection algorithms is better than traditional methods. Isolation Forest, while competitive in precision for legitimate accounts, demonstrated lower recall, suggesting it may miss some legitimate activities. These findings suggest that leveraging graph-based methodologies can enhance the detection of complex fraud patterns within financial transactions.

Keywords Ontology · SWRL rules · Graph · Fraud detection · Finance

The authors "Hamza Chergui, Hamid Ahaggach, and Nicolas Cabioch" contributed equally to this work.

L. Abrouk (✉) · H. Ahaggach
LIB, University of Burgundy, Dijon, France
e-mail: lylia.abrouk@u-bourgogne.fr; hamid.ahaggach@u-bourgogne.fr

H. Chergui · N. Cabioch
SKAIZen Group, Paris, France
e-mail: hchergui@skaizengroup.fr; ncabioch@skaizengroup.fr

M. Kaya et al. (eds.), *Social Network Analysis and Mining Applications in Healthcare and Anomaly Detection*, Lecture Notes in Social Networks,
https://doi.org/10.1007/978-3-031-75204-9_11

1 Introduction

This paper is an extended version of our original conference paper, 'OntoFiC: An Ontology for Financial Fraud Detection and Customer Behavior Modeling', presented at The 2023 IEEE/ACM International Conference on Advances in Social Networks Analysis and Mining [1]. While the original article focused on the development of the *OntoFiC* ontology for modeling SWIFT transactions and actors, employing a rules-based approach for identifying fraudulent activities, this new version significantly extends our research. We have refined and corrected the ontology with a comprehensive process for its construction, added SWRL rules with input from experts, and developed a new hybrid approach that combines the ontology with graph-based fraud detection techniques.

The relentless evolution of financial fraud techniques poses an ever-increasing challenge to financial institutions worldwide. Effective fraud detection is not just a matter of safeguarding assets, but also a crucial aspect of maintaining customer trust and regulatory compliance.

Fraud detection poses a significant challenge for financial institutions, given that while fraudulent transactions are relatively rare, their potential impact can be substantial. These impacts range from the need to reimburse affected customers to potentially incurring severe penalties, especially in cases involving money laundering. As central entities in financial exchanges, banks must exercise due diligence in monitoring transactions that could be related to money laundering or terrorism financing, underscoring the necessity for effective tools in fraud prevention and detection.

The SKAIZen Group is spearheading a research and innovation initiative focused on creating models of customers and financial institutions by consolidating a knowledge base from diverse data sources. This initiative is designed to enhance fraud detection capabilities within financial transactions. Our contribution to this article is part of a collaborative effort with SKAIZen Group under the "France Relance" project, which aims to develop a knowledge base enriched with transactional data. This base considers various types of financial data, such as customer and account information, and the relationships between entities (e.g., beneficiary, debtor, and the connections between accounts and customers).

In our research, we introduce a dedicated ontology *OntoFiC* for financial information that models both the transactions within the SWIFT network and the related parties, including customers and financial institutions. This framework is informed by the SWIFT model, now recognized as the ISO 20022 standard, and builds upon our prior work on a KYC (Know Your Customer) knowledge base. The ontology serves to pinpoint unusual behaviors by enforcing predefined SWRL rules. Our ontology is populated with transactions from a real dataset. Our approach leverages the semantic richness of the ontology to encode intricate relationships and rules that govern financial transactions. This semantic layer facilitates advanced reasoning over the data, allowing for the identification of potential instances of fraud.

Following this, we construct a graph representation to detect fraudulent customers and transactions. Finally, we visualize the results of our fraud detection efforts in order to facilitate the analysis of relationships between different actors and offering a robust solution for financial institutions in their fight against fraud.

This paper is organized as follows: Sect. 2, presents a comprehensive review of the existing literature on financial fraud detection, including a discussion on ontology-based approaches across various domains and graph anomaly techniques, highlighting the gaps our study aims to address. In Sect. 3, we delve into the details of our research methodology, a novel hybrid approach for financial fraud detection. This includes a detailed explanation of the ontology construction process, a description of the graph anomaly detection approach, and how we combine the both to enhance results. Section 4 presents the results of our experimentation including ontology and graph construction. We analyze the implications of our findings, discussing both the strengths and weaknesses of our approach. Finally, the paper concludes with Sect. 5, where we summarize the key insights from our research and suggest directions for future work.

2 Literature Review

2.1 Ontology

For several years, ontologies have been used to represent knowledge in various domains, including commerce, health, biology, and finance. We define the ontology O as a 4-tuple $\{\mathcal{C}, \mathcal{P}, \mathcal{J}, \mathcal{A}\}$ in which $\mathcal{C}$ is a set of classes, $\mathcal{P}$ is a set of properties, $\mathcal{J}$ is a set of instances, and $\mathcal{A}$ is a set of axioms. Classes represent the real-world entities or objects; properties accompany classes (i.e., as an attribute) or represent relations between classes; instances denote the class individuals; and we specify by axioms additional constraints involving classes and properties.

2.1.1 Ontology Construction

Numerous studies have explored the development of ontologies, focusing on constructing structured representations of knowledge for various applications. Ontology construction encompasses multiple critical tasks, including defining the domain of interest, identifying pertinent terms and concepts, formulating rules and axioms, utilizing representation languages such as the Resource Description Framework (RDF), RDF Schema (RDFS), or the Web Ontology Language (OWL) for encoding, integrating existing ontologies, and assessing the quality of the resulting ontologies.

Researchers [2–4] have explored three primary approaches to ontology construction: manual construction, cooperative construction, and (semi-) automatic construction. Manual construction entails domain experts directly creating the ontology, whereas collaborative construction involves experts in overseeing the majority, if not all, of the tasks within the construction process. Conversely, (semi-)automatic construction seeks to minimize human input, striving towards more automated methods while recognizing the challenges of achieving complete automation.

2.1.2 Financial Ontology

For many years, ontologies have served as a framework for representing knowledge across diverse fields such as commerce, health, biology, and finance. Recent advancements in the financial domain have seen a growing use of ontologies for detecting fraud by representing domain knowledge effectively. Ontologies offer a structured way to define rules and analyze transactions for suspicious activities. For instance, Attigeri et al. [5] introduced an ontology aimed at modeling banking frauds, employing the TF-IDF technique and the Latent Dirichlet Allocation (LDA) model to identify key terms and define relationships using the WordNet thesaurus, enhancing fraud detection capabilities.

Elorche et al. [6] proposed using an ontology to improve the detection and prevention of fraud in electronic payment systems. Their ontology includes definitions of activities, rules, risks, and transactions, although details on its construction are not extensively discussed. Bo and Xinfei [7] propose OntoLFR, a logistics financial risk ontology model designed to address the variability, complexity, and relevance of risks in the logistics finance field. This model aids in early warning and pre-control by enabling risk-related reasoning and analysis.

In another contribution, Ahmed et al. [8] developed the Financial Fraud Detection (FFD) ontology, incorporating severity-ranked rules and an alert generation algorithm to combat money laundering, showcasing the practical application of ontologies in alerting systems.

Hussaini et al. [9] also developed an ontology focused on financial frauds, aiming to identify and prevent fraudulent patterns by modeling user behavior and validating their approach with multiple datasets, further demonstrating the effectiveness of ontologies in the financial security arena.

2.2 Machine Learning-Based Techniques

Recent studies have extensively compared machine learning models, focusing on their effectiveness in fraud detection based on diverse datasets and variables [10–12]. In the realm of fraud detection, supervised learning techniques are predominantly employed to identify suspicious or fraudulent transactions. Varmedja et al. [13] explored the use of four distinct algorithms for credit card fraud detection, alongside the Synthetic Minority Oversampling Technique (SMOTE) to mitigate the issue of data imbalance that arises from the low frequency of fraudulent transactions [13]. Mehbodniya et al. [14] utilized multiple algorithms for credit card fraud detection, including Logistic Regression, Random Forest (RF), K-Nearest Neighbors (KNN), and neural networks, finding that the KNN algorithm yielded the best results on real-world data [14]. More et al. [15] employed the Random Forest algorithm to detect fraudulent transactions and classify alerts by severity [15].

Unsupervised learning approaches are also utilized for detecting fraudulent transactions. Larik et al. [16] presented an approach to detect rare activities related to money laundering, proposing a clustering algorithm and calculating an Anomaly Index Calculation for Anti-Money Laundering (AICAF) index based on principal component analysis and the K-means algorithm. The objective is to model user behavior and detect suspicious behavior [16]. Porwal et al. [17] used the K-means algorithm to create fraudulent and legitimate classes for credit card transactions [17].

Semi-supervised learning approaches leverage unsupervised learning techniques to label data with classes generated by the model. These labeled data are then used to feed a supervised learning algorithm, combining the strengths of both supervised and unsupervised learning methods for enhanced fraud detection [18–20].

2.3 Graph Anomaly Techniques

Ontologies serve as powerful tools for representing knowledge and relationships between entities within a domain. Leveraging the models provided by ontologies, we can harness graph techniques such as community detection and graph anomaly algorithms. These techniques are instrumental, particularly in fields like fraud detection, where understanding complex relationships within data is crucial. Pourhabibi et al. [21] conducted a comprehensive survey on graph-based anomaly detection approaches, highlighting the diverse range of techniques available, including community-based and probabilistic-based methods, designed to detect anomalies at various levels such as nodes, edges, or entire subgraphs.

In recent years, deep learning approaches have gained significant traction in the realm of graph analytics. *Pygod* [22], a Python library dedicated to graph outlier detection, has emerged as a comprehensive resource encompassing state-of-the-art techniques for graph anomaly detection. However, despite the advancements in methodology and tooling, there remains a notable gap in the exploration of these techniques within the financial domain. The construction of graphs from financial data and the application of sophisticated anomaly detection algorithms in this context have yet to be fully explored. Closing this gap could unlock valuable insights for fraud detection and risk mitigation within financial systems.

Additionally, Huang et al. [23] introduced DGraph, a dynamic graph dataset sourced from real-world financial data. DGraph addresses limitations in existing Graph Anomaly Detection (GAD) datasets by offering a comprehensive dataset with millions of nodes, dynamic edges, and ground-truth nodes. The authors provide insights into the structural, neighbor distribution, and temporal dynamics of anomalous nodes in financial networks. The experiments conducted showcase the efficacy of DGraph in advancing GAD research.

Similarly, Chen et al. [24] presented the AntiBenford subgraph framework, designed to identify anomalous subgraphs in financial networks based on deviations from Benford's Law. The framework is grounded in statistical principles and offers an efficient algorithm for detecting AntiBenford subgraphs. Empirical evaluations demonstrate the framework's effectiveness in uncovering anomalies in cryptocurrency transaction networks, outperforming existing graph-based anomaly detection methods.

2.4 *Discussion*

Machine learning approaches train models on existing data to detect fraud patterns and anomalies. These approaches can handle large volumes of data, making them suitable for large-scale fraud detection tasks, and adapt to new patterns of fraud over time with high accuracy, provided there is sufficient training data. However, machine learning approaches heavily rely on the quality and quantity of the training data. Models can be difficult to interpret and don't explain why a transaction is fraudulent or not. Graph anomaly detection approaches create graphs where nodes represent entities (such as users and transactions) and edges represent the relationships or transactions between these entities. These approaches identify complex fraudulent schemes that might not be apparent when analyzing transactions in isolation, making it easier to understand fraudulent transactions. However, for large datasets, analyzing graphs can become computationally intensive.

Graph anomaly detection approaches are particularly well-suited for detecting fraud in SWIFT transactions for several key reasons: Graph anomaly detection excels at analyzing complex relationships and interactions, while SWIFT transactions involve a complex network of banks and financial institutions. Additionally, graph analysis can uncover hidden relationships and networks, such as groups of accounts collaborating to commit fraud. SWIFT transactions are often targeted fraud schemes involving multiple accounts and cross-border transactions. Graph analysis can visualize the flow of funds across accounts, identifying suspicious patterns that might indicate money laundering or other complex fraudulent activities.

Combining ontology-based approaches with graph approaches for fraud detection leverages the strengths of both methodologies for uncovering complex and sophisticated fraud schemes. The graph is adept at mapping out SWIFT transactions, while the ontology explains why a transaction is flagged as fraudulent by the graph analysis. This hybrid approach not only identifies but also interprets fraudulent transactions, offering a comprehensive and nuanced understanding of fraud that is essential for prevention. By integrating the precision of graph analysis with the contextual insights of ontology, this methodology enhances the detection of sophisticated fraud schemes, making it a powerful tool for financial institutions in their fight against fraud.

3 Methodology

In this section, we present the detailed methodology employed in our research to develop a robust financial ontology and integrate it with graph-based fraud detection techniques. As illustrated in Fig. 1, our methodology begins with the construction of the $OntoFIC$ ontology based on SWIFT transactions, incorporating domain-specific knowledge provided by SWIFT experts. This foundational design ensures that the financial ontology accurately reflects the complex structure and nuanced details of financial transactions. Additionally, we incorporate a knowledge base from Know Your Customer (KYC), enriching the ontology with detailed client information and thus creating comprehensive customer profiles.

Following this, the ontology is populated with real transaction data from the SWIFT network. This is succeeded by the meticulous integration of SWRL rules, that apply logical reasoning to identify potential fraud.

Concurrently with the reasoning process, a graph-based model is constructed from the transactional data to identify anomalies and outliers. These detected anomalies are then interpreted by the ontology to ascertain the reasons behind their classification as potential fraud, determining which rules–if any–contributed to this assessment. In cases where the existing rules do not account for the detected anomalies, the ontology provides a structured framework that enables experts to interpret the underlying reasons for suspected fraud. With that, all instances of fraud are visualized to provide clear and interpretable insights, offering clear and interpretable insights that assist in identifying potential fraud clusters and in

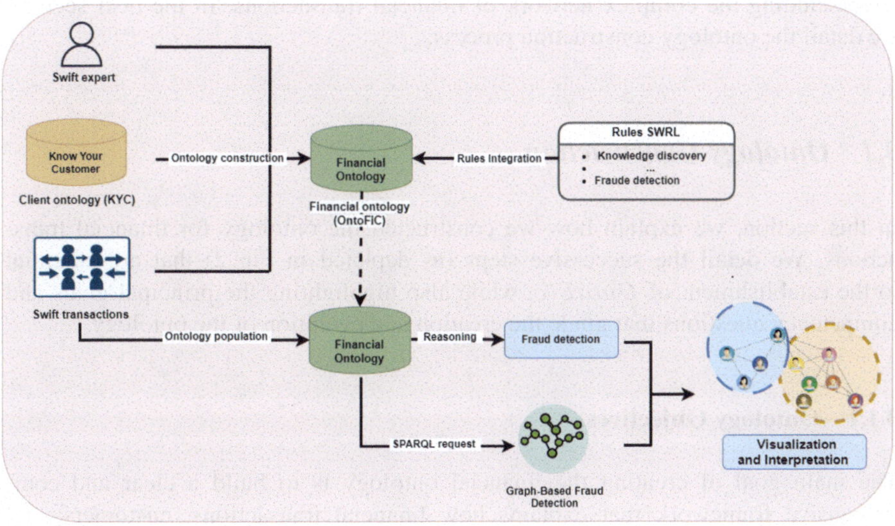

Fig. 1 Overview of the proposed methodology

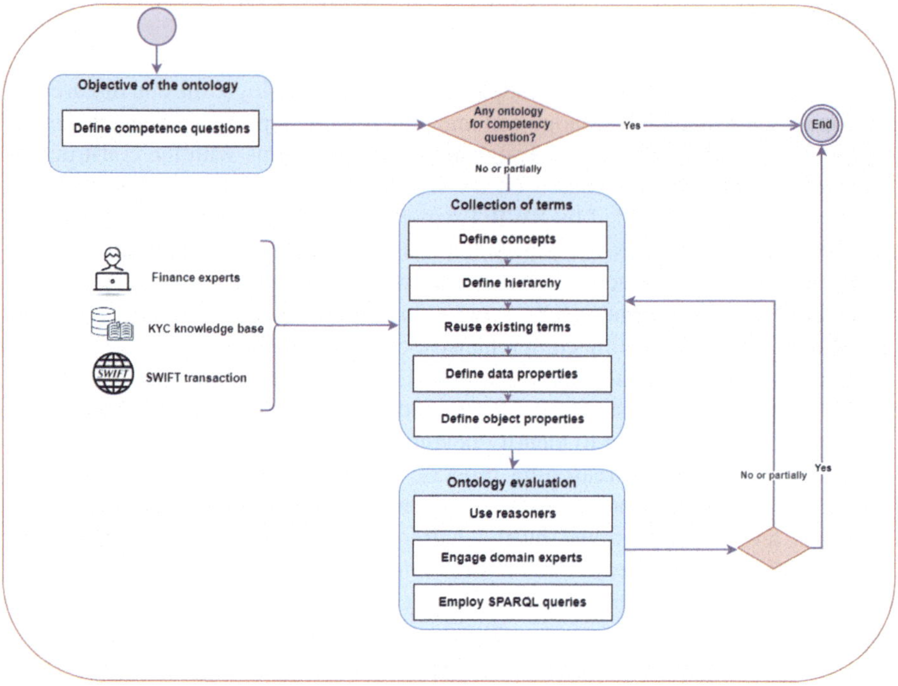

Fig. 2 Steps in the creation of the ontology OntoFic

understanding the complex network of financial transactions. In the next section, we detail the ontology construction process.

3.1 Ontology Construction

In this section, we explain how we constructed the ontology for financial transactions. We detail the successive steps (as depicted in Fig. 2) that are essential to the establishment of $OntoFic$, while also highlighting the principal goals and competency questions that guide the creation and evolution of the ontology.

3.1.1 Ontology Objectives

The main goal of creating the financial ontology is to build a clear and comprehensive framework that explains how financial transactions, customers, and banks interact, especially within the SWIFT network. This framework aims to make it easier for different banking systems to work together and to automatically understand and use financial information from various sources.

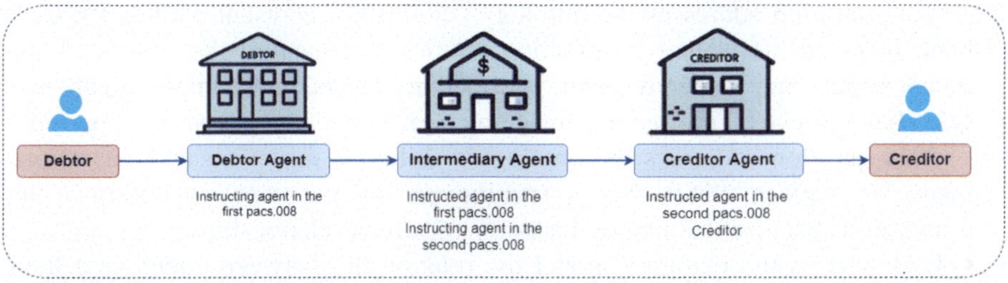

Fig. 3 Transaction in the SWIFT network

The initial phase of our research involves developing an ontology that captures the essence of the financial domain, focusing on the intricacies of transactions and the roles of various participants. This ontology leverages the groundwork laid by the SKAIZen Group, which specialized in distilling knowledge from financial texts to enrich a Know Your Customer (KYC) ontology tailored for banking institutions. Central to our study are SWIFT transactions, which adhere to a globally recognized standard known as ISO. This standard outlines the formatting guidelines for transaction messages. Specifically, our analysis is concentrated on international banking transactions governed by the ISO 20022 standard, exemplified by "*pacs.008*" messages within the MX message suite. Figure 3 illustrates the flow of transactions within the SWIFT network.

3.1.2 Competency Questions

In this section, we introduce our competency questions, which are designed to validate the ontology's capacity to address specific inquiries, as detailed in Sect. 3.1.7. We employed SPARQL queries to test the ontology's ability to respond to these questions, with the results presented in the ontology evaluation section (refer to Table 3).

- **Q1:** How does the ontology detail the specific components of a SWIFT transaction, such as the BIC code, MT code (Message Type), and message fields?

  This question addresses the ontology's ability to accurately represent and organize the essential elements that constitute a SWIFT financial transaction. This question is crucial for evaluating the ontology's effectiveness in capturing the intricacies of financial communication and operations within the global banking network.
- **Q2:** How can we trace the complete route of a SWIFT transaction through intermediary banks to its final destination ?

This question addresses the ontology's ability to represent entities for each bank involved, as well as transaction entities that capture the details of the transfer, including sender, receiver, intermediary banks, timestamps, and status.

- **Q3:** How retrieve all transactions made by a given client over a specific period?
  This question addresses the ontology's ability to retrieving all transactions made by a given client over a specific period and captures not only the transactions but also the temporal aspects and client relationships.
- **Q4:** How does the ontology model the relationship between clients and their respective banks? How identify relationships between clients and banks and describe the nature of these relationships?
  This question addresses the ontology's ability to accurately represent the relationship between clients and their respective banks by establishing entities and defining relationships that reflect the nature of their association.
- **Q5:** How does the ontology support the application of Know Your Customer (KYC) requirements?
  This question addresses the ontology's ability to supports KYC requirements by integrating entities and attributes that capture essential client data for identity verification. This includes personal information, transaction behaviors, and compliance status.
- **Q6:** How can we analyze transaction trends over time for a specific sector or group of clients?
  This question addresses the ontology's ability to accurately represent relevant criteria, such as industry sector or client demographics. By applying temporal filters, we can identify patterns and anomalies in transaction behaviors over time.
- **Q7:** How does the ontology adapt to regulatory changes in the financial sector? Does it allow for easy updating of rules and concepts to remain compliant?
  This question addresses the ontology's ability to evaluate by allowing for dynamic updates to its structure. As regulations evolve, new entities, attributes, and rules can be added to the ontology to reflect these changes.
- **Q8:** How does the ontology manage the representation of sensitive data to ensure the confidentiality and security of client information?
  This question addresses the ontology's ability to implement mechanisms for data protection. This includes defining access control policies that restrict sensitive data visibility based on user roles and applying encryption to data stored within the ontology.
- **Q9:** How does the ontology help experts to detect fraudulent activities ?
  This question addresses the ontology's ability to help experts in detecting fraudulent activities by modeling transaction patterns, client behaviors, and anomaly detection criteria.

3.1.3 Concepts

In *OntoFic* ontology, we have three main concepts: "Agent", "Customer", and "Transaction". The concept of "Agent" represents financial institutions playing various roles in financial transactions. The concept of agent can be further categorized into three main subconcepts: CreditorAgent, DebtorAgent and IntermediaryAgent:

- *Agent:CreditorAgent:* Refers to financial institutions associated with the creditor customer, essentially representing the receiving end of a transaction.
- *Agent:DebtorAgent:* Represents financial institutions associated with the debtor customer, indicating the sending end of a transaction.
- *Agent:IntermediaryAgent:* Denotes financial institutions that act as intermediaries, facilitating transactions between two other financial institutions. These agents are crucial in transactions that require a mediator to process transfers between the debtor and creditor agents.

The concept *Customer* describes the individuals or entities engaging in transactions, distinguished by their roles and nature. The customer is categorized into three main sub-concepts:

- *Customer:Organization:* This sub-category includes entities engaged in selling goods and services, further categorized into *Customer:Organization:Association:* encompasses organizations, associations, and NGOs. *Customer:Organization: Company:* covers both public and private companies, representing the corporate participants in financial transactions.
- *Customer:Person:* Identifies individual participants in financial transactions, highlighting the personal banking aspect within the financial domain.

The concept *Transaction* captures the essence of the financial interactions between customers, defined as money transfers. Transactions represent the flow of funds from one customer to another, encapsulating the core activity within this ontology. Figure 4 provides a snapshot of the classes present in the ontology.

3.1.4 Object Properties

The *OntoFic* ontology includes several object properties that define the relationships between the classes.These object properties include: s:

- *hasActivity*: This property links an organization to its associated domain of activity, indicating the organization's operations scope. It links organizations (Domain: *Organization*) to their respective fields of activity (Range: *Activity*).
- *hasCreditor*: Identifies the creditor in a financial transaction, specifying which customer receives payment (Domain: *Transaction*, Range: *Customer*).
- *hasDebtor*: Pinpoints the debtor in a transaction, the party making the payment (Domain: *Transaction*, Range: *Customer*).
- *hasCreditorAgent*: Specifies the financial agent associated with the creditor in a transaction, highlighting the agent facilitating the transaction for the creditor (Domain: *Transaction*, Range: *Agent*).
- *hasDebtorAgent*: Indicates the agent involved from the debtor's side, ensuring the debtor's payments are processed (Domain: *Transaction*, Range: *Agent*).

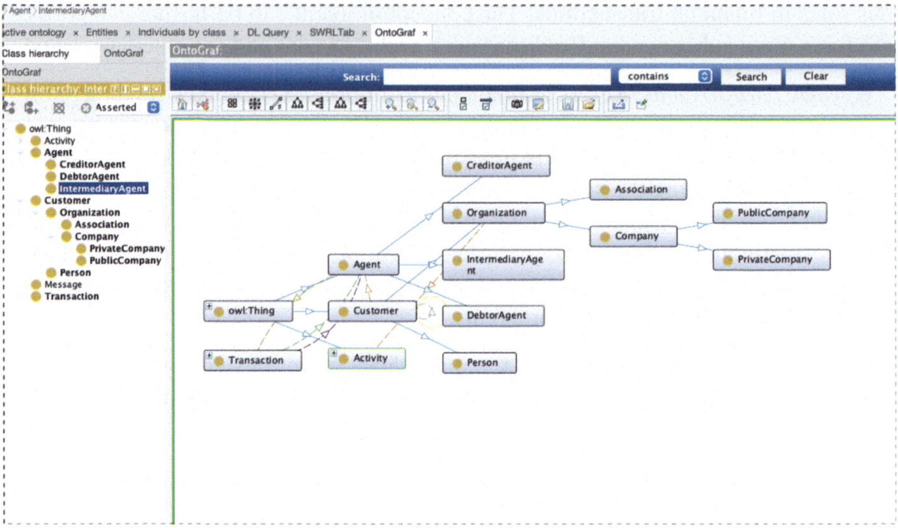

Fig. 4 A snapshot of the classes present in the *OntoFIC* ontology

- *hasInstructedAgent*: Identifies any intermediary agents in a transaction, denoting the intermediary agent's involvement (Domain: *Transaction*, Range: *Agent*).

3.1.5 Data Properties

The *OntoFic* ontology incorporates a variety of data properties designed to characterize the distinct attributes of Agents, Customers, and Transactions. Table 1 provides a detailed summary of these data properties.

3.1.6 Rule with SWRL for Fraud Detection

We present in Table 2 some inference rules using the SWRL language that we defined with the experts.

3.1.7 Ontology Evaluation

The ontology was developed using Protégé 5.5.0. Ensuring the validity and coherence of our ontology was imperative prior to its application. To this end, we verified the ontology's consistency and confirmed that it was error-free by employing reasoners such as FaCT++ and HermiT. Furthermore, the ontology underwent a thorough evaluation by financial experts who reviewed its vocabulary, concepts, data hierarchy, and semantic structure. Additionally, the ontology's capability to address

Table 1 Data properties

Data property	Concept	Type	Description
Amount	Transaction	Numeric	Amount exchanged between two customers
BICFI	Agent	String	Code representing an Agent
ClrSysMmbId	Agent	String	Identifier of the system members
CreDtTm	Transaction	DateTime	Creation date and time
CtryOfRes	Customer	String	Country of residence
Currency	Transaction	String	Currency used in the transaction
EndToEnd	Transaction	String	End-to-end identifier for the transaction
hasPersonalData	Customer	Boolean	Indicates presence of personal data
Id	Customer	String	Customer identifier
InstrId	Transaction	String	Instruction identifier, a point-to-point reference
LEI	Agent	String	Legal Entity Identifier for the Agent
Name	Agent, Customer	String	Name of the agent or customer
PmtId	Transaction	String	Payment identifier
UETR	Transaction	String	Unique end-to-end transaction reference

predefined competency questions was validated through the execution of SPARQL queries, the results of which are documented in Table 3. This comprehensive evaluation process was instrumental in establishing the ontology's reliability and relevance in the financial domain.

3.2 *Graph Anomaly Detection Approach*

In our methodology for anomaly detection within graph-based structures, we begin by utilizing a domain-specific ontology to construct a comprehensive graph representation. This graph intricately maps agents and customers as nodes, interconnected through transactions represented as edges. Such a graph provides a detailed depiction of the complex web of interactions and relationships among entities within our domain.

Subsequently, we extract pertinent features from the nodes, derived from their transaction histories. These features encompass statistical measures such as minimum, maximum, average, and count, enabling us to characterize the behavior of each node based on its transactional activity.

To detect anomalies within this graph, particularly leveraging the rich features of nodes and edges, we employ graph outlier detection algorithms from the *Pygod* library. These algorithms leverage sophisticated techniques to identify anomalous patterns within the graph structure. Unlike other approaches in the literature that focus on specific types of anomalies, our utilization of Deep Learning algorithms allows us to exploit the entirety of available information, encompassing features

Table 2 Rules for fraud detection

Rs.	Description	SWRL rule
R1	High transaction amount: flags transactions where the amount is greater than a certain threshold	`Transaction(?t) ∧ amount(?t, ?amt) ∧ swrlb:greaterThan(?amt, 10000) → IsFraud(?t, true)`
R2	Unusual transaction time: identifies transactions made outside of normal business hours (9 AM to 5 PM) as suspicious.	`Transaction(?t) ∧ hasMessage(?t, ?m) ∧ CreDtTm(?m, ?dt) ∧ swrlb:notEqual(swrlb:hour(?dt), [9-17]) → IsFraud(?t, true)`
R3	International transactions : the creditor's country of residence and the creditor agent's country do not match, indicating a possible international fraud scheme.	`Transaction(?t) ∧ hasCreditor(?t, ?c)∧ Customer(?c) ∧ CtryOfRes(?c, ?ccRes) ∧ hasCreditorAgent(?t, ?ca) ∧ Agent(?ca) ∧ AgentCountry(?ca, ?acRes) ∧ swrlb:notEqual(?ccRes, ?acRes) → IsFraud(?t, true)`
R4	Repeated UETR: checks for different transactions having the same UETR, which could indicate a cloning or duplication fraud attempt.	`Transaction(?t1) ∧ UETR(?t1, ?uetr1) ∧ Transaction(?t2) ∧ UETR(?t2, ?uetr2) ∧ swrlb:equal(?uetr1, ?uetr2) ∧ swrlb:notEqual(?t1, ?t2) → IsFraud(?t1, true) ∧ IsFraud(?t2, true)`
R5	Transactions in High-Risk Countries: flags transactions where the creditor resides in a country that is considered high-risk for financial fraud.	`Transaction(?t) ∧ hasCreditor(?t, ?c) ∧ Customer(?c) ∧ CtryOfRes(?c, ?ccRes) ∧ swrlb:memberOf(?ccRes, HighRiskCountries) → IsFraud(?t, true)`
R6	Rapid Succession of Transactions: This rule looks for two transactions by the same creditor where the creation times of the transactions are less than one hour apart	`Transaction(?t1) ∧ CreDtTm(?t1, ?dt1) ∧ hasCreditor(?t1, ?c) ∧ Transaction(?t2) ∧ CreDtTm(?t2, ?dt2) ∧ hasCreditor(?t2, ?c) ∧ swrlb:lessThan(swrlb:subtractDates(?dt1, ?dt2), PT1H) ∧ swrlb:notEqual(?t1, ?t2) → IsFraud(?t2, true)`

(continued)

Table 2 (continued)

Rs.	Description	SWRL rule
R7	New Account with Large Transaction: This rule flags large transactions (e.g., over 5000 units) that are made by new customers (assuming lower IDs indicate newer accounts).	`Customer(?c) ∧ ID(?c, ?id) ∧ Transaction(?t) ∧ hasCreditor(?t, ?c) ∧ amount(?t, ?amt) ∧ swrlb:greaterThan(?amt, 5000) ∧ swrlb:lessThan(?id, 1000) → IsFraud(?t, true)`
R8	Transaction with Invalid BIC or LEI: This rule flags transactions where the creditor agent involved does not have valid BICFI or LEI identifiers.	`Transaction(?t) ∧ hasCreditorAgent(?t, ?ca) ∧ Agent(?ca) ∧ (¬BICFI(?ca, ?bic) ∨ ¬LEI(?ca, ?lei)) → IsFraud(?t, true)`
R9	Transactions in Unsupported Currency: This rule identifies transactions made in currencies that are not supported	`Transaction(?t) ∧ currency(?t, ?curr) ∧ swrlb:notMemberOf(?curr, SupportedCurrencies) → IsFraud(?t, true)`
R10	Customer Country and Transaction Currency Mismatch: This rule flags transactions where the transaction currency does not match the official currency of the customer's country of residence.	`Transaction(?t1) ∧ UETR(?t1, ?uetr1) ∧ Transaction(?t2) ∧ UETR(?t2, ?uetr2) ∧ swrlb:equal(?uetr1, ?uetr2) ∧ swrlb:notEqual(?t1, ?t2)→ IsFraud(?t1, true) ∧ IsFraud(?t2, true)`

of both actors and edges. This holistic approach enhances our ability to predict anomalies in nodes and edges effectively.

Upon obtaining predictions from the outlier detection algorithms, we significantly enhance our ontology by integrating the fraudster status derived from the analysis. This process involves not only updating the ontology with the status of entities identified as potential fraudsters by the graph analysis but also incorporating additional information that give the reasons behind their classification as fraudulent.

By adding information from the graph analysis into the ontology, we enrich the ontology with a deeper layer of insight, including not just the identification of fraudulent actors and transactions, but also the relationships and patterns that signify fraudulent behavior. The ontology provides explanations for why specific patterns or behaviors are indicative of fraud, based on the properties. This approach serves as a decision-support tool for experts. It aids them in making informed decisions by presenting a comprehensive view of each fraudulent case.

Table 3 Competency questions and SPARQL queries

Qs.	Competency question	SPARQL query
Q1	Specific components of a SWIFT transaction	SELECT ?swiftTransaction ?bicCode ?message WHERE { ?swiftTransaction rdf:type :Transaction . ?swiftTransaction :hasBIC ?bicCode . OPTIONAL { ?swiftTransaction :hasMessage ?message. }}
Q2	Complete route of a SWIFT transaction	SELECT ?transaction ?sender ?receiver ? intermediaryBanks ?timestamp ?status WHERE {?transaction ont:hasDebtor ?sender. ?transaction ont:hasCreditor ?receiver. OPTIONAL { ?transactionont:hasInstructingAgent ?intermediaryBanks. } ?transaction ont:CreDtTm ?timestamp. ?transaction ont:SttlmInf ?status.}
Q3	Transactions made by a given client over a specific period	SELECT ?transaction WHERE { ?client ont:ID ?clientId. ?client ont:hasTransaction ?transaction. ?transaction ont:CreDtTm ?date. FILTER (?clientId = "ClientID" && ?date >= xsd:dateTime("StartDateTime") && ?date <= xsd:dateTime("EndDateTime"))}
Q4	Relationship between clients and banks	SELECT ?client ?bank ?relationshipType WHERE { ?client ont:hasCreditorAgent ?bank. BIND("Creditor Agent" AS ?relationshipType) UNION {?client ont:hasDebtorAgent ?bank. BIND("Debtor Agent" AS ?relationshipType)}}
Q5	Support for KYC requirements	SELECT ?client ?personalData WHERE { ?client ont:hasPersonalData ?personalData. }

(continued)

Table 3 (continued)

Qs.	Competency question	SPARQL query

Q6	Analyze transaction trends over time	`SELECT ?sector (COUNT(?transaction) AS ?`
		`transactionCount) WHERE {`
		`?client ont:hasActivity ?activity.`
		`?activity rdf:type ?sector.`
		`?client ont:hasTransaction`
		`?transaction.`
		`?transaction ont:CreDtTm ?date.`
		`FILTER (?date >=`
		`xsd:dateTime("StartDate`
		`Time") && ?date <=`
		`xsd:dateTime("EndDate`
		`Time"))`
		`} GROUP BY ?sector`

Q7	Updating the ontology and rules to remain compliant?	This question addresses the ontology's update, the forthcoming version of our ontology will be accessible on the industry portal site:
		`(http://industryportal.enit.fr/ontologies`
		`/ONTOFIC)`

Q8	Confidentiality and security of client information?	This question pertains to the ontology's security protocols and data handling policies. Details on these protocols and policies should be consulted in the ontology's documentation or security framework section on the industry portal.

Q9	Detecting fraudulent activities (After applying rules SWRL)	`SELECT ?transaction`
		`WHERE {`
		`?transaction ont:IsFraud true.}`

4 Experimentation

The experiments were conducted using a dataset of 1,000,000 transactions from the SWIFT network. These transactions were SWIFT messages from which we extracted relevant fields related to the transaction and the client.

Furthermore, we employed the reasoners Fact++ and HermiT to verify the consistency and coherence of our financial ontology. The reasoners were used to confirm that the data had been appropriately linked and that the logical inferences were consistent with the data within the ontology.

4.1 Ontology Population

Populating the financial ontology was a crucial step for analyzing financial data and identifying suspicious and fraudulent transactions. This process involved creating instances, concepts, object properties, and data properties within the ontology. Using *Owlready2*,[1] we populated our ontology with 1,000,000 financial transactions.

4.2 Graph Construction

From the ontology, we queried all the actors and created our nodes. Then, with queries on the transactions, we constructed the edges between the nodes. If a transaction has no intermediary, we add an edge between the originator and the beneficiary. If it has one, we add two edges: one from the originator to the intermediary, and another from the intermediary to the beneficiary. Next, we compute five features for each actor based on their transaction history (sum, min, max, average, count). Finally, we apply state-of-the-art graph anomaly detection algorithms to identify anomalous actors, which we then compare with the Isolation Forest algorithm. It's worth noting that the Isolation Forest algorithm is designed for tabular data and may not be optimal for graph data.

4.3 Results

To assess the efficacy of our approach, we employed four anomaly graph detection algorithms utilizing Deep Learning (DOMINANT, GADNR, ONE, and CoLA), Alongside these, we implemented the Isolation Forest algorithm, which is also unsupervised. We optimized the hyperparameters using grid search and for evaluation, we employed the following metrics.

$$Precision = \frac{TP}{TP + FP}; \; Recall = \frac{TP}{TP + FN};$$

$$F1\;Score = \frac{2 \times TP}{2 \times TP + FP + FN};$$

The analysis of the results presented in Table 4 suggests that the anomaly graph detection algorithms, excluding Isolation Forest, exhibit a marginal improvement in performance metrics compared to traditional methods. While Isolation Forest demonstrates competitive precision in detecting legitimate accounts, its relatively

[1] http://owlready2.readthedocs.io.

Table 4 Summary table of algorithms results

	Fraudulent account			Legitimate account			Average		
Algorithm	Précision	Rappel	F1	Précision	Rappel	F1	Précision	Rappel	F1
DOMINANT	**0.80**	0.12	0.21	**0.46**	**0.96**	**0.62**	**0.63**	0.54	0.42
GADNR	0.74	**0.19**	**0.30**	**0.46**	0.91	0.61	0.60	**0.55**	**0.46**
ONE	0.80	0.12	0.21	**0.46**	0.93	**0.62**	0.53	0.46	0.42
CoLA	0.71	0.15	0.25	0.45	0.92	0.61	0.58	0.53	0.43
Isolation forest	0.76	0.12	0.20	0.45	0.95	0.61	0.61	0.53	0.41

Bold values indicate the highest values in each column

lower recall indicates a tendency to miss some instances of legitimate activity. In contrast, DOMINANT, GADNR, ONE, and CoLA algorithms show slightly enhanced precision, recall, and F1 scores across both legitimate and illegitimate accounts.

The marginal improvement observed with anomaly graph detection algorithms underscores their potential in effectively capturing complex patterns and relationships within the data. By leveraging graph-based methodologies, these algorithms can improve financial fraud transactions or account detection. This improvement suggests that anomaly graph detection approaches hold promise in addressing the nuanced challenges inherent in identifying both legitimate and illegitimate behavior within diverse datasets.

While the enhancement in performance is noteworthy, it's essential to acknowledge that anomaly detection remains a multifaceted task influenced by various factors such as data quality, feature selection, and algorithm parameters. Therefore, while anomaly graph detection algorithms exhibit promising results, further research and experimentation may be warranted to optimize their performance for specific use cases and datasets. Nonetheless, the observed improvement underscores the potential of leveraging graph-based methodologies in augmenting anomaly detection capabilities and advancing the field towards more accurate and robust detection techniques.

4.4 *Visualization and Interpretation*

After populating the ontology and applying the *SWRL* rules defined in Table 2, we illustrate an example of fraud detection based on rule number 1. This example, depicted in Fig. 5, demonstrates how applying these rules enables the ontology reasoning to flag the transaction "$trans352773A23E89D4EA$" as fraudulent ($IsFraud$ property set to true). This specific identification of fraudulent transactions is based on criteria of the transaction amount exceeding 10,000. To further validate and explore these instances of fraud, $SPARQL$ queries are executed to retrieve detailed information about the transactions. This information is then utilized

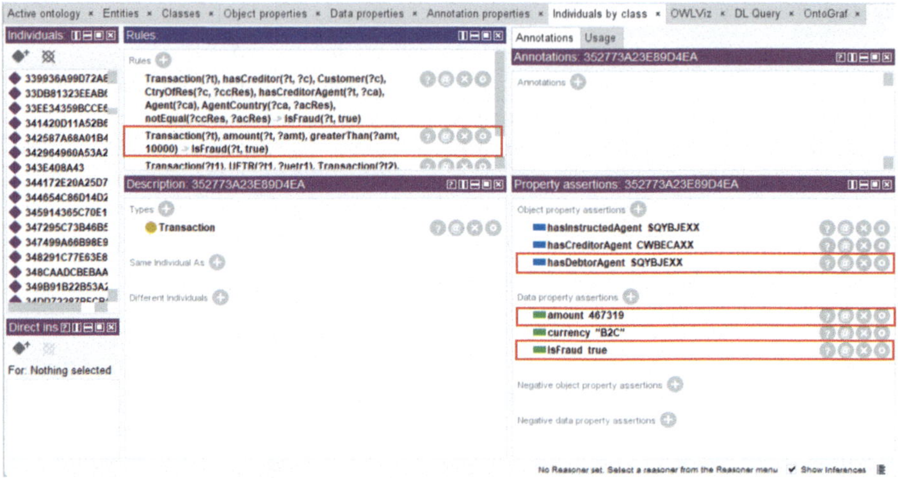

Fig. 5 Visualization of fraudulent transactions detected by the *OntoFic* ontology

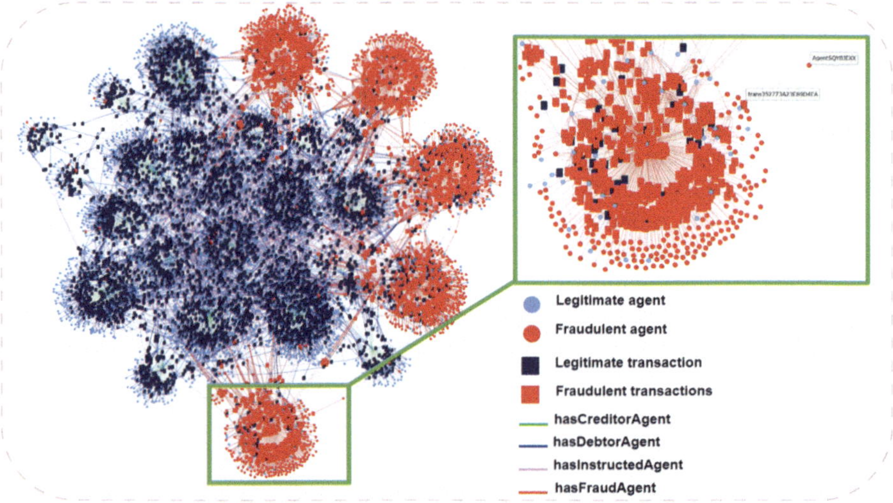

Fig. 6 Visualization of fraudulent transactions

to construct a graph, which serves as the basis for applying our anomaly detection algorithms.

The application of these algorithms allows for the identification of fraudulent transactions, as illustrated in Fig. 6. Notably, we are able to detect communities of fraud, where both the transactions and the agents flagged by the ontology reasoning are also identified by the algorithms as suspicious. This dual detection mechanism enhances the robustness of our fraud detection framework, allowing for a more comprehensive and accurate identification of fraudulent activities.

The visualization of these fraudulent communities and transactions is crucial for interpreting the results of our anomaly detection efforts. By integrating graphical representations using *Pyvis* library[2] with algorithmic analysis, we can offer intuitive insights into the patterns and networks underlying fraudulent activities. This approach not only facilitates a deeper understanding of how fraud manifests within the dataset but also provides a clear rationale for why certain transactions or agents are deemed suspicious.

Moreover, the ability to visually interpret these findings enables stakeholders to make informed decisions regarding fraud prevention and intervention strategies. It underscores the importance of a holistic approach to fraud detection, combining rule-based reasoning, algorithmic analysis, and visual interpretation to effectively combat financial fraud.

5 Conclusion

This paper introduces a novel approach to enhancing the detection of financial fraud, particularly within the SWIFT network. By integrating a dedicated financial ontology with advanced graph anomaly detection techniques, our approach that not only identifies fraudulent transactions, also provides insights into the underlying patterns of such activities. Our ontology, $OntoFiC$, is crafted to model the details of financial transactions, capturing the nuances of customer and bank interactions, and is enriched with real transactional dataset to ensure its relevance and applicability.

The application of graph-based anomaly detection algorithms further augments our methodology, allowing us to uncover complex fraudulent schemes that might not be detectable through traditional methods. The experimental results demonstrate the effectiveness of our approach, showcasing its potential in accurately identifying fraudulent transactions and offering a robust solution for financial institutions in their fight against fraud.

Future work will focus on refining the ontology and the anomaly detection algorithms to enhance their precision and recall rates. We also plan to explore the integration of other machine learning models to improve the adaptability and effectiveness of our fraud detection system. Additionally, extending our framework to incorporate real-time transaction monitoring and developing a more dynamic model that can evolve with emerging fraud tactics are among our key objectives. Through continuous improvement and adaptation, we aim to provide a state-of-the-art solution for financial fraud detection, contributing to the security and integrity of the financial industry.

[2] https://pyvis.readthedocs.io.

Appendix: Online Resources

The supplementary online material supports the comprehension and reproduction of this study. It includes: an OWL file representing the ontology (*OntoFic*), accessible on industry portal site (http://industryportal.enit.fr/ontologies/ONTOFIC).

References

1. Abrouk, L., Chergui, H., Ahaggach, H.: Ontofic: an ontology for financial fraud detection and customer behavior modeling. In: Proceedings of the 2023 IEEE/ACM International Conference on Advances in Social Networks Analysis and Mining. ASONAM '23, pp. 509–513. ACM, New York, NY, USA (2024). https://doi.org/10.1145/3625007.3631503
2. Buitelaar, P., Cimiano, P., Magnini, B.: Ontology Learning from Text: Methods, Evaluation and Applications vol. 123. IOS press
3. Mishra, S., Jain, S.: A study of various approaches and tools on ontology. In: 2015 IEEE International Conference on Computational Intelligence & Communication Technology, pp. 57–61 (2015). IEEE
4. Browarnik, A., Maimon, O.: Ontology learning from text: why the ontology learning layer cake is not viable. International Journal of Signs and Semiotic Systems (IJSSS) **4**(2), 1–14 (2015)
5. Attigeri, G., M M, M., Pai, R., Kulkarni, R.: Knowledge base ontology building for fraud detection using topic modeling. Procedia Computer Science **135**, 369–376 (2018) https://doi.org/10.1016/j.procs.2018.08.186
6. El Orche, A., Bahaj, M., Ain Alhayat, S.: Ontology based on electronic payment fraud prevention. Faculty of Sciences & Technologies HASSAN 1 (2018)
7. Bo, Y., Xinfei, W.: Construction and application of risk ontology in logistics finance from the perspective of risk correlation. Journal of Physics: Conference Series **1288**(1), 012060 (2019) https://doi.org/10.1088/1742-6596/1288/1/012060
8. Ahmed, M., Ansar, K., Muckley, C.B., Khan, A., Anjum, A., Talha, M.: A semantic rule based digital fraud detection. PeerJ Computer Science **7**, 649 (2021)
9. Hussaini, A., Guessoum, Z., Laurent, E.: Elaboration of financial fraud ontology, pp. 277–285 (2022). https://doi.org/10.15439/2022F35
10. Zhang, Y., Trubey, P.: Machine learning and sampling scheme: An empirical study of money laundering detection. Computational Economics 54(3), 1043–1063 (2019)
11. Lorenz, J., Silva, M.I., Aparício, D., Ascensão, J.T., Bizarro, P.: Machine learning methods to detect money laundering in the bitcoin blockchain in the presence of label scarcity. In: Proceedings of the First ACM International Conference on AI in Finance, pp. 1–8 (2020)
12. Bestami Yuksel, B., Bahtiyar, S., Yilmazer, A.: Credit card fraud detection with nca dimensionality reduction. In: 13th International Conference on Security of Information and Networks, pp. 1–7 (2020)
13. Varmedja, D., Karanovic, M., Sladojevic, S., Arsenovic, M., Anderla, A.: Credit card fraud detection - machine learning methods. In: 2019 18th International Symposium INFOTEH-JAHORINA (INFOTEH), pp. 1–5 (2019). https://doi.org/10.1109/INFOTEH.2019.8717766
14. Mehbodniya, A., Alam, I., Pande, S., Neware, R., Rane, K.P., Shabaz, M., Madhavan, M.V.: Financial fraud detection in healthcare using machine learning and deep learning techniques. Security and Communication Networks **2021** (2021)
15. More, R., Awati, C., Shirgave, S., Deshmukh, R., Patil, S.: Credit card fraud detection using supervised learning approach. International Journal of Scientific & Technology Research **9**, 216–219 (2021)

16. Larik, A.S., Haider, S.: Clustering based anomalous transaction reporting. Procedia Computer Science **3**, 606–610 (2011)
17. Porwal, U., Mukund, S.: Credit card fraud detection in e-commerce: An outlier detection approach. arXiv preprint arXiv:1811.02196 (2018)
18. Le Khac, N.A., Kechadi, M.-T.: Application of data mining for anti-money laundering detection: A case study. In: 2010 IEEE International Conference on Data Mining Workshops, pp. 577–584 (2010). IEEE
19. Raza, S., Haider, S.: Suspicious activity reporting using dynamic bayesian networks. Procedia Computer Science **3**, 987–991 (2011)
20. Carcillo, F., Le Borgne, Y.-A., Caelen, O., Kessaci, Y., Oblé, F., Bontempi, G.: Combining unsupervised and supervised learning in credit card fraud detection. Information sciences **557**, 317–331 (2021)
21. Pourhabibi, T., Ong, K.-L., Kam, B.H., Boo, Y.L.: Fraud detection: A systematic literature review of graph-based anomaly detection approaches. Decision Support Systems **133**, 113303 (2020)
22. Liu, K., Dou, Y., Zhao, Y., Ding, X., Hu, X., Zhang, R., Ding, K., Chen, C., Peng, H., Shu, K., et al.: Pygod: A python library for graph outlier detection. arXiv preprint arXiv:2204.12095 (2022)
23. Huang, X., Yang, Y., Wang, Y., Wang, C., Zhang, Z., Xu, J., Chen, L., Vazirgiannis, M.: Dgraph: A large-scale financial dataset for graph anomaly detection. Advances in Neural Information Processing Systems **35**, 22765–22777 (2022)
24. Chen, T., Tsourakakis, C.: Antibenford subgraphs: Unsupervised anomaly detection in financial networks. In: Proceedings of the 28th ACM SIGKDD Conference on Knowledge Discovery and Data Mining, pp. 2762–2770 (2022)

A Study of Firm-Switching of Inventors in Big Tech Using Public Patent Data

Yidan Sun and Mayank Kejriwal

Abstract Complex systems research and network science have recently been used to provide novel insights into economic phenomena, such as patenting behavior and innovation in firms. Studies have found that increased inventor mobility, through firm switching or *transitioning*, is associated with higher overall productivity. This paper proposes a structural study of transitioning inventors and their role in patent co-authorship networks within a cohort of highly innovative and economically influential companies, namely the five Big Tech firms (Apple, Microsoft, Google, Amazon, and Meta) during the post-recession period (2010–2022). Using Big Tech patent data, we empirically investigate three research questions. Our findings indicate that transitioning inventors exhibit a higher degree of centrality than average, and their removal results in greater network fragmentation than expected by chance. The transition rate over the 12-year study period was highest between 2015–2017, indicating non-trivial shifts in the Big Tech innovation ecosystem during that period. We also find moderate evidence of increased estimated impact, on average, of patents co-authored by an inventor following transition, compared to those co-authored before transition.

Keywords Complex systems · Co-authorship networks · Inventor mobility · Productivity · Big Tech

---

Y. Sun · M. Kejriwal (✉)
University of Southern California, Los Angeles, CA, USA
e-mail: yidans@isi.edu; kejriwal@isi.edu

M. Kaya et al. (eds.), *Social Network Analysis and Mining Applications in Healthcare and Anomaly Detection*, Lecture Notes in Social Networks,
https://doi.org/10.1007/978-3-031-75204-9_12

1 Introduction

Innovation[1] has long been acknowledged in economics and social sciences as a key driver of long-term productivity and economic measures of aggregate income, such as the Gross Domestic Product (GDP) [2–5]. In a knowledge-based economy [6, 7], which is prevalent in much of the industrialized world, innovative products and services developed and commercialized by private organizations can be a significant factor in determining the firm's valuation [5, 8]. Moreover, innovation can also contribute to positive societal benefits through higher corporate social responsibility exhibited by more innovative firms. In a seminal work, Mishra analyzed a sample of more than 13,000 US 'firm-years' over 15 years starting from the early 1990s and discovered that, mediated by high corporate social responsibility, more innovative firms ultimately achieved significantly higher valuation following a period of innovation [9]. As with any complex system, it bears noting that the relationship between innovation and valuation is itself a complex one, and not always significant (some instances of negative association for specific sectors and types of innovations may be found in, for example, [10]). Both the sector and geography can play a role. Most studies have found support for the claim that for technology and 'science-based' firms (to quote the terminology used in [8]), there is a positive relationship.

The positive impact of innovation on valuation is particularly pronounced in technology sectors, such as fintech [11], and for early-stage companies, such as start-ups [12]. While not the only measure of an organization's *innovation productivity*, the quantity of patents filed by a company is a widely used objective measure among researchers and policymakers [13–15]. Currently, there exists a vast body of literature on various aspects of patent analysis, including the construction and examination of patent networks, valuation estimation based on patent analysis, textual analysis of patents, and numerous qualitative studies on patents [16–19].

Our study contributes to this broad body of literature on patent analysis by examining the unique behavior and structural properties of *firm-switching* or *transitioning* inventors in a 'patent co-authorship network'. Such a network depicts the collaborative relationships among inventors based on their co-authorship of patents, where individual inventors are represented by nodes, and the edges connecting these nodes indicate that the inventors have jointly authored at least one patent. Specifically, we construct and analyze such networks for five 'Big Tech' firms—Apple, Google, Meta, Microsoft, and Amazon—which outperformed the broader market post-2008 financial crisis and became some of the world's most valuable

[1] This article is an extended version of our previous work presented at the 2023 International Conference on Advances in Social Networks (ASONAM 2023) [1]. Along with making significant additions to the experimental study and results with new figures and tables, we also have expanded the methods section and provide broader context and discussion on the findings in a new *Discussion* section, including through new qualitative results not published before.

companies.[2] Our study spans from 2010 to 2022, a pivotal period during which these tech giants innovated in response to changing market conditions and underwent significant transformations in the technology world. In this study, we consider an inventor a 'co-author' on a patent where one of these five one Big Tech firms is the 'assignee' organization, i.e., the entity filing the patent and holding legal ownership of the intellectual property. We define a 'transitioning inventor' as an individual who initially works for one Big Tech firm (e.g., Apple) and co-authors patents filed by that company, but later moves to another (e.g., Amazon) and begins co-authoring patents filed by the new firm.

There is increasing evidence that such firm-switching or 'transitioning' inventors may play an under-appreciated role in boosting innovation potential within the technology ecosystem [20]. Intuitively, inventor 'mobility' [21] represents the ability to transition, and even for general workers (not just inventors), evidence suggests that mobility can lead to productivity gains and better incentive alignment in the overall economy [22]. Highly productive inventors are also more likely to be 'poached' by a rival company seeking to innovate in a parallel field. These rival companies may be motivated to offer greater benefits to the inventor, such as higher pay and more freedom in developing and publishing their ideas, many of which the organization can potentially patent. As poaching is usually targeted, this can further motivate the inventor due to better alignment between the company's incentives and the inventor's goals. While firm switching behavior has received some theoretical and empirical attention in the economics literature [20, 22, 23], it has never before been studied from a structural perspective (i.e., from the standpoint of *economic complexity* [24]), focusing on the five Big Tech organizations in the post-recessionary era (2010–2022).

We formulate and investigate three specific research questions (RQs) to better understand the structural role and other properties of these transitioning inventors in the broader Big Tech ecosystem during this period:

RQ1: How do the structural properties of transitioning inventors in the patent co-authorship network compare with those of other inventors, and does their removal lead to lower connectivity and more fragmentation than expected by chance?

RQ2: Does the rate of inventor transition remain constant over time, or is there a specific period during which the majority of transitions occur?

RQ3: Is transition associated with an increase in the estimated impact of co-authored patents *after* transition, compared to the impact of patents co-authored *before* transition?

In RQ1, we use usual network science tools to explore the structural properties of transitioning inventors within the entire co-authorship network, which includes all Big Tech patent authors during the research period, as well as within a sub-network consisting only of transitioning inventors. In RQ2, we evaluate how the transition rate evolves over the research period—whether it remains stable, fluctuates, or

[2] https://www.cnbc.com/2020/01/28/sp-500-dominated-by-apple-microsoft-alphabet-amazon-facebook.html.

displays a more complex pattern. We also examine if certain Big Tech firms have experienced higher transition rates compared to others or if the transition-mixture is relatively even among the five companies. RQ3 aims to study whether the transition is associated with an estimated measure of 'excess' impact due to transition. While we only consider one measure of 'excess' impact, our definition attempts to control for potential biases, such as the length of time elapsed since the patent was granted.

2 Materials and Methods

Our study examines patents filed by five major technology companies: Google, Meta (formerly Facebook), Apple, Amazon, and Microsoft. The patent data was retrieved using the 'Query Builder' feature from PatentsView [25], a powerful tool developed with the support of the Office of the Chief Economist at the U.S. Patent & Trademark Office (USPTO) for visualizing and analyzing intellectual property (IP) data. The Query Builder offers a user-friendly interface that allows users to search the PatentsView database for patent information based on a wide range of criteria, including patent title, inventor names, assignee names, dates, and classifications, among others. Once a query is constructed, users can execute the search and download the patent data in various formats, including spreadsheets, etc.

To obtain the relevant patent data for this study, we issued the following search criteria to the Query Builder: '*Assignee Organization* contains *[Organization Name]*.'[3] Here, *[Organization Name]* is a placeholder for each of the five Big Tech companies targeted, and *Assignee Organization* is a field name in the PatentsView dataset. Additionally, we applied a time constraint to focus on patents filed by these companies between 2010 and 2022 (inclusive) and granted within the same period.

During the extended study period, the Query Builder tool (that we used for querying the patent database and downloading the data) was temporarily unavailable due to scheduled improvements. As an alternative, we provide an illustration of the search functionalities available through the 'Advanced Search' feature of PatentsView (particularly for readers) in Fig. 1. While its search function is similar to that used via the Query Builder, Advanced Search is limited to viewing individual patents and does not support bulk downloading of patent data. Users can conduct searches using options such as the 'Assignee, At-Issue' function, specifying parameters like 'all these words' or 'at least one of these words', and filtering patents based on their filing or grant dates. Upon executing a search, the system presents a list of patents meeting the entered criteria, displaying details such as patent titles, citations, and filing dates. Users can then explore a more detailed view

[3] The 'contains' search option returns patents where the assignee organization name includes the specified organization name as a substring. For example, patents assigned to 'Google LLC' will be returned if the [Organization Name] is 'Google.' While the 'equals' search option could be used, it is less robust and may not capture subsidiary organizations, as discussed subsequently.

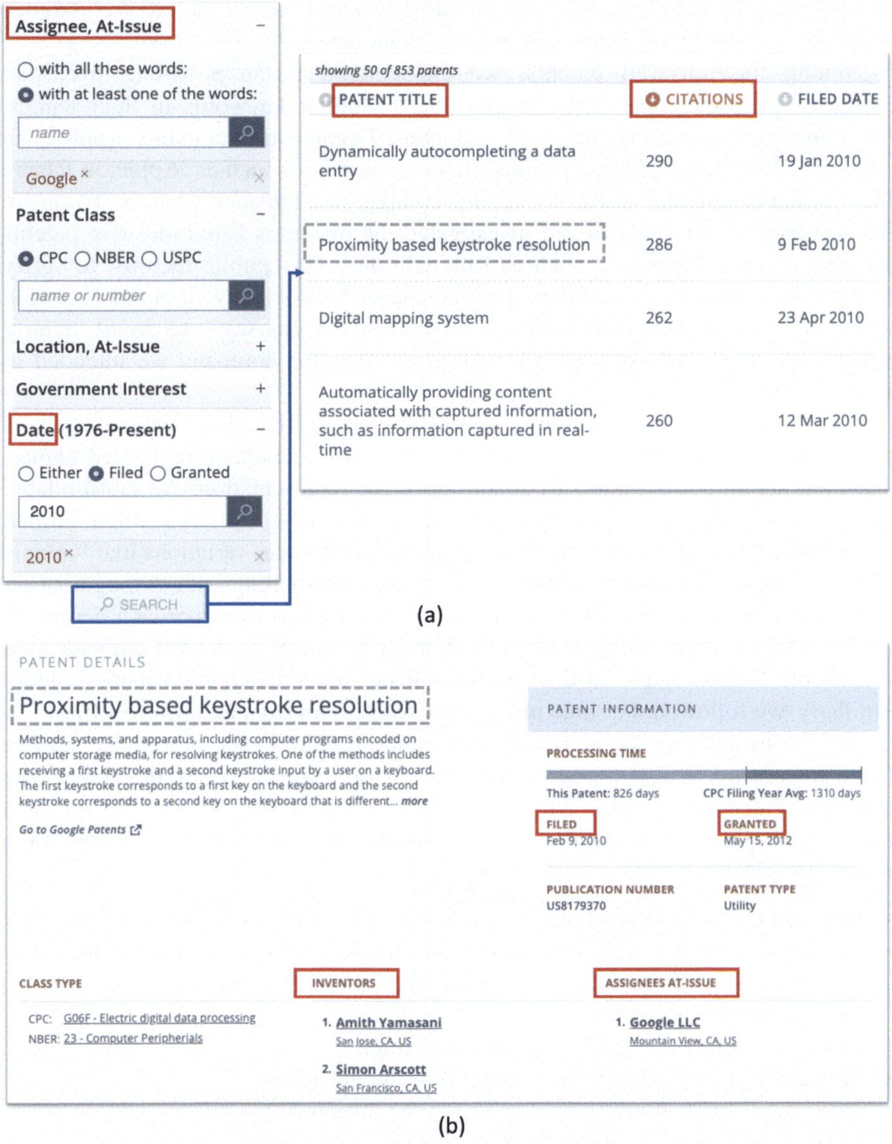

Fig. 1 Illustration of the PatentsView [25] Advanced Search Interface. (**a**) The 'Assignee, At-Issue' feature allows users to enter assignee names, offering options to search using 'all these words' or 'at least one of these words', and to select patents based on the filing or grant date. The system retrieves patents that meet the criteria by displaying a list that includes patent titles, citations, and filing dates. (**b**) Detailed view of a selected patent from the returned list, showing the inventor names, specific name of the assignee at issue, filing date, grant date, and additional details

of any selected patent from this list, including inventor names, the precise assignee name, filing dates, grant dates, and other relevant details.

Among the retrieved patents, we encountered instances where irrelevant assignees were included in the results due to similar keywords in their names. For example, when using the query 'Assignee Organization contains Apple', the results inadvertently included patents filed by companies such as 'Appleton Papers Inc.', which is unrelated to Apple Inc., the company we intended to study. To ensure the accuracy of our analysis, we investigated the inventors listed on these patents utilizing external resources, such as LinkedIn and other public records, to verify whether the inventors were affiliated with the intended company, or in fact belonged to an unrelated organization with a similar name. In this way, we could identify whether the retrieved assignee was indeed the genuine company we intended to study.

After identifying the genuine assignees, we found that these technology corporations often have numerous branches, subsidiaries, alternate registered names, and even spelling variations. To ensure accurate representation, we consolidated all patents filed by subsidiary branches and alternate names under a single unified name for each company. For instance, all patents filed under variations like 'Google LLC', 'Google Technology Holdings LLC', and misspellings like 'Google LCC' were assigned to the unified name 'Google'. We applied this approach across all five companies in our study. Patents filed under assignees such as 'Facebook' and 'Facebook Technologies, LLC' were combined under the unified name 'Meta'. Similarly, we followed the same process for Apple, Amazon, and Microsoft.

After consolidating the assignees and gathering all patents filed under the five companies of interest, we focused our analysis on a subset of key fields from the extensive PatentsView data. While the complete set of fields[4] available for each patent in the PatentsView can be quite extensive, we restricted our analysis to the following selected fields:

- `app_date`: Date of patent application filing.
- `assignee_organization`: Patent rights holder (Google, Meta, Apple, Amazon, Microsoft). In the patents we examine, each patent only have one assignee organization associated.
- `inventor_key_id`: Unique inventor identifier.
- `inventor_first_name`: First name(s) of the inventor(s).
- `inventor_last_name`: Last name(s) of the inventor(s).
- `patent_title`: The title given to the invention covered by the patent.
- `patent_date`: Patent's grant date.
- `patent_number`: Unique patent ID.
- `citedby_patent_number`: Count of patents citing this patent.

[4] A data dictionary describing all of these fields may be accessed at https://patentsview.org/query/data-dictionary.

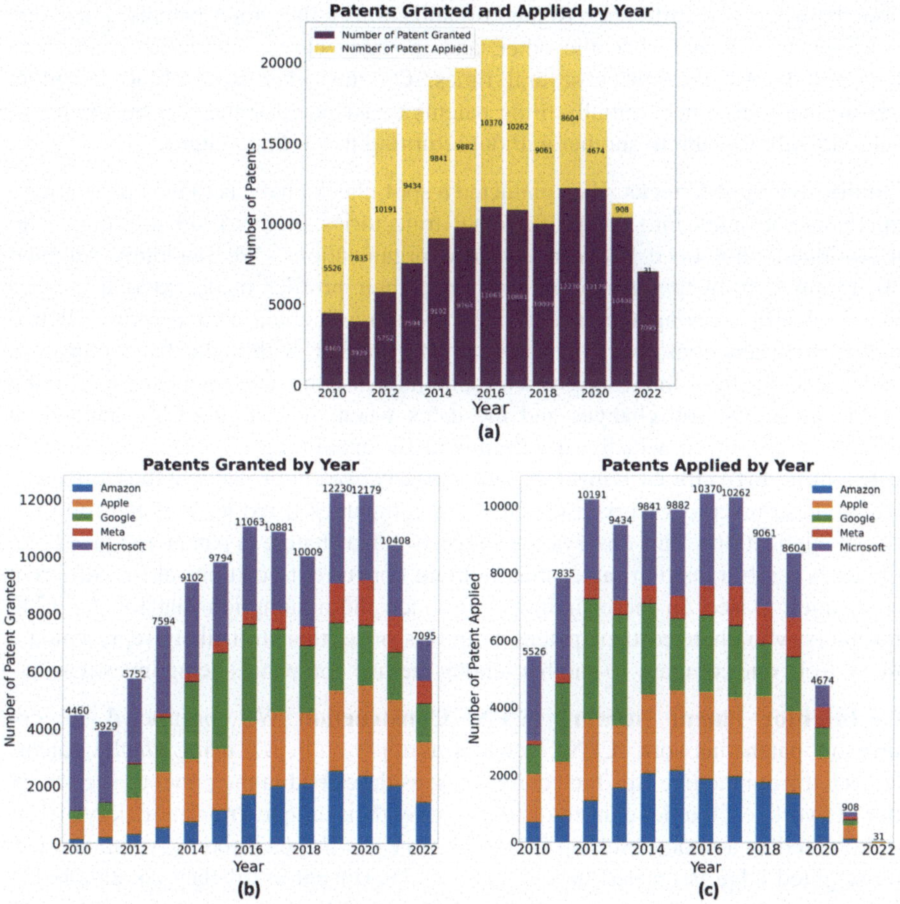

Fig. 2 (**a**) The distribution of granted patents and filed patents; (**b**) distribution of patents granted per year, by company; (**c**) distribution of patents applied for by each company per year

Basic Descriptive Statistics Between 2010 and 2022, a total of 2329 inventors were granted patents with more than one assignee organization among the five Big Tech companies. Figure 2 illustrates the distribution of patents filed and granted across these organizations during this time period. Among these 2329 inventors, 2213 had patents associated with exactly two different assignee organizations. In relative terms, the number of individuals authoring patents with multiple assignee organizations represents a small but non-trivial fraction of the total number of individuals who authored patents for these five companies during the same period (74,637 inventors).

We ordered the patents submitted by each of these 2213 inventors chronologically based on their application dates. Interestingly, we observed two types of transitioning behavior among these inventors. 873 inventors had multiple transitions between two different assignee organizations—they filed patents under one assignee, then switched to the other, and in many cases, continued to alternate between the two assignees several times. On the other hand, 1340 inventors transitioned only once, initially filing patents under one assignee organization and subsequently moving to another without returning to the first assignee.

Qualitative Spot-Checks We conducted a spot-check analysis to gain preliminary qualitative insights into the professional trajectories of the 1340 inventors who transitioned only once between assignee organizations. We randomly sampled 30 inventors from this group and examined their profiles using external sources like LinkedIn. Among the inventors for whom we could find records, all had undergone transitions from one company to another within the five companies under investigation. Interestingly, we found a clear connection between the timing of the inventors' job changes and the dates when they started filing patents at their new employer, which we determined by examining the patent application dates (`app_date`) for each inventor. Additionally, we confirmed that the companies where these inventors worked matched the companies listed as assignees on their patent applications. This observation suggests that a change in patent assignee often indicates a job transition rather than holding concurrent positions at two different companies. Based on these findings, we made the assumption that for the 1340 inventors who changed their patent assignees once, this shift likely represented a move from one company to another among the five companies being investigated.

Co-Inventor Patent Network (CPN) Construction We constructed the co-inventor patent network (CPN), denoted as $C_1 = (V, E)$, using *all* the patents collected from the five Big Tech companies, as described in the previous section. In this network, each unique inventor (denoted by their unique `inventor_key_id`) is represented as a node, resulting in a total of $|V| = 74,637$ nodes. An undirected, unweighted edge is created between two nodes (inventors) if they co-authored at least one patent together as employees of any of the five companies during the period of interest (2010–2022).

Figure 3 illustrates an example ego sub-network of CPN centered on inventor Jane T. Kim (indicated by the red node) and Jane's co-authorship with eight other inventors (each represented by a blue node). Every node beside Jane T. Kim represents an inventor who has filed at least one patent with Jane during the period of interest. Each node is uniquely identified by the inventor's ID. Thicker edges denote direct co-authorship with Jane T. Kim, while thinner edges represent co-authorship among Jane's co-inventors.

Recall that the subset of these inventors who transitioned just once between different organizations from 2010 to 2022 consists of 1340 inventors. To understand the structural properties of these transitioning inventors within the overall co-inventor network, we constructed a subgraph $C_2 \subset C_1$. The nodes in C_2 consist of these 1340 inventors, and the edges are a subset of edges from C_1 that exist only between these nodes. The purpose of constructing C_2 is to study the unique collaboration dynamics of inventors who have experienced a transition in their organizational affiliation.

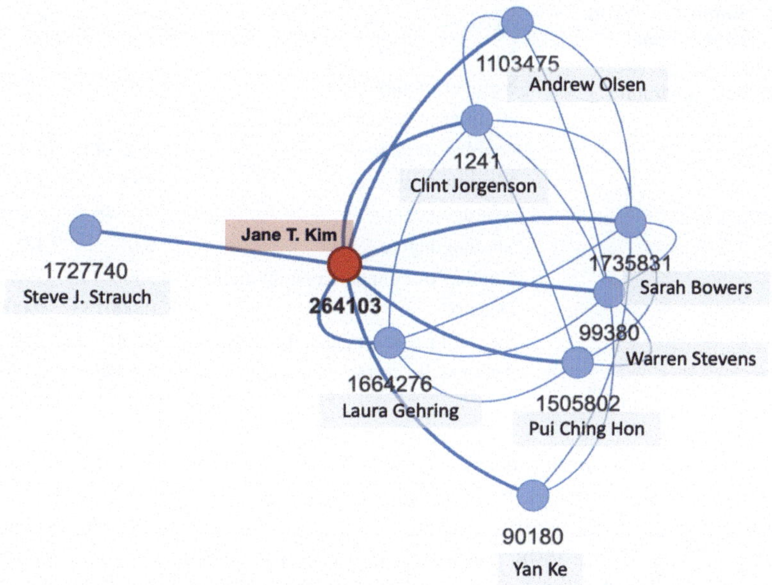

Fig. 3 Illustration of an inventor's (Jane T. Kim) ego sub-network within the Co-Inventor Patent Network (CPN), where each node, identified by a unique inventor key ID, represents a co-inventor who has collaborated with Kim on one or more patents

Finally, to investigate the fragmentation aspect of RQ1, we consider the network C_r, which is obtained by removing all nodes in C_2 (i.e., the 1340 transitioning inventors) from C_1, along with all edges in C_1 that were incident on at least one of the 1340 inventors.

3 Results

3.1 RQ1

In Table 1, we present the network statistics of both the original CPN (C_1) and its subgraph C_2, which exclusively includes the 1340 inventors who transitioned only once from 2010 to 2022. The original CPN (C_1) consisting of 74,637 inventors (as nodes) is connected by 372,245 edges or unique co-authorships.[5] The degree distribution of C_1 follows a power-law distribution with a gamma value of -2.32. Despite the large number of inventors, only a small fraction (~2.5% or 1900

[5] Because the CPN is undirected, a co-authorship relation is counted only once. In the future, we will also consider the weighted version of this network.

Table 1 Summary network statistics of the original co-inventor patent network (CPN) C_1 and subgraph C_2

Network statistics	C_1	C_2
Number of nodes	74,637	1340
Number of singletons	1900	652
Number of non-singletons	72,737	688
Number of edges	372,245	710
Maximum degree	460.0	13.0
Average degree	9.9748	1.0597
Median degree	6.0	1.0
Number of connected components	3598	792
Density	0.000133	0.000791
Size of largest connected component	66,818	239
Average clustering coefficient	0.6754	0.0986

nodes) are singletons, indicating a relatively well-connected network. On average, each inventor in this network has co-authored patents with approximately 10 other inventors, with the most prolific inventor having co-authored with 460 others. The network is divided into 3598 connected components (including singletons), with the largest connected component consisting of 66,818 inventors. The density of the network is relatively low ($\sim$0.000134), implying that it is still quite sparse, despite the inventors being divided only among five unique organizations. However, as expected from the social nature of such collaborations, the average clustering coefficient is moderately high ($\sim$0.675), which indicates substantial clustering and transitivity among the inventors.

We also computed the degree distribution of the nodes corresponding to the 1340 inventors who transitioned only once from 2010 to 2022 within the network graph C_1. Figure 4a and b illustrate the overall degree distribution (all nodes) in C_1 as well as the degree distribution of the subset of 1340 nodes in C_1. We then ranked these degrees and compared the ranks with respect to the overall network. We found that 80.61% of the transitioning inventors are in the top quartile (25%) of all nodes, and 95.07% of the transitioning inventors are within the top half (50%) of all nodes, which are significantly higher than would be expected for a random sample of 1340 nodes selected from the network. These numbers suggest that the majority of transitioning inventors have high degree centrality, indicating some degree of influence (at least in a local sense) within the network. However, by calculating the clustering coefficient for each of the transitioning inventors in C_1 and subsequently averaging these coefficients, we derive an average local clustering coefficient of approximately 0.379 for these transitioning inventors, which is lower than the network average of 0.675. This suggests that transitioning inventors are structurally embedded in a more star-like structure: all collaborators of transitioning inventors do not themselves collaborate on the same patents as often. In other words, transitioning inventors co-author patents with groups of inventors, the only connection being the transitioning inventors themselves.

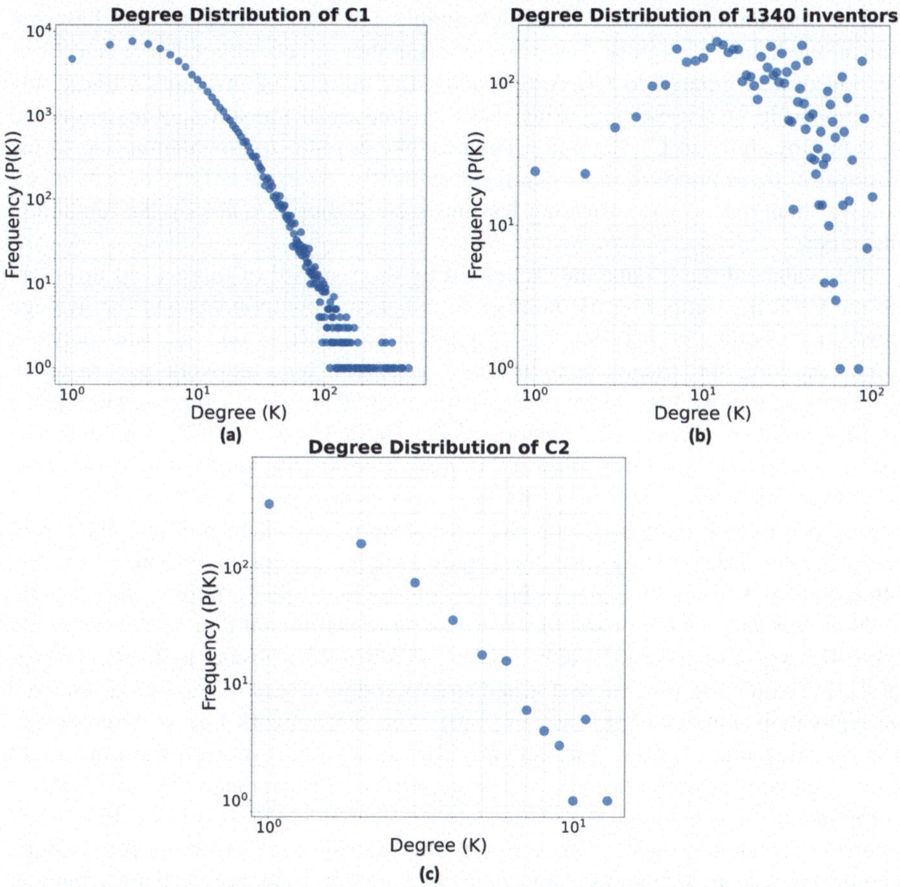

Fig. 4 (**a**) The degree distribution of all nodes in the CPN C_1; (**b**) degree distribution of the subset of 1340 transitioning inventor nodes in C_1; (**c**) degree distribution of all nodes in C_2

Recall that we had also constructed the subgraph C_2 that only contains as nodes the 1340 inventors who transitioned just once from 2010 to 2022. We found that C_2 is denser ($\sim$0.000791) than C_1 while having a lower average clustering coefficient (0.0986) than C_1. Among the 1340 inventors, there are 710 co-authorship connections. However, nearly half of the 1340 inventors have not co-authored patents with any others in C_2 (although they have co-authored patents with inventors in the larger network C_1). These transitioning inventors, therefore, have fewer co-authorship connections on average, as evidenced by an average degree of approximately 1.06 and a maximum degree of 13. The shape of this degree distribution is illustrated in Fig. 4c. While the data is too small to interpret the shape conclusively as that of a scale-free distribution, it is also not inconsistent with such a distribution.

The 'remaining' network, C_r, which mainly consists of inventors who have not transitioned, has a slightly lower average number of co-authorship connections per inventor compared to C_1. Additionally, the number of inventors without any co-authorship increases, suggesting that the removal of transitioning inventors led to some inventors in C_1 becoming isolated. We explore fragmentation due to the removal of these nodes in more detail subsequently. As expected, the density of C_r is lower than that of C_1, indicating less intense collaboration among the remaining inventors.

We evaluated the fragmentation caused by the removal of these 1340 inventors on the CPN by comparing the number of connected components and the average clustering coefficient between the original network (C_1) and C_r (the network after removing the transitioning inventors) as well as a network generated by randomly removing 1340 inventors from the original network. Compared to C_1, the average number of connected components in C_r increases to 3952. This indicates that transitioning inventors play a bridging role in the innovation ecosystem, which was also suggested earlier by their lower clustering coefficient (but higher degree centrality) compared with the overall network. There are now (i.e., after removing the transitioning inventors) more isolated groups of inventors who are interconnected within their groups but not connected to other groups in the network.

Note that this degree of fragmentation is more significant than what one would typically expect to occur randomly, lending an affirmative answer to the second part of RQ1. To quantify this, we performed an experiment where we *randomly* removed an equivalent number of inventors (1340) from the network C_1, as noted above. We repeated this process independently 100 times and averaged the number of connected components across these 100 iterations. This average (3897.1 connected components) is found to be significantly lower than 3952 ($N=100$, $p = 1.46 \times 10^{-9}$, one-sided Student's t-test). This suggests that transitioning inventors play a more significant role in maintaining the network's global connectivity than a random group of inventors embedded in the same environment (the five Big Tech firms), as their removal results in slightly increased fragmentation compared to removing a random set of inventors.

Similarly, the average clustering coefficient exhibits interesting behavior upon the removal of inventors. The average clustering coefficient in the remaining network (C_r) is 0.674. This suggests that, on average, the remaining inventors in C_r still tend to form moderately interconnected groups. Despite the network fragmentation caused by the removal of the 1340 inventors, collaboration among groups of inventors remains largely unaffected, as indicated by the similar average clustering coefficient in C_r and C_1.

We illustrate the removal of a transitioning inventor from the CPN using an example in Fig. 5. On the left-hand side, we present the ego sub-network within C_1 for Michal Hlavac, who is among the 1340 inventors who transitioned just once between 2010 and 2022. In this example, Michal is connected to approximately five different groups of co-authors with whom he collaborated on patents. Following Michal's removal, along with all edges linked to him, the ego sub-network fragmented into four connected components, as shown on the right-hand side. Despite

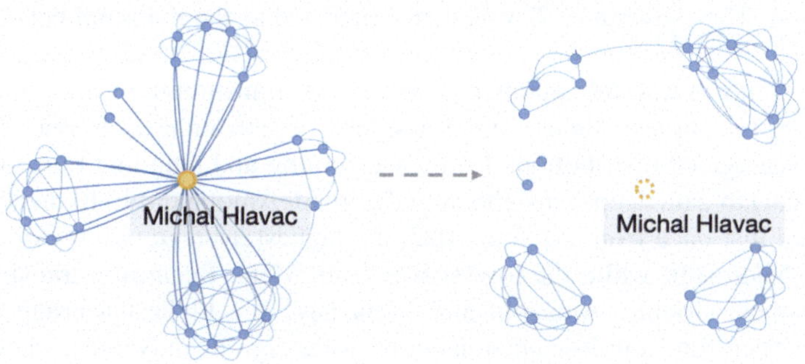

Fig. 5 Illustration of removing a transitioning inventor from CPN. On the left-hand side is the ego sub-network within CPN for Michal Hlavac, one of the 1340 inventors who transitioned just once between 2010 and 2022. On the right-hand side is the resulting ego sub-network after removing Michal and all edges connected to Michal

Michal's exclusion, we can observe that the collaboration among the groups of inventors remains mostly preserved.

In contrast, when we repeatedly remove a random set of 1340 inventors from the network, the average clustering coefficient of the nodes in the remaining network is slightly lower, at 0.660. This value is also found to be significantly lower than 0.674 (N=100, $p = 4.074 \times 10^{-20}$, one-sided Student's t-test). This indicates that the removal of the specific group of transitioning inventors results in a network (C_r) that maintains slightly higher transitivity as compared to the network resulting from the random removal of inventors.

3.2 *RQ2*

The primary focus of RQ2 is to examine if the rate of transition of the 1340 inventors from 2010 to 2022 is relatively stable over the period of study, or if it peaks (or shows other irregularities) during some periods. We also seek to investigate if transitioning occurred uniformly often between the five organizations or if some organizations are, in fact, over-represented in terms of out-transitions or in-transitions than would be expected through chance alone. As a first step toward these investigations, we determined an estimator for the transition time T_t when an inventor transitioned from the first organization to the second organization. To do so, we identified when a transitioning inventor filed their *last* patent with the first assignee organization and when they filed their *first* patent with the second assignee organization. The estimate of T_t was then calculated as the midpoint between these two points.[6]

Figure 6 illustrates the number of inventors transitioning from their initial assignee organization to their second assignee organization each year. We show company-segregated distributions for both incoming and outgoing transitions (and for each year) to gain deeper insights into the trend. Among the 1340 inventors who transitioned just once from 2010 to 2022, the highest average outflow of inventors was from Microsoft, while the lowest was from Meta. Regarding transitions into the companies, Google, Amazon, and Meta have the highest average influx of inventors. Therefore, outflowing transitions were significantly more skewed than incoming transitions, which were more evenly divided. Furthermore, the annual rate of inventor transitions suggests that there is a peak from 2015 to 2017 for both outgoing and incoming transitions. Together, the figure shows a concentrated transitioning period between the assignee organizations, which further implies that the innovation ecosystem within these organizations underwent a non-trivial shift (with the greatest changes suggested for Microsoft) during a relatively brief 3-year period.

While the results in Fig. 6 are illustrative, they are tabulated at the granularity of years. To gain further insight into these transitions at a finer granularity (which is also useful because the rate of transition increases during a relatively narrow time period of 2–3 years), we compute two additional variables for each transitioning inventor: first, we record the time when they first filed a patent with their first assignee organization as their 'innovation start' time T_s. Similarly, we marked the time when they last filed a patent with their second assignee organization as their 'innovation end' time T_e. This period between the start and end times is referred to as the 'innovation period.'[7] Given these additional variables, we sought to identify the periods during which transitions occurred most frequently at a finer granularity (quarters or 3-month periods rather than years). To achieve this, we utilized a moving three-month window that starts from January 2010 and is incrementally rolled (in increments of one day) all the way until December 2022. Within each such window, we determined how *long* each inventor was associated with the first or second assignee.

---

[6] For clarity, we use the term T_t as an estimator, representing the approximate, rather than the exact, time an inventor transitioned between organizations. Due to the lack of direct sources pinpointing the exact transition time, we considered T_t, i.e., the midpoint between the last patent filed with the first organization and the first patent filed with the second, as a reasonable estimate. While platforms like LinkedIn may provide detailed timelines, obtaining this data was challenging in our context and we leave a fuller investigation for future research.

[7] It bears noting that these terms should only be interpreted in the context of this study and time period, e.g., some inventors may have been innovating in other organizations (e.g., startups acquired by some of these organizations, or research labs) before or after the time period of study. The 'innovation end' time, therefore, should not be 'literally' taken to imply that the inventor has stopped innovating or filing patents.

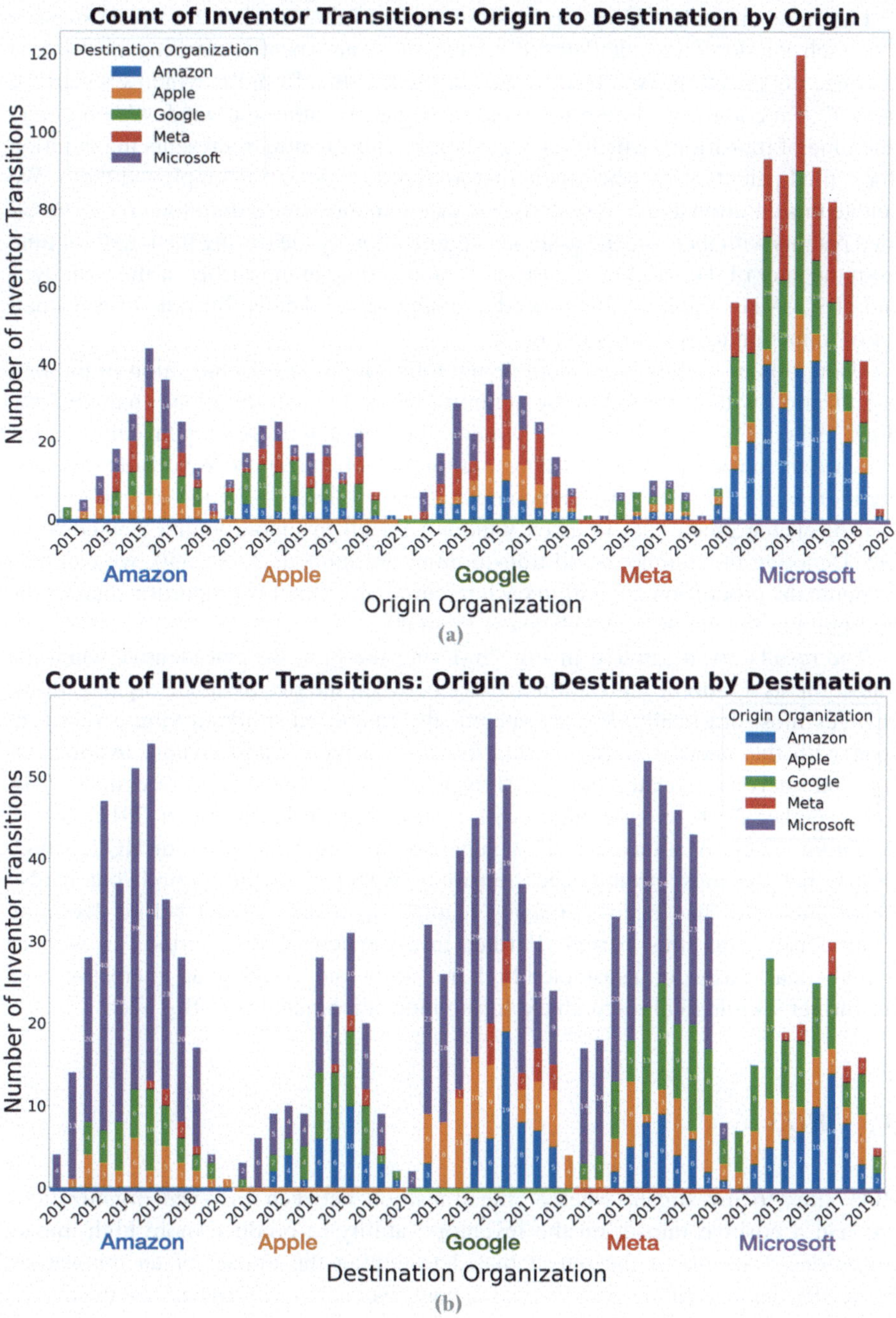

Fig. 6 The number of inventor-transitions from their first assignee organization to their second assignee organization each year from 2010 to 2022. (**a**) The number of inventor-transitions outflow by company, with the color in each bar indicating the destination company the inventor transitioned to. (**b**) The number of inventor-transitions inflow by company, with the color in each bar indicating the source company the inventor transitioned from

Formally, this calculation may be described as follows: First, for every inventor i in each window, we calculated the length of time spent innovating in the first assignee organization. We do so by measuring the time from the window's start (or from T_s if it commenced after the window began) to either the window's end or T_t (the time of transition), whichever was sooner. This quantity represents the duration that i filed patents with when their first assignee organization employed them. We denote this duration as D_i^1. Similarly, we can compute such a duration (D_i^2) where i filed patents with their second assignee organization by measuring the length of time from the later of the window's start, or T_t, and ending at the earlier of the window's end or T_e. An example of this procedure using actual data is illustrated for a small set of transitioning inventors in Fig. 7a.

Using this procedure, we calculate the total 'duration' of innovation in the first organization within a window by summing all individual durations (namely., the 'blue' bars in Fig. 7a within a 'red' window, but for all transitioning inventors rather than just the ones shown in the figure) for the first organization. We denote this total duration as $D1$. Similarly, we can compute the total duration for the second job (the sum of all the green bars in a red window) for all inventors within a window as $D2$. Denoting the number of all transitioning inventors as $I = 1340$, we can now compute the proportion $\frac{D2}{D1}$ within each window, and plot this proportion against the mid-point of the window (which spans 3 months).

The results are illustrated in Fig. 7b. Using the plot, we can identify when the transition, as a ratio of innovation activity between the two assignee organizations, changes most drastically. We are specifically interested in identifying a two-year span with the steepest slope, as this indicates a more rapid change in the ratio $\frac{D2}{D1}$. Our analysis indicated that the derivative of the segment from December 2014 to November 2016 remains high (with a short blip in late summer 2016) before declining secularly afterward. This supports the previous result in RQ2, which shows that the most pronounced transition happened in this period, but it also shows that rates had been increasing leading up to this period before declining continuously after this period. Further investigation of this period, as well as hypothetical causes for a sustained high transition rate, could be an interesting area for further sociological research exploring innovation patterns in Big Tech.

3.3 RQ3

RQ3 aims to investigate whether the transition between assignee organizations has had a positive impact on the inventors' ability to produce more high-impact inventions. We note at the outset that determining the impact of an innovation, especially in the technology industry, is a controversial topic [26] because the impact could occur over long time horizons, be an indirect enabler of other technologies, and is not always measurable using simple metrics. Nevertheless, one way of examining the impact is by considering the citation count of an inventor's patents before and after an inventor transitions. Done in aggregate across all patents filed

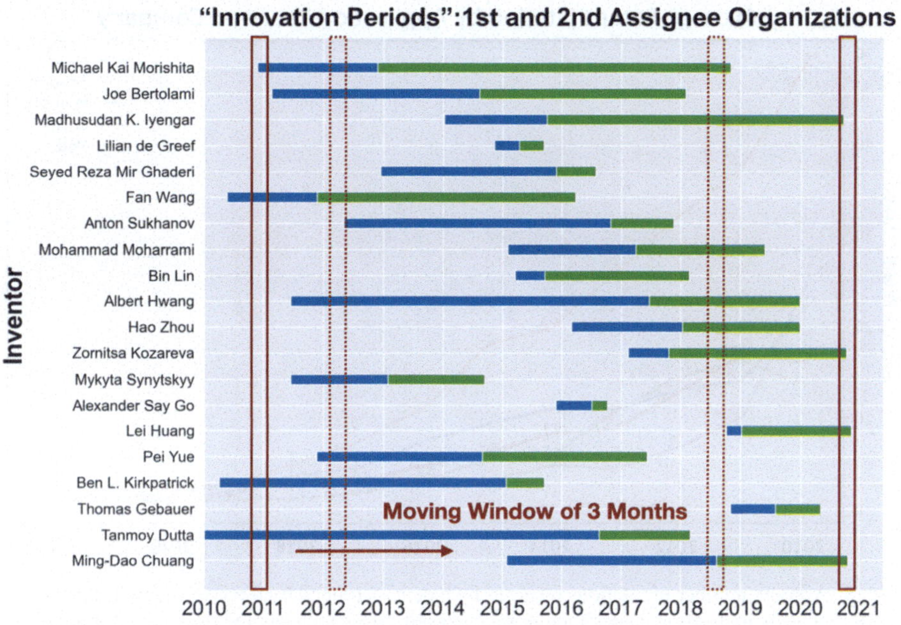

(a)

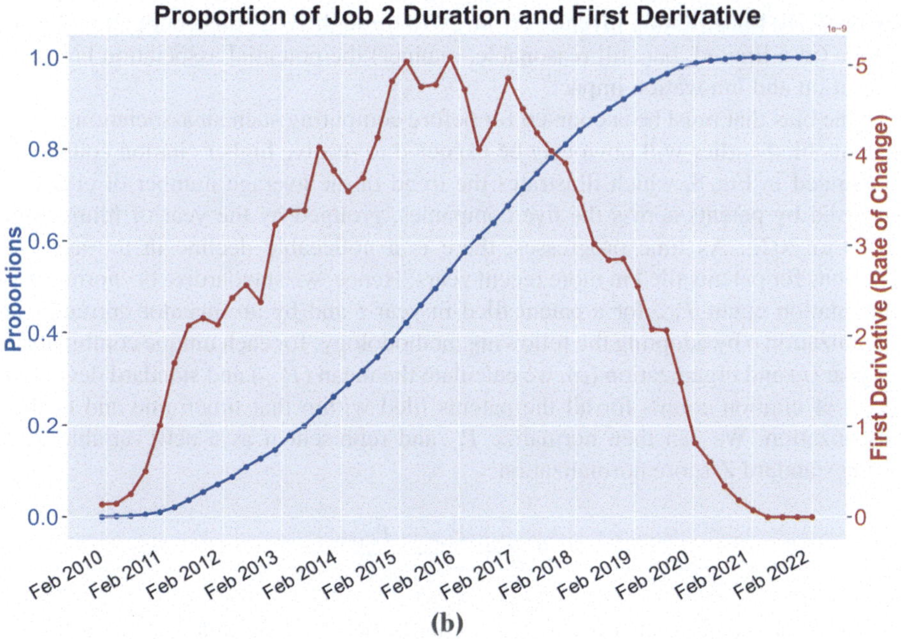

(b)

Fig. 7 (**a**) An illustration of the 3-month moving window for a set of 20 inventors. The start of the blue bar (T_s) marks the beginning of the inventor's 'innovation start' time. The transition time to the second organization is denoted by T_t, where the blue bar ends and the green bar begins. The end of the green bar (T_e) marks the 'innovation end' time; (**b**) The trend of the ratio $\frac{D2}{D1}$ ('proportion of the job 2 duration') between 2010 and 2022, and its first derivative

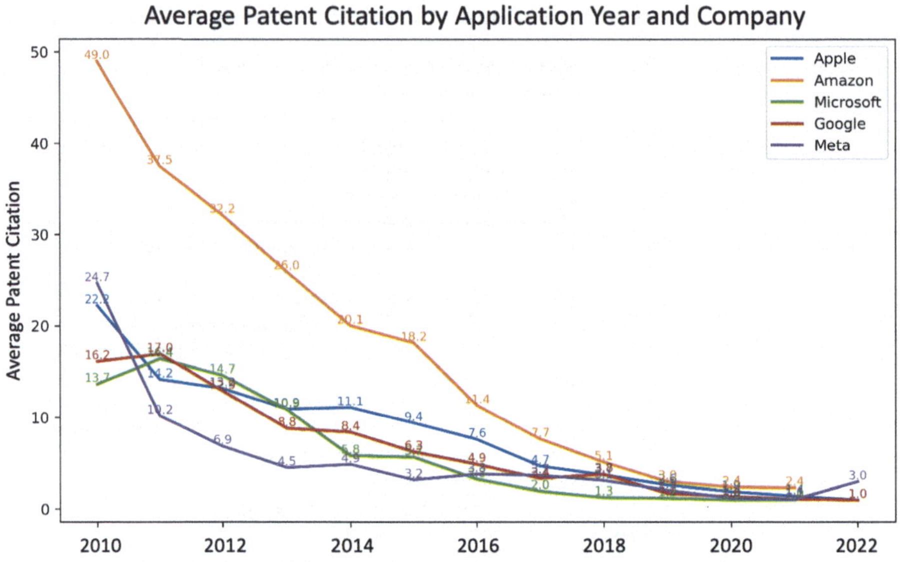

Fig. 8 Average number of citations received by patents, grouped by the year of application since 2010. For each application year, citations are averaged across patents filed by different companies

by the 1340 transitioning inventors from 2010 through 2022, this count allows us to gauge (in a limited, but still reasonable, manner) the potential association between transition and innovation impact.

One bias that must be accounted for before computing such an association is that patents filed earlier will obviously be expected to receive higher citation counts, as illustrated in Fig. 8, which illustrates the trend in the average number of citations received by patents across the five companies, grouped by the year of filing from 2010 to 2022. As time progresses, there is a noticeable decline in the average citations for patents filed in more recent years. Hence, we standardize or 'normalize' the citation count $P_{t,o}$ for a patent filed in year t and by an inventor currently in organization o by adopting the following methodology: for each unique combination of year (t) and organization (o), we calculate the mean ($\bar{P}_{t,o}$) and standard deviation ($s_{t,o}$) of citation counts for all the patents filed within that timeframe and in that organization. We can then normalize P_{t_o} and represent it as a new variable $Z_{t,o}$ using standard Z-score normalization:

$$Z_{t,o} = \frac{P_{t,o} - \bar{P}_{t,o}}{s_{t,o}} \tag{1}$$

By implementing such a Z-score normalization, we are able to derive a normalized citation count, or estimated impact, for each patent within our dataset. Similarly, we can calculate the estimated impact for an *inventor* over a given time period by averaging the estimated impacts of all patents filed in that time period

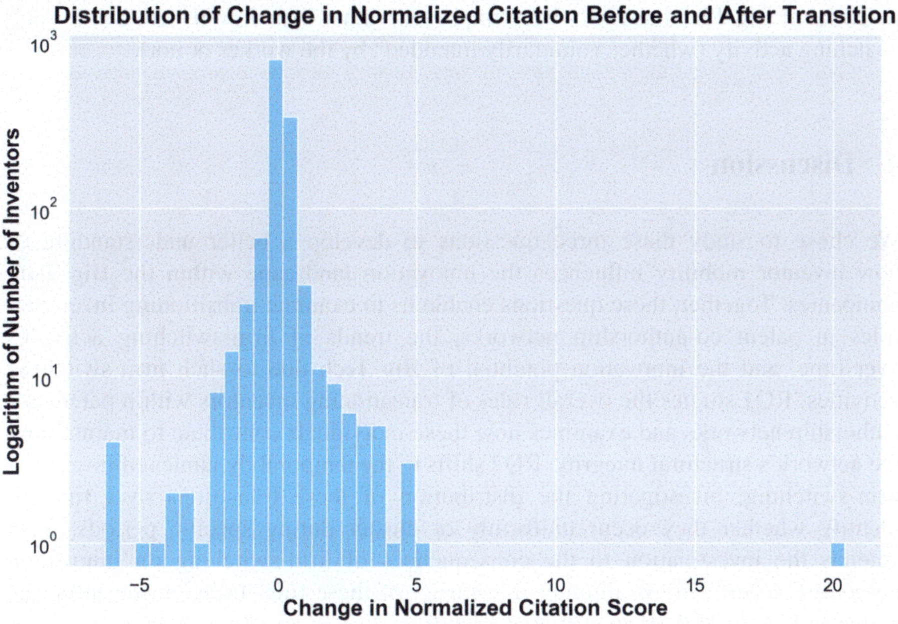

Fig. 9 Distribution of estimated excess impact, using the methodology described in the main text, for the 1340 transitioning inventors. Note that the y-axis is on the log scale

where that inventor was a co-author. With these measures of estimated impact, we investigated RQ3 by first calculating the average estimated impact for each inventor using the patents filed in the entire time period *before* the inventor transitioned,[8] as well as the inventor's average estimated impact *after* the transition. Because these two estimates are obtained for each of the 1340 transitioning inventors, we obtain two 'paired lists' (representing before and after impacts for the same inventor). Subtracting the 'before transition' estimated impact from the 'after transition' impact, we obtain a single vector containing the estimated *excess* impact (due to transition) for each of the 1340 inventors. We plot the distribution of this estimated excess impact as a histogram in Fig. 9. A paired Student's t-test showed evidence in favor of the research hypothesis that the after-transition impact is greater than the before-transition impact (i.e., we were able to reject the null hypothesis convincingly; N=1340; p= 0.00025).

While this result would need to be replicated for other measures of estimated impact, and other normalization procedures, it does suggest that the innovation

[8] Using the terminology introduced earlier for RQ2, this would be the average estimates impact of all patents where the inventor was a co-author in the period $T_t - T_s$; recall that both of these estimators apply individually to each inventor.

potential of Big Tech has likely been improved, rather than diminished, due to such switching activity (whether voluntarily intended[9] by the worker or not).

4 Discussion

We chose to study these three questions to develop a better understanding of how inventor mobility influences the innovation landscape within the Big Tech companies. Together, these questions enable us to examine transitioning inventors' roles in patent co-authorship networks, the trends of firm-switching activities over time, and the innovation potential of Big Tech due to such firm-switching activities. RQ1 studies the overall roles of transitioning inventors within patent co-authorship networks and examines how these individuals contribute to maintaining the network's structural integrity. RQ2 shifts to the temporal dynamics of inventors' firm-switching, investigating the distribution of these transitions over time to identify whether they occur uniformly or cluster during specific periods. RQ3 extends the investigation to the consequences of firm-switching on innovation outcomes, specifically examining the impact of these transitions on the influence and productivity of their co-authored patents.

Summarizing our results, in investigating RQ1, we found that transitioning inventors can play key structural roles in patent co-authorship networks in Big Tech firms in the period of study, much greater than would be predicted by chance. For example, their removal leads to more significant fragmentation, as measured by the change in the number of connected components, compared to the chance of removal of an equivalent number of nodes. Results for RQ2 showed that transitioning over this period did not exhibit a regular or 'secular' trend; instead, there was a significant outflow of inventors from Microsoft and a prominent inflow into Google, Amazon, and Meta. The rate of transition peaked between 2015 and 2017 and stayed high consistently during this period, suggesting a marked shift in the innovation ecosystem of these organizations during this period.[10] Following this period, the transition rate declined and ultimately reached a low level by the time of the pandemic. Finally, in investigating RQ3, we found that estimated excess impact, as measured using a normalized citation score of patents that a transitioning inventor co-authored (before and after transition), was positive and statistically

[9] Transitioning or switching doesn't always indicate the worker's choice. Sometimes, the first organization may have terminated the worker, while in other cases, the worker may have been persuaded to leave and join the second organization. Accounting for volition in these analyses is a crucial yet challenging aspect that future sociological research may want to consider.

[10] During this timeframe, Google experienced an average year-over-year growth exceeding 15% in employee numbers, while Meta and Amazon surpassed 30% [27]. Besides, several significant acquisitions also took place, such as Facebook's (now Meta) acquisition of WhatsApp in 2014 and Amazon's acquisition of Whole Foods in 2017. The underlying reason for this peak remains an interesting direction for exploration.

significant. This finding suggests that the transition did not diminish the productivity of transitioning innovators, on average, across Big Techs.

In comparing our work with other similar research, Toth et al. [28] constructed a weighted and time-decayed co-inventor network utilizing patent data within the IT sector to evaluate the influence of co-inventor networks on firm-level innovation performance and examine how inventors transitioning between firms facilitate knowledge transfer. Their study indicates that 'broker inventors,' who bridge disconnected parts of the co-inventor network, play an important role in boosting innovation by fostering diverse connections between firms and introducing external knowledge. Furthermore, they also suggest that when the collaboration network of inventors inside the company is cohesive–meaning it is tightly knit and interconnected–new knowledge can more easily be combined with the existing knowledge within the company. Additionally, they suggest that the "small-world" nature of inventor collaboration networks within firms enhances the future impact of innovation when firms hire new broker inventors. Chemmanur et al. [29] find that hiring a greater number of higher-quality inventors (defined as those with a history of past citations per patent surpassing the median inventor in their dataset) is an important pathway for firms to enhance their innovation output, measured by metrics including the number of patents, total citations, and citations per patent. Additionally, this study also reveals that incoming inventors joining firms with higher-quality management teams tend to have substantially higher average citations per patent compared to outgoing inventors from such firms.

Citing other studies, Steil et al. [30] and Guha et al. [31] explored the experiences and motivations of transitioning employees in technology organizations through survey-based investigations. Steil et al. [30] conducted a survey within technology organizations in Santa Catarina, Brazil. They found that both managers and technicians who participated in their survey exhibited significant positive correlations between perceived learning opportunities and the intention to stay and significant negative correlations with the intention to leave the organization. Guha et al. [31] surveyed employees working in 17 different reputed IT firms in Kolkata, India. They observed that a prestigious company brand name strongly influences the turnover propensity of employees prioritizing work. Additionally, turnover propensity tends to be higher among younger employees, largely influenced by the appeal of higher salaries offered by other organizations.

One limitation of our study is that it only considers inventors who have transitioned once between two companies, excluding those who have transitioned more than once between companies or have filed patents with multiple companies. While we found evidence that these transitioning inventors play an important structural role in the CPN, we did not assess whether inventors with multiple transitions hold even greater structural significance than those who transition only once within the CPN. One interesting avenue for future work is to investigate how the removal of such multi-transition inventors might lead to even greater fragmentation in CPNs, as studied in RQ1. Additionally, although our results indicate an increase in the estimated excess impact of patents co-authored by transitioning inventors, further investigation can seek to determine if inventors who underwent multiple transitions exhibit greater productivity compared to those who transitioned only once, as studied in RQ3. It would also be interesting to explore whether an inventor's productivity and the impact of their contributions increase with each subsequent transition.

Another limitation of this study lies in the challenge in establishing causality of the relationship between inventor transitions and productivity. While our findings suggest a positive association between transitions and increased productivity, we cannot conclusively determine that transitions themselves are the cause of this productivity boost. For example, we cannot rule out the possibility of productivity gains being influenced more by inventors *joining* high-impact teams rather than the act of transitioning *per se*.

One final limitation that we note is that our analysis aggregates patents filed by the five Big Tech firms from 2010 to 2022, without distinguishing among different patent sub-categories. It is possible that the focus on patent development varies among these companies, e.g., Apple has filed a higher proportion of design-related patents compared to the other four firms according to our dataset. It is possible that the impact (including of transitioning inventors) of patent co-authors depends on the specific sub-category in some non-trivial way, with certain categories possibly receiving more citations and, consequently, reflecting greater estimated impact. Future work could aim to tease apart these differences, but we note that it is not always clear how to separate the sub-categories of patents in a meaningful way, especially considering the inter-disciplinary nature of both research and innovation today.

However, as an example of how such sub-categorization and analysis could occur, we point to the Artificial Intelligence Patent Dataset [32] from the USPTO website, which categorizes over 13.2 million patents and pre-grant publications based on whether they incorporate AI technology. Our preliminary analysis, employing a two-way layout ANOVA (Analysis of Variance) with control for the assignee organization, revealed a significant positive correlation between AI-related patents in our patent dataset and their estimated impact (Two-way ANOVA, $F = 26.9$, $p < 0.001$). Furthermore, we observed a significant interaction effect between the assignee organization and AI classification, suggesting that the impact of an AI patent on its estimated impact varies by company (Two-way ANOVA, $F = 17.16$, $p < 0.001$). This evidence suggests that the perceived increase in inventors' productivity may not *solely* be attributed to the transition itself but may also be due to the inherent high-impact associated with the sub-category of the patent they file after transitioning, which an extended version of RQ3 might help reveal.

5 Future Work

Innovation in Big Tech is clearly an important economic phenomenon in, not just the United States, but the larger technology ecosystem in industrialized nations. Our study suggests many interesting avenues for future research. One intriguing possibility is to investigate some of the same research questions through a causal lens, using additional data (e.g., survey) and statistical inference techniques, to address a key challenge in our study: establishing a causal link between inventor transitions and subsequent productivity. While our findings suggest a positive association between transitions and increased productivity, determining whether transitions directly cause this boost in productivity warrants further causal exploration. Furthermore, future studies could examine other aspects of innovation and collaboration within Big Tech firms beyond patent data. This may include analyzing financial resources allocated to R&D projects, the number of employees assigned, and the duration of the projects. Additionally, researchers could explore non-patent measures of innovation, such as the frequency and impact of new product releases, the adoption rates of new services, and the introduction of novel features.

Another aspect worth exploring is to better understand organizational strategies related to talent acquisition and retention, particularly in the context of the increasing prevalence of 'scooping' or 'poaching' talent among tech companies [33, 34]. One hypothesis is that it is not uncommon for companies to hire employees from other companies to work on projects aligned with their current development interests. This can be studied by investigating whether transitioning inventors maintain their focus within their original fields upon transitioning to new companies. To address this question preliminarily, we conducted Latent Dirichlet Allocation (LDA) analysis on the titles of patents within our dataset. We uncovered distinct themes such as *User Interface, Object Tracking*, and *Machine Learning*, each characterized by a unique set of keywords reflecting their specific focus areas. Using this method, future research can compare the thematic focus of patents before and after an inventor's transition to investigate whether inventors tend to remain within their established areas of expertise, or venture into new areas post-transition. Additionally, it would be insightful to observe how patent themes evolve over time across various companies, which might suggest any shifts in technological focus evidenced by the patents they file. Additional longitudinal studies can be further used to examine the thematic evolution of patents to elucidate how these trends align with major shifts in the entire technology industry, such as strategic pivots, acquisitions, or the emergence of novel technologies.

Finally, another direction that could be explored is to investigate the same research questions using a broader array of analytical techniques. For instance, we could evaluate more definitions of estimated impacts by giving greater weight to highly influential patents or those associated with popular trends. Moreover, exploring additional metrics, such as the number of patent licenses granted, can also be valuable as it reflects a patent's commercial value and real-world applicability, providing greater insight into how innovations are utilized in the market. Additionally, the co-patent network itself presents an opportunity for more detailed investigation. Future research could benefit from employing more advanced network analysis techniques, such as Exponential Random Graph Models (ERGM), for a more extensive exploration of networks at the micro-level [35]. ERGM would allow us to model and evaluate the 'propensity' for collaboration among inventors.

By integrating additional data, such as the patent topics that inventors' co-authors worked on in both their previous affiliations and after transition across various periods, future researchers can dive deeper into the reasons or patterns behind the mobility phenomenon. The data could also be used in a link prediction framework [36] to identify potential future transitions based on observed tendencies within the network.

6 Conclusion

In this work, we quantified and modeled the impacts of inventor transitions within five Big Tech companies (Apple, Microsoft, Google, Amazon, and Meta) during the crucial post-recession period of 2010–2022. Concentrating on this significant era of technological advancement, our research explored the effects of mobility among inventors across these five firms by utilizing publicly available patent data and modeling it as a network. Through three research questions, our study aimed to reveal new insights into how the mobility of inventors influences the landscape of technological innovation and collaboration in a fiercely competitive and swiftly changing environment today. We also discussed potential extensions of the study based on content analysis of patents and causal inference and laid out promising avenues for future research.

References

1. Y. Sun and M. Kejriwal, "A structural study of big tech firm-switching of inventors in the post-recession era," in *Proceedings of the International Conference on Advances in Social Networks Analysis and Mining*, 2023, pp. 670–677.
2. B. H. Hall, "Innovation and productivity," National bureau of economic research, Tech. Rep., 2011.
3. C. Freeman, *The economics of innovation.* Edward Elgar Publishing, 1990.
4. J. Courvisanos and S. Mackenzie, "Innovation economics and the role of the innovative entrepreneur in economic theory," *Journal of Innovation Economics & Management*, no. 2, pp. 41–61, 2014.
5. M. Gürler, "Innovation as an accelerating effect on gross domestic product (gdp) per capita," *The European Journal of Research and Development*, vol. 2, no. 3, 2022.
6. R. G. Harris, "The knowledge-based economy: intellectual origins and new economic perspectives," *International journal of management reviews*, vol. 3, no. 1, pp. 21–40, 2001.
7. J. H. Dunning, *Regions, globalization, and the knowledge-based economy.* OUP Oxford, 2000.
8. C. Greenhalgh and M. Rogers, "The value of innovation: The interaction of competition, r&d and ip," *Research Policy*, vol. 35, no. 4, pp. 562–580, 2006.
9. D. R. Mishra, "Post-innovation csr performance and firm value," *Journal of Business Ethics*, vol. 140, pp. 285–306, 2017.

10. G. Rubera and A. H. Kirca, "You gotta serve somebody: the effects of firm innovation on customer satisfaction and firm value," *Journal of the Academy of Marketing Science*, vol. 45, pp. 741–761, 2017.
11. J. Kabulova and J. Stankevičienė, "Valuation of fintech innovation based on patent applications," *Sustainability*, vol. 12, no. 23, p. 10158, 2020.
12. G. Greenberg, "Small firms, big patents? estimating patent value using data on israeli start-ups' financing rounds," *European Management Review*, vol. 10, no. 4, pp. 183–196, 2013.
13. J. B. Sørensen and T. E. Stuart, "Aging, obsolescence, and organizational innovation," *Administrative Science Quarterly*, vol. 45, no. 1, pp. 81–112, 2000.
14. M. Burhan, A. K. Singh, and S. K. Jain, "Patents as proxy for measuring innovations: A case of changing patent filing behavior in indian public funded research organizations," *Technological Forecasting and Social Change*, vol. 123, pp. 181–190, 2017.
15. Y. Chen, Z. Yang, F. Shu, Z. Hu, M. Meyer, and S. Bhattacharya, "A patent based evaluation of technological innovation capability in eight economic regions in pr china," *World Patent Information*, vol. 31, no. 2, pp. 104–110, 2009.
16. B. Yoon and Y. Park, "A text-mining-based patent network: Analytical tool for high-technology trend," *The Journal of High Technology Management Research*, vol. 15, no. 1, pp. 37–50, 2004.
17. J. Yoon, S. Choi, and K. Kim, "Invention property-function network analysis of patents: a case of silicon-based thin film solar cells," *Scientometrics*, vol. 86, no. 3, pp. 687–703, 2011.
18. G. Greenberg, "Small firms, big patents? estimating patent value using data on israeli start-ups' financing rounds," *European Management Review*, vol. 10, no. 4, pp. 183–196, 2013.
19. Y. Choi and S. Hong, "Qualitative and quantitative analysis of patent data in nanomedicine for bridging the gap between research activities and practical applications," *World Patent Information*, vol. 60, p. 101943, 2020.
20. G. A. Crespi, A. Geuna, and L. Nesta, "The mobility of university inventors in europe," *The Journal of Technology Transfer*, vol. 32, pp. 195–215, 2007.
21. K. Hoisl, "Tracing mobile inventors–the causality between inventor mobility and inventor productivity," *Research Policy*, vol. 36, no. 5, pp. 619–636, 2007.
22. H. S. Farber, "The analysis of interfirm worker mobility," *Journal of Labor Economics*, vol. 12, no. 4, pp. 554–593, 1994.
23. A. Stoyanov and N. Zubanov, "Productivity spillovers across firms through worker mobility," *American Economic Journal: Applied Economics*, vol. 4, no. 2, pp. 168–198, 2012.
24. C. A. Hidalgo, "Economic complexity theory and applications," *Nature Reviews Physics*, vol. 3, no. 2, pp. 92–113, 2021.
25. PatentsView, "Patentsview," https://patentsview.org, Accessed 2023.
26. A. B. Jaffe and G. De Rassenfosse, "Patent citation data in social science research: Overview and best practices," *Journal of the Association for Information Science and Technology*, vol. 68, no. 6, pp. 1360–1374, 2017.
27. CNBC, "Apple had slower headcount growth than tech peers, no layoffs yet," January 18 2023.
28. G. Tóth and B. Lengyel, "Inter-firm inventor mobility and the role of co-inventor networks in producing high-impact innovation," *The Journal of Technology Transfer*, vol. 46, pp. 117–137, 2021.
29. T. J. Chemmanur, L. Kong, K. Krishnan, and Q. Yu, "Top management human capital, inventor mobility, and corporate innovation," *Journal of Financial and Quantitative Analysis*, vol. 54, no. 6, pp. 2383–2422, 2019.
30. A. V. Steil, D. de Cuffa, G. H. Iwaya, and R. C. d. S. Pacheco, "Perceived learning opportunities, behavioral intentions and employee retention in technology organizations," *Journal of Workplace Learning*, vol. 32, no. 2, pp. 147–159, 2020.
31. S. Guha and S. Chakrabarti, "Differentials in attitude and employee turnover propensity: A study of information technology professionals." *Global Business & Management Research*, vol. 8, no. 1, 2016.
32. United States Patent and Trademark Office (USPTO), "Artificial intelligence patent dataset," https://www.uspto.gov/ip-policy/economic-research/research-datasets/artificial-intelligence-patent-dataset, accessed: [Insert Date Accessed].

33. The Wall Street Journal, "Startups are scooping up big tech's cast-off workers," *The Wall Street Journal*, January 2022. [Online]. Available: https://www.wsj.com/articles/startups-are-scooping-up-big-techs-cast-off-workers-981f7d35
34. SFGate. (2020, June) Openai, google pay top salaries, poach talent. [Online]. Available: https://www.sfgate.com/tech/article/openai-google-pay-salaries-poach-18489070.php
35. G. Robins, P. Pattison, Y. Kalish, and D. Lusher, "An introduction to exponential random graph (p*) models for social networks," *Social networks*, vol. 29, no. 2, pp. 173–191, 2007.
36. L. Lü and T. Zhou, "Link prediction in complex networks: A survey," *Physica A: statistical mechanics and its applications*, vol. 390, no. 6, pp. 1150–1170, 2011.

Measuring the Echo-Chamber Phenomenon Through Exposure Bias

Nathan Bartley, Keith Burghardt, and Kristina Lerman

Abstract Online social platforms use recommender algorithms to collate and sort the universe of messages users see, which is distorted in how popular content will be perceived before any personalization. We call this "exposure bias," and we focus on evaluating different recommendation and personalization approaches using diverse exposure bias metrics to understand how ranked content affects user perception. Similarly we simulate user activity in a social network to assess the influence of such ranking approaches on exposure bias. Furthermore, we are working on parsimonious agent-based models to explore intervention effects over time. Our empirical findings reveal that users exposed to personalized feeds from various recommender system types experience more exposure bias than reverse chronological and popularity-based feeds.

Keywords Recommender systems · Social networks · Personalized timelines · Exposure bias

1 Introduction

Online social networks (OSNs) play a pivotal role in information dissemination, encompassing a wide spectrum of knowledge and news, from innovations to job opportunities, and even during emergencies like natural disasters [19, 33, 37]. However, the burgeoning popularity of OSNs has led to an unprecedented surge in user-generated content, resulting in information overload. To manage this deluge, OSNs have built recommendation systems to curate personalized feeds for users, wherein content is reordered to optimize various metrics, e.g., engagement and user time spent on the platform. While personalized feeds offer significant advantages, recent evidence suggests that recommendation systems may inadvertently constrict

N. Bartley (✉) · K. Burghardt · K. Lerman
Information Sciences Institute, Marina Del Rey, CA, USA
e-mail: nbartley@usc.edu

M. Kaya et al. (eds.), *Social Network Analysis and Mining Applications in Healthcare and Anomaly Detection*, Lecture Notes in Social Networks,
https://doi.org/10.1007/978-3-031-75204-9_13

the range of information users encounter, potentially fostering echo chambers [32] and intensifying partisanship [10, 35].

While these problems prove pernicious and difficult to study, other areas of research, namely social sensing and social psychology literature, provide a complementary perspective to these problems. Research shows that a human's capacity for social sensing, i.e., their ability to perceive their immediate social network and make judgements about it, is useful for forecasting elections [15] and the signals they get from their environment can impact their own behavior [9, 16]. An important aspect of this human social sensor however is that it is susceptible to scale-based cognitive biases: individuals can be fairly accurate in making inferences about their immediate social circle, however skews appear when making inferences about broader populations [14]. This suggests that how people are exposed to their environment impacts how they extrapolate trends and norms from their local social network [29].

We treat personalized feeds as a ranking and filtering method that will skew users' perception of their network, and therefore content popularity. What this means is that a user who follows a set of accounts where some may be much more active than others will have a skewed inventory of possible messages to serve that user. With a skewed inventory, there will likely be an over-representation of these highly-active users' opinions in a user's feed. Moreover, users themselves differ in when and how much time they allocate to social media, resulting in varying degrees of content consumption during their sessions. These disparities, coupled with the recommendation algorithm's content ordering within the feed, invariably impacts the information users encounter. We introduce the term "content exposure bias" or simply "exposure bias" to describe these potential feed distortions stemming from the content posted by followed accounts. In prior research, we delineated and quantified this bias within the context of an algorithmic sock-puppet audit [5, 6].

To briefly introduce the idea of exposure bias: we treat the problem as the difference between the potential network (all edges between users based on who follows who) and the aggregated feed network formed by the feeds of all individual users (all edges actually observed by users in their finite length sessions). These feed networks are subsets of the activated network (the network formed by edges that actually could be observed based on user activity). Minimizing this difference should be important to mitigate possible cognitive biases individuals might experience when perceiving their social environment.

This report describes a series of projects addressing the following research questions:

RQ1. Can we observe exposure bias in empirical online social networks like Twitter?
RQ2. Do different feed recommendation algorithms affect exposure bias?
RQ3. Do different session lengths affect the level exposure bias?
RQ4. Do interventions in recommender algorithms change the level of exposure bias over time in a simulated online social network?

We extend the conference version of this report in Bartley et al. [7] primarily through the addition of new results, namely the integration of more complex recommender systems in the analysis and preliminiary results around our agent-based models[7].

2 Related Work

2.1 *Cognition and Social Networks*

In the realm of cognitive sciences, extensive research has shown the prevalence of cognitive biases in human decision-making. In particular we discuss the salience bias, which compels individuals to pay more attention to surprising or unexpected stimuli. In social psychology this salience bias often leads to the heightened perception of minority groups, resulting in an overestimation of their prominence. This phenomenon closely resembles a statistical bias known as the "majority illusion," which emerges within network structures, distorting the visibility of uncommon opinions [26]. This highlights a connection between perceptual biases and the dynamics of social networks, namely information diffusion. Past studies have unveiled the role of repeated stimulus exposure in fostering simple contagion, the significance of high-degree nodes in facilitating information spread, and the impact of cognitive overload on information transmission [23, 27, 36]. While these insights are valuable, the current research endeavors shift focus toward examining different feed "queue" strategies and exploring the intricacies of information exposure in session-based social networks.

Building upon these insights, recent work in the statistical and theoretical domains has further expanded our understanding. Experiments were carried on with complex contagion model of information diffusion on Twitter data, demonstrating that repeated exposures from diverse sources offer a more comprehensive explanation of Twitter behavior than simplistic contagion models [31]. Meanwhile, other lines of theoretical work explored a graph theoretical perspective to address the majority illusion in social networks, including grappling with the NP-hardness of both its identification and elimination, and the classification of various types of networks that experience the effect [18, 30]. In the current set of studies, the focus shifts toward partial observations within session-based social networks and the upstream facets of information diffusion, particularly the dynamics of information exposure.

2.2 *Algorithmic Audits of Online Social Networks*

Since the pioneering work by Sandvig, Hamilton, Karahalios, & Langbort in 2014 there has been a growing interest in algorithmic audits, where researchers investigate and probe online algorithms for potential discriminatory behaviors, spanning various sectors, from e-commerce platforms [25] to search engines [39] and online social networks (OSNs) [2, 4, 6, 38].

2.2.1 Content Recommendations

On Youtube, Tomlein et al. [41] evaluated a "filter bubble popping" strategy to reconfigure recommended videos [41]. Although our work doesn't pertain to YouTube, incorporating exposure biases alongside measures like Search Engine Results Pages (SERP) could complement their analyses. Similarly, Beattie et al. [8] examined social "Who to Follow" recommendations on Twitter, proposing a method to break echo chambers through user embeddings, offering valuable intervention tools [8]. In contrast, Ramaciotti et al. [34] employed simulations and empirical Twitter data to examine different recommender systems' effects on the social graph. Through this they identified the co-evolution of the social graph and users' ideological positions [34]. Our work is more focused on user activity and connecting it to their positions within the social graph.

2.2.2 Social Recommendations

In a study related to ours, Huszár et al. [24] investigated the algorithmic amplification of different countries' political parties on Twitter [24]. They considered different global sets of users and relevant political tweets that those users left lingering impressions on, whereas our studies focus on the exposure within an individual user's feed.

Along the dimension of agent-based models, Donkers and Ziegler [12] used agent-based models in a opinion dynamics scenario to assess ideological demarcation in social media networks, allowing for a more nuanced understanding of echo chambers and how they might form. Interestingly they do not explicitly consider a user's perceptions of their network as a whole so much as consider a user's perception of each individual user's tweets that they are recommended [12]. This differs from our work as we more consider multiple different recommendation algorithms and different measures of network perceptions.

Similar work in auditing link recommendations has been done, however they are focused on social network recommendations and not as concerned with possible perception related biases users might experience [21, 40].

The most relevant news feed research to this set of studies comes from Meta researchers. Starting with Bakshy et al. [3] researchers studied how users with different ideologies were exposed to political news from different ideological slants [3]. They find that by analyzing URL diversity partisan users were getting exposed to cross-ideological content (albeit asymmetrically). This result is a primary study suggesting that user choices are in part responsible for the content users see. Guess et al. [20] showed significant differences in what content the personalized and reverse chronological based feeds exposed to users on Instagram and Facebook (e.g., the fraction of posts in users' feeds that friends posted was higher in the personalized versus the chronological feeds). While there are reported significant differences between the feeds, there was no reported impact on political attitudes or outcomes related to the 2020 US presidential elections [20]. Similar to Guess et al. [20] and Gonzalez-Bailon et al. [17] studied the feedback loop between algorithm and user via the spread of political URLs on Facebook, showing an ideological separation [17]. Our work differs in that we study the prevalence of traits across users' friends, which would impact the perceived prevalence of such traits. In other words we think that exposure bias is driven by *who* users are exposed to rather than simply *what* they are exposed to.

Another relevant Meta study is Yan et al. [42] which surveyed Facebook users' and asked if they are satisfied with their friend counts; with this survey they attempts to explain that satisfaction with a measure of weighted perception bias [42]. Their work extended the bias measure introduced originally by Alipourfard et al. by incorporating heterogeneous weighted user information, e.g., a user embedding of an interaction graph [1]. Our work differs from this in that ours is focused on explaining this local perception bias and how it differs between feed algorithms and biased user behavior types.

2.3 Practical Concerns

Previous work has been carried out by Twitter itself into its own content recommendation system [28], detailing both the components of the system and how they measure the behavior of the system overall [13]. Lazovich et al. [28] in particular outlines different criteria practitioners might use to decide how to measure bias within their own recommendation systems. Our work differs in that this work does not choose metrics that explicitly account for the social graph structure of the system: the metrics instead focus on tweets being categorized as "in-network" or "out-of-network". However, the criteria of adjustability, scale invariance, and interpretability are relevant for our analyses [28].

3 Technical Challenges

There have been several technical challenges pertaining to this line of work. Originally we were focused on expanding the sock puppet audits, and while creating the sock puppets and running them was relatively scaleable, getting them to operate from within university-related computing infrastructure was difficult, and justifying the costs for externally hosted VMs was difficult as well.

In addition to empirical data we are pursuing simulations in two ways, both of which have posed scaling problems: the first way is by statically generating activity for each user in a network and constructing their feeds from a global perspective.

This has posed scaling problems primarily in the number of nodes in the network as the number of potential friends to sort through and construct feeds for increases.

The second way is using agent-based simulations, where each node interfaces with a model to get served content from other nodes. The Repast library lends itself well to parallelizing agent-based models, however it requires high-performance computing resources. We have since implemented a model using the Repast library to scale our simulations on an archival empirical network consisting of $100,000$ nodes and 1.5 million edges.

Clean experimentation has also posed a challenge: not only for the sock-puppet auditing and comparing black-box systems appropriately, but also for simulations as well. We try to control as many factors as possible comparing two different feed-sorting approaches like graph size, assortativity, allocation of binary traits across the population, and degree-attribute correlation (i.e., correlation between binary trait X and degree sequence).

Finally, the last of the larger technical challenges has been getting performant recommendations. If we are trying to simulate recommender systems in OSNs, it makes intuitive sense to emulate the production recommender systems as much as possible, however doing so while simulating user activity and any necessary simulation state changes is computationally expensive. Recommender system libraries used for benchmarking systems also do not tend to provide models appropriate for constructing news feeds (i.e., online model that can rank content unseen in the training set); the most relevant we could find involve suggesting new connections (e.g., Who to follow suggestions). We have since implemented PyTorch versions of two deep learning based models, however to hold them in memory we used few features.

4 Originality

We believe this is original work as it suggests the utility of incorporating the passive exposure to information as a part of the overall measure of bias in an OSN. Not only does the structure of a network manner in determining who you get exposed to, but the activity of your friends (and through that the work of the News Feed mediating your exposure to said activity). We do not believe that this gets adequate treatment in the study of OSNs especially in the context of echo chambers and (mis)information diffusion.

We believe that this work also suggests ample opportunity for intervention from a platform level for addressing concerns of misinformation. Rather than having to adjust the visibility of certain accounts across the entire platform, a dial could be set for each individual account (potentially controlled by the user as well) adjusting who they see post-recommendations (perhaps client-side).

5 Outline of Proposed Solutions

We propose the following outline for a research agenda pertaining to exposure bias in OSNs:

1. For RQ1 we measure the existence of exposure bias in a production OSN ecosystem with sock-puppet audits. Additional work would consist of more sock-puppet accounts and the use of data donations from users.
2. For RQ2 and 3 we use simulations and Twitter data from 2014 before any production recommender system was implemented, gathered by Alipourfard et al., [1]. Among several metrics we extend and utilize the measure of local perception bias B_{local} described in their work:

$$B_{\text{local}} = \mathbb{E}\{q_f(\mathrm{X})\} - \mathbb{E}\{f(\mathrm{X})\} \tag{1}$$

   where

$$\mathbb{E}\{q_f(\mathrm{X})\} = \bar{d} * \mathbb{E}\{f(U)A(V)|(U,V) \text{ Uniform}(E)\} \tag{2}$$

   $f(U)$ is the value of the binary trait of friend U, and $A(V)$ is the attention node V pays to friend U. This measure can be described as the expected difference in how frequent a user sees the trait $X = 1$ in their network versus the true prevalence/frequency of the trait.
3. For RQ4 we use agent-based simulations and control recommendations to see dynamics of exposure bias in artificial scenarios. We can use real data to generate the graphs and activity patterns and see if interventions can significantly change different measures of exposure bias.

6 Preliminary Experimental Evaluation

6.1 RQ1

For RQ1 we refer to a previous report [6]. To summarize, we can observe a skew in popularity of what is observed from the inventory of tweets between the personalized and reverse chronological feeds, but a study with eight sockpuppets do not identify a skew in exposure bias between the activity network and the networks observed in the feeds (measured by Gini coefficient).

We performed an additional more expansive auditing study on Twitter from 05-2021 until 02-2022 with approximately twenty-four sock puppets. Each account followed the same set of 100 users, and similar to the previous report logged in several times a day to get exposed to a fix amount of tweets. In this secondary study however we allow for the sock puppets to possibly like the tweets they get exposed to, allowing for a possible additional dimension of personalization.

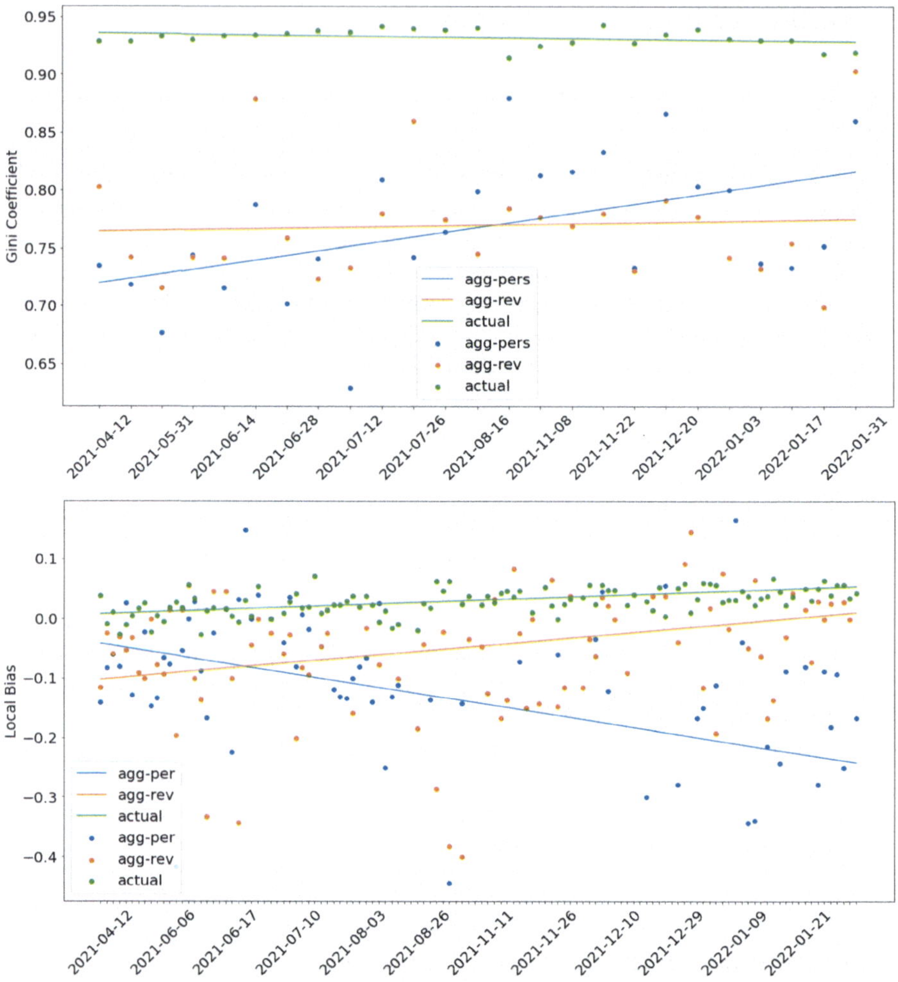

Fig. 1 Sock-puppet audit Gini Coefficient & B_{local} over time. Bias refers to the measurement of Local Bias described in [1]. This figure is combined and modified from two figures reported in Bartley, Burghardt and Lerman, 2024 [5]. Actual activity refers to the measurements calculated from the actual number of tweets and retweets the 100 friends posted during the time window (as gathered from the X/Twitter API). Agg-rev refers to the aggregate reverse chronological timeline (computed by the aggregating all the reverse-chronological sock puppet timelines), and agg-per reefers to the aggregate personalized timeline

We observe in Fig. 1 that while the aggregated sock puppet accounts using reverse chronological feeds seem to stay relatively stable over time (or increasing as in the B_{local} measure), the aggregate of the sock puppets using personalized feeds experience increased perception bias in both Gini and B_{local}. The results for the two sets of aggregate sets of accounts were tested under paired t-tests, with significant differences between personalized and reverse chronological (B_{local} t-statistic: -135.91, p-value: $< 10^{-10}$, Gini t-statistic: -176.58, p-value: $< 10^{-10}$). While there are caveats in the data we evaluated, we believe these differences to be significant enough to merit further study. We also tested several imputation methods for the time-series analysis to ensure robustness; we find as reported in Bartley, Burghardt and Lerman, 2024 that all imputations yield similar trends for the aggregate-personalized and aggregate-reverse chronological feeds suggesting robustness [5].

6.2 RQ2

For RQ2 we utilize both empirical Twitter data and simulations of user activity and feed-construction schemes to evaluate the effect of different algorithms on exposure bias. We observe in the empirical data reported in Figs. 2 and 3 significant difference in the bias especially as we vary the degree-attribute correlation ρ_{kx} (t-statistic: -4.96, p-value: $< 10^{-10}$).

We further simulate user activity under potential personalized recommender system-based feeds as reported in Figs. 4, 5, 6 and 7. Under the logistic regression system users are presented feeds that are rank ordered on the probability that user will retweet/interact with the friend's tweet. Similarly the non-negative matrix factorization system simulates a collaborative filtering method where tweets are re-ordered by the feed user's affinity for that friends' tweets. Both the deep learning models NCF and Wide & Deep were significantly greater than the popularity based feed, however the NCF model was much more biased than the Wide & Deep model. We observe under paired t-tests that the logistic regression based feeds were most biased under B_{local}, followed by NCF feeds, reverse chronological feeds, non-negative matrix factorization, Wide & Deep, then popularity.

As we could not reasonably model reverse chronological timelines with the static numerical simulations, we simulate other timelines and assess their difference under a Mann-Whitney U test. We find the correlated and popularity timelines presented are both significantly different than a random baseline (not reported here). The correlated timeline, not used in other simulations, reflects sampling the friends directly based on out-degree rather than sorting as in popularity. We also examine other metrics in Fig. 8 including the fraction of positive friends seen each day (i.e., $X_i = 1$ for friend i) and Gini coefficient as a measure of visibility inequality.

6.3 RQ3

For RQ3 we utilize similar empirical and simulated data to evaluate different lengths. Variance in the results seem to suggest that only in a few conditions do finite

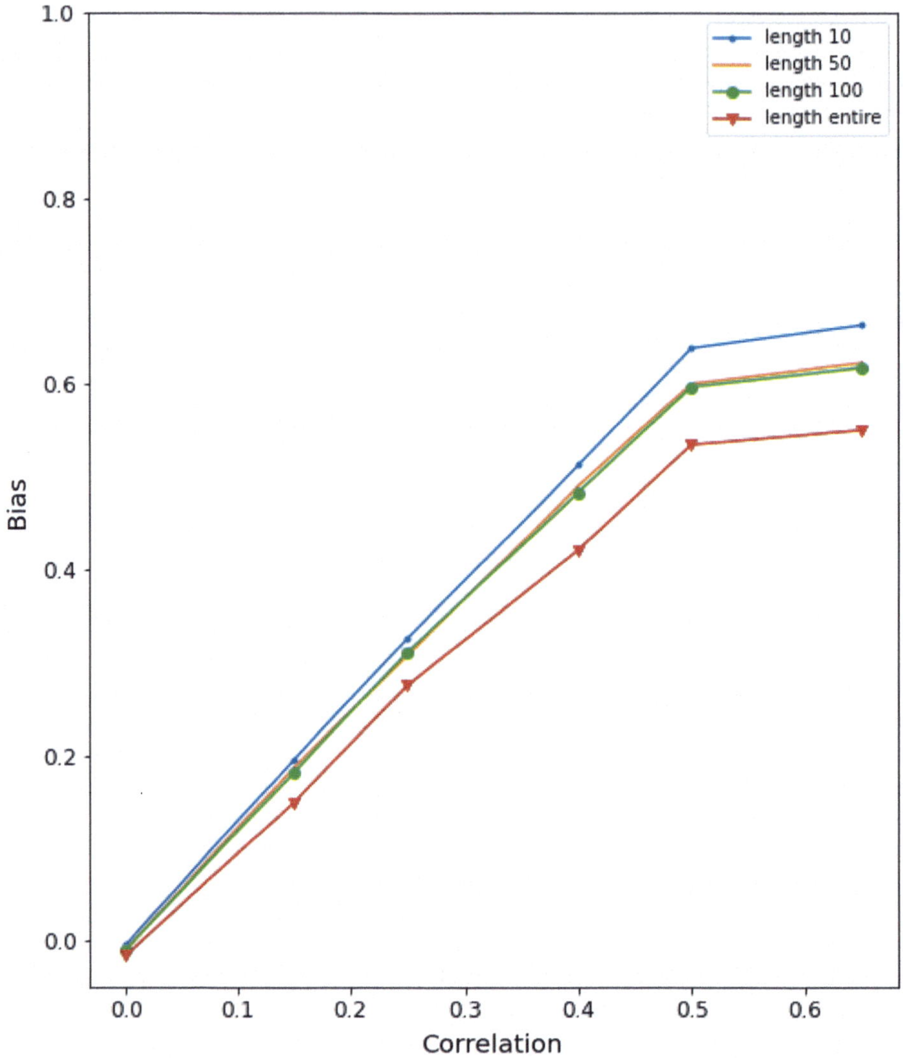

Fig. 2 Empirical Popularity Local Bias versus degree-node correlation. Bias refers to the measurement of Local Bias described in [1]. Increasing correlation increases the probability higher degree nodes have the trait $X = 1$

length sessions demonstrate different effects of exposure bias. Intuitively, in the empirical data, longer sessions seem to present less bias according to the local bias measure in each Figs. 2, 3, 4, 5, 6, and 7, which can be explained by the saturation of observed edges leading to a less biased estimator.

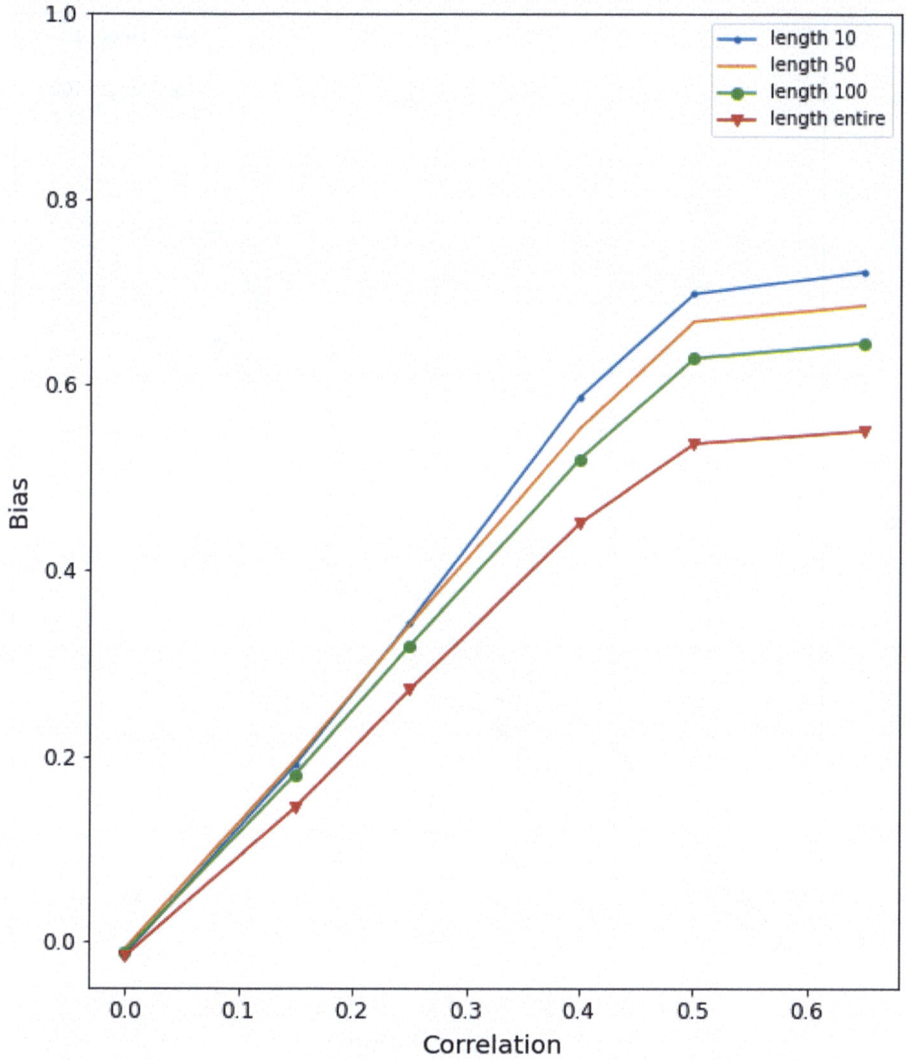

Fig. 3 Empirical Reverse Chronological Local Bias versus degree-node correlation. Bias refers to the measurement of Local Bias described in [1]. Increasing correlation increases the probability higher degree nodes have the trait $X = 1$

6.4 RQ4

We are currently evaluating agent-based models to assess the impact of interventions in the level of exposure bias over time. We are using two different deep learning models of a recommendation system, one a Neural Collaborative Filtering model described by He et al. [22] and one a Wide & Deep model describe by Cheng et

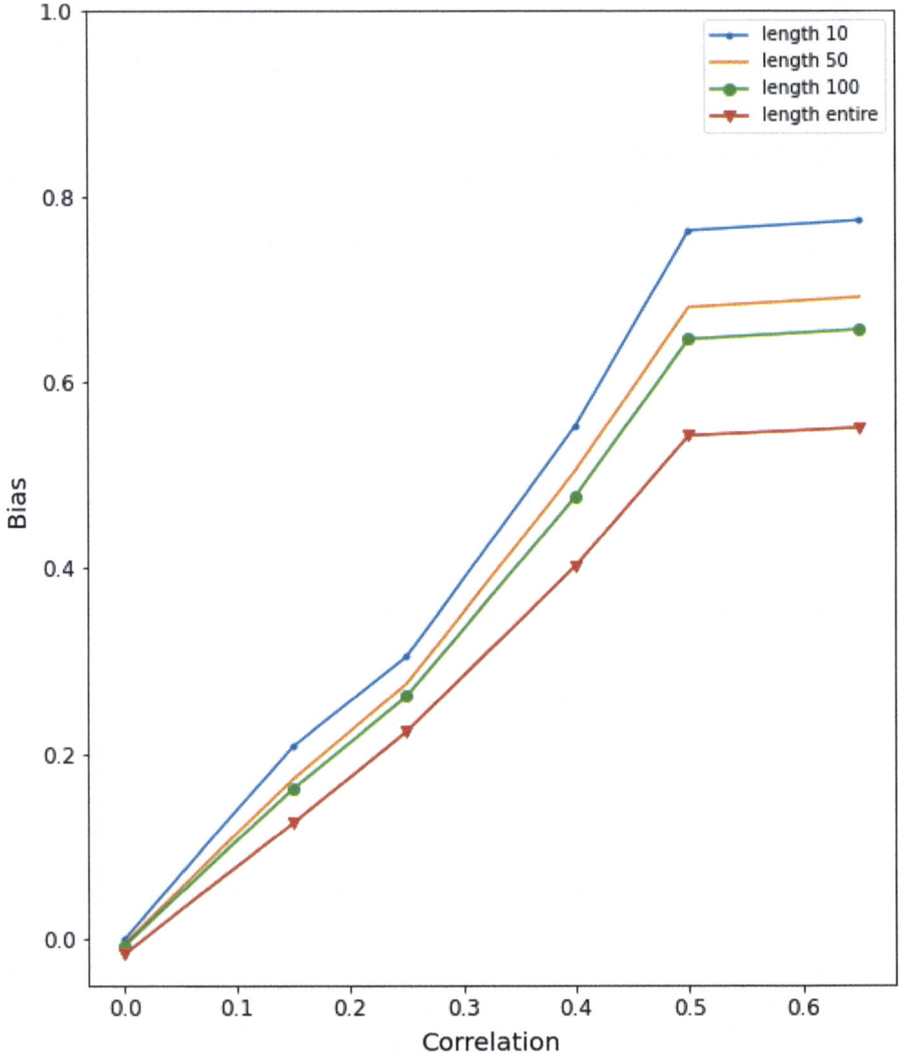

Fig. 4 Empirical Logistic Regression Local Bias versus degree-node correlation. Bias refers to the measurement of Local Bias described in [1]. Increasing correlation increases the probability higher degree nodes have the trait $X = 1$

al. [11] trained for each user. We are also using a reverse chronological algorithm, random and popularity-based feed for each user. The model parameters and steps can be described as follows:

1. Activate user i with uniform probability 0.083
2. If activated, user i then produces N tweets, where $N \sim Lognormal(0, 1)$ and adds to central inventory of tweets

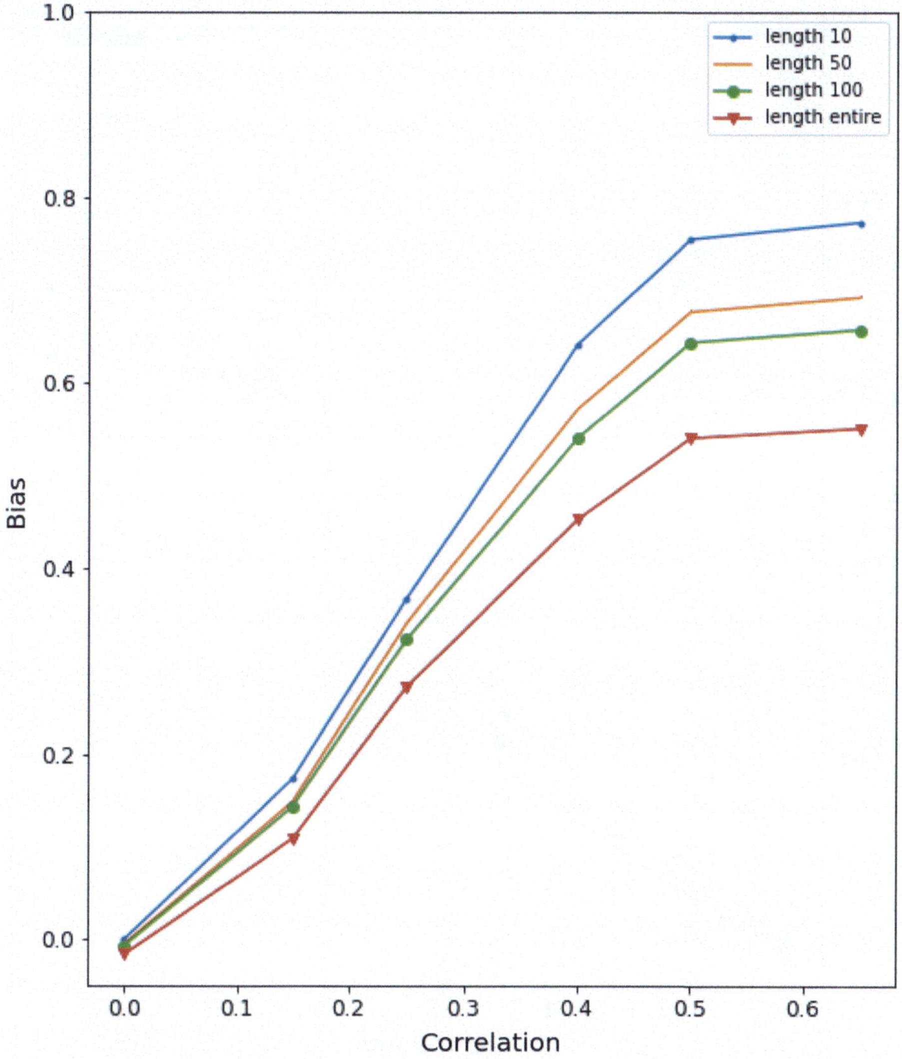

Fig. 5 Empirical Non-negative Matrix Factorization Local Bias versus degree-node correlation. Bias refers to the measurement of Local Bias described in [1]. Increasing correlation increases the probability higher degree nodes have the trait $X = 1$

3. "Backend" model serves possible tweets to user i if appropriate
4. User i likes tweet from another user with same label with probability 0.20, probability 0.05 otherwise

We run the agent-based models based on network connection data from RQ3 and Alipourfard et al. [1], with approximately 5600 users interacting with a recommender system that is exposing them to a subgraph of their network through ranked ordered feeds for at leat 24 timesteps. We present preliminary results in

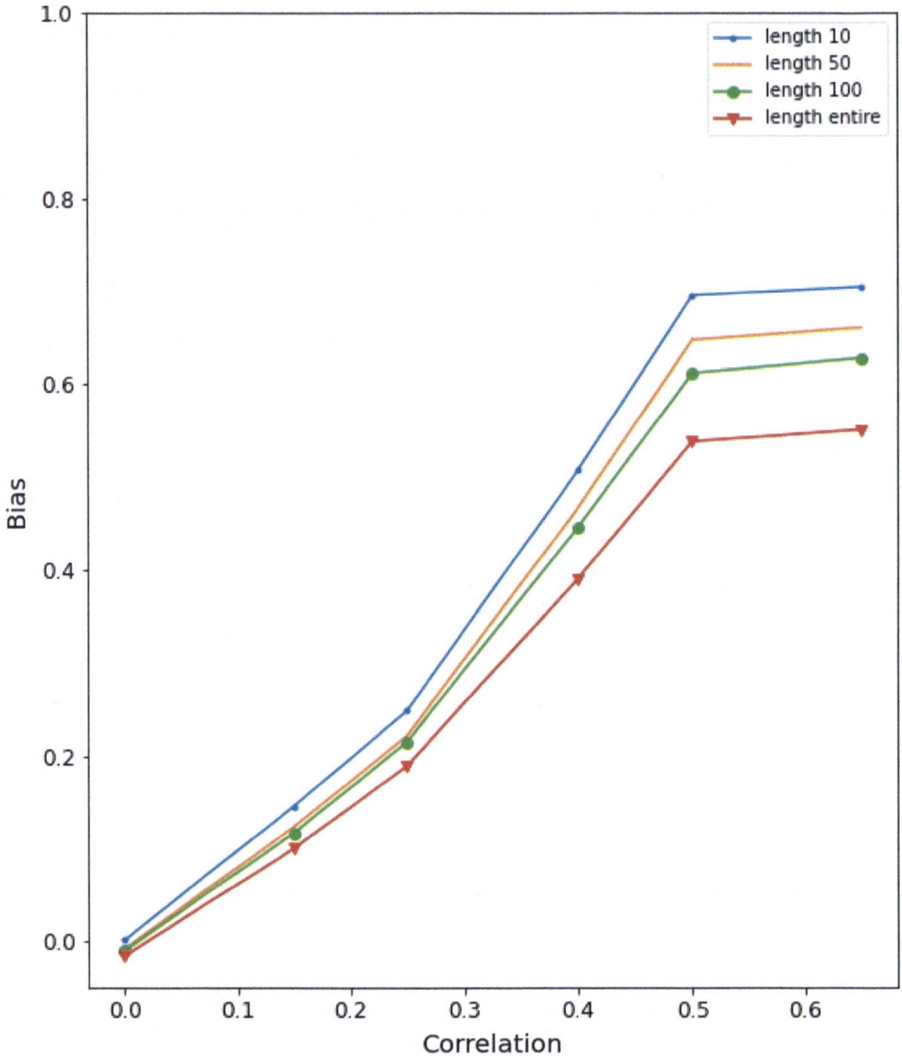

Fig. 6 Empirical Neural Collaborative Filtering (NCF) Local Bias versus degree-node correlation. Bias refers to the measurement of Local Bias described in [1]. Increasing correlation increases the probability higher degree nodes have the trait $X = 1$

Fig. 9. We observe relatively low local bias across all models, but in particular we observe that the recommender system based feeds consistently under-reports the active trait X, even as the prevalence of the binary trait goes up, whereas the rest of the conditions experience varying levels of low bias. Interestingly, the greedy algorithmic approach MinimizeRho seems to correlate strongly with the random feed, minimizing the absolute value of the local bias measure relative to the other models.

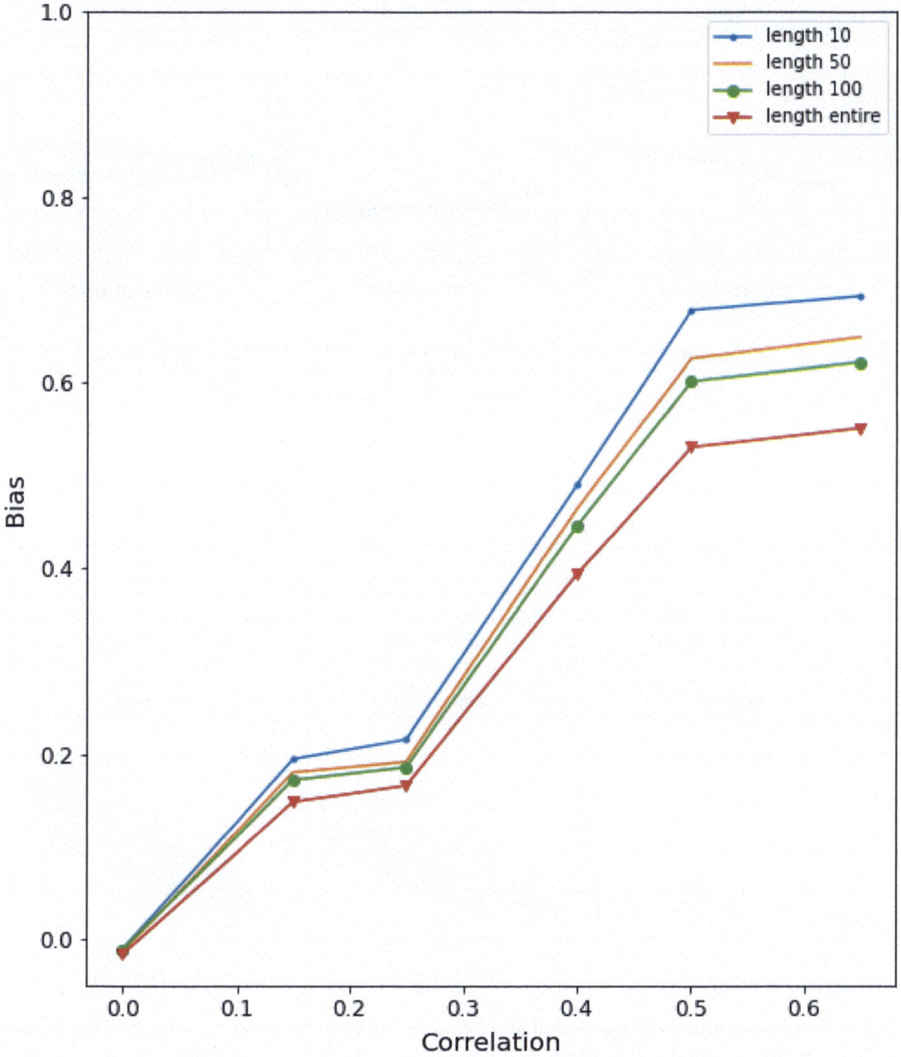

Fig. 7 Empirical Wide & Deep Local Bias versus degree-node correlation. Bias refers to the measurement of Local Bias described in [1]. Increasing correlation increases the probability higher degree nodes have the trait $X = 1$

7 Conclusion

In this study, we investigate the phenomenon of exposure bias in social networks through four main research questions.

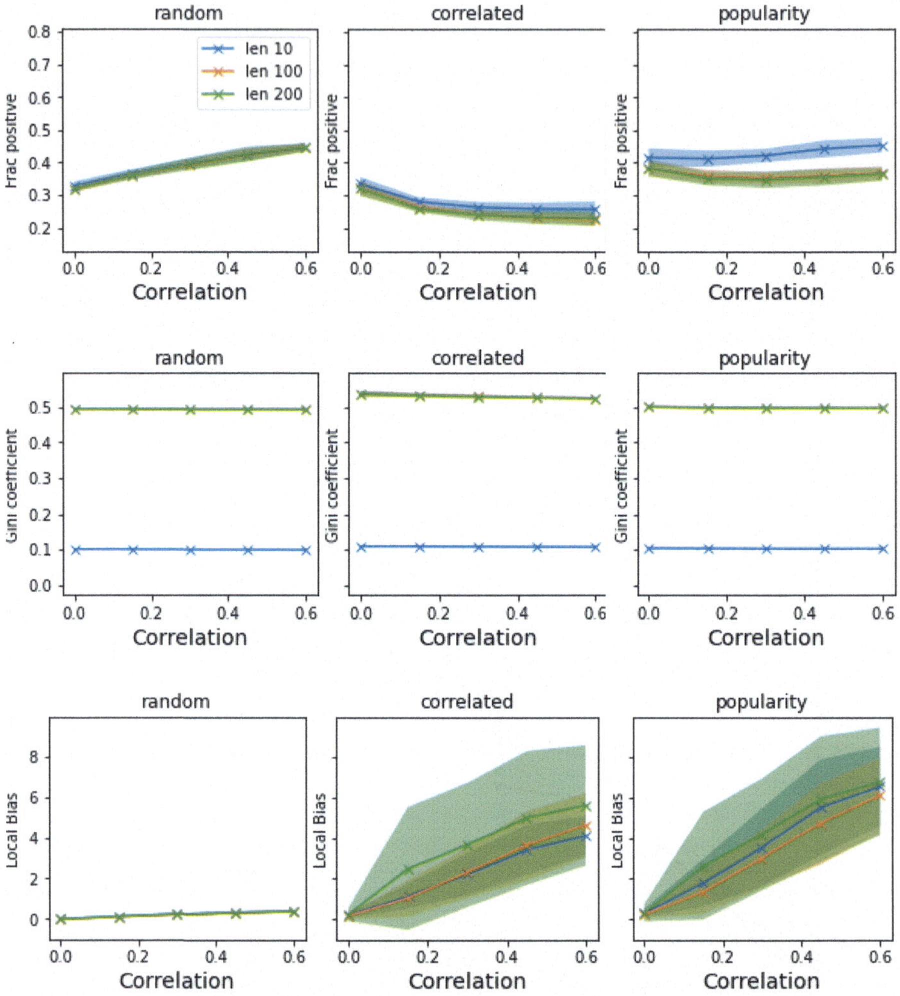

Fig. 8 **Power-law simulations**. Plotted are the mean values of each metric, with bars being one standard deviation. We plot F_{ti} and not F_{ui} as they reported nearly identical data

7.1 Addressing Research Questions

RQ1 Can we observe exposure bias in empirical online social networks like Twitter?

Our empirical audits, utilizing both initial and expanded sock-puppet studies, strongly suggest the presence of exposure bias in Twitter. We observed that personalized feeds, compared to reverse chronological feeds, significantly skew the visibility of content. This indicates that the algorithmic curation of content

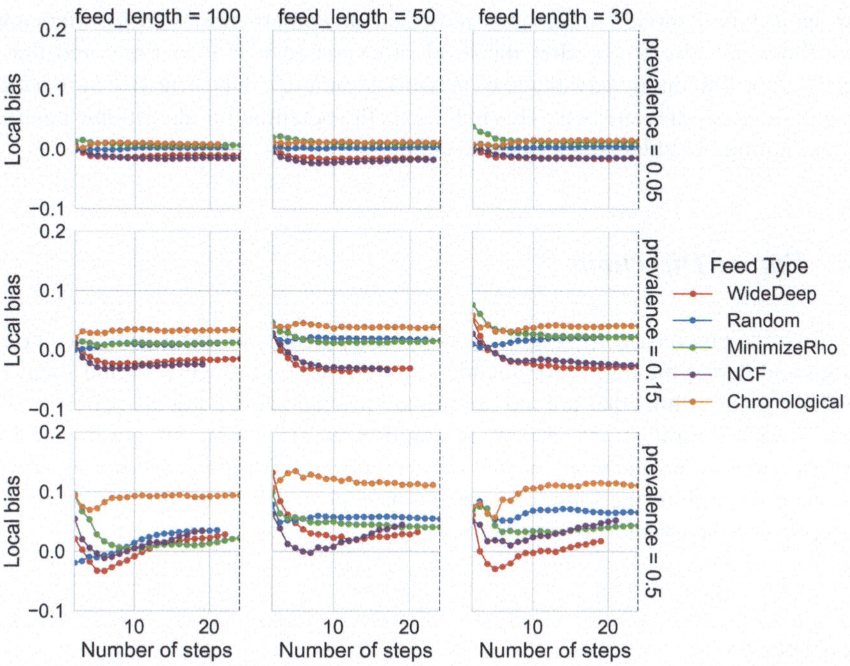

Fig. 9 Agent-based model simulation of approx. 5600 users and a sample of their friends. Bias refers to the measurement of Local Bias described in [1]

(and therefore of users) can indeed create an echo-chamber effect, where users are exposed to a narrower range of perspectives.

RQ2 Do different feed recommendation algorithms affect exposure bias?

Our simulations and analysis of empirical data demonstrated that different recommendation algorithms have varying impacts on exposure bias. Logistic regression-based feeds exhibited the highest levels of bias, followed by NCF, reverse chronological, non-negative matrix factorization, Wide & Deep, and popularity-based feeds. This finding indicates the role recommendation algorithms can have in reacting to users and shaping their experience of their network.

RQ3 Do different session lengths affect the level of exposure bias?

We found that session length plays a statistically significant role in the level of exposure bias experienced by users. Longer sessions generally resulted in reduced bias, as users were able to encounter a more diverse set of content. This suggests that session length can act as a mitigating factor against the narrowing effects of personalized feeds.

RQ4 Do interventions in recommender algorithms change the level of exposure bias over time in a simulated online social network?

Our agent-based model simulations indicated that interventions in recommender algorithms can effectively alter the level of exposure bias over time, and that a greedy algorithm taking advantage of network structure can be effective at reducing our measures of exposure bias. This highlights the potential for algorithmic changes for facilitating healthier online discourse.

7.2 Future Directions

Our findings emphasize the importance of transparency and accountability in the design and deployment of recommendation systems. Future work should focus on developing algorithms that not only optimize for engagement but also consider the broader social implications of content curation, namely *who* you get exposed to as a user and the implications of that on perception. Additionally, further research is needed to explore the long-term effects of exposure bias on user behavior and perception of their social environments.

References

1. Alipourfard N, Nettasinghe B, Abeliuk A, Krishnamurthy V, Lerman K (2020) Friendship paradox biases perceptions in directed networks. Nature communications 11(1):707
2. Angwin J, Larson J, Mattu S, Kirchner L (2016) Machine bias. In: Ethics of data and analytics, Auerbach Publications, pp 254–264
3. Bakshy E, Messing S, Adamic LA (2015) Exposure to ideologically diverse news and opinion on facebook. Science 348(6239):1130–1132
4. Bandy J, Diakopoulos N (2021) More accounts, fewer links: How algorithmic curation impacts media exposure in twitter timelines. Proceedings of the ACM on Human-Computer Interaction 5(CSCW1):1–28
5. Bartley BK N, Lerman K (2024) Auditing exposure bias on social media for a healthier online discourse. In: Workshop Proceedings of the 18th International AAAI Conference on Web and Social Media
6. Bartley N, Abeliuk A, Ferrara E, Lerman K (2021) Auditing algorithmic bias on twitter. In: 13th ACM Web Science Conference 2021, pp 65–73
7. Bartley N, Burghardt K, Lerman K (2023) Evaluating content exposure bias in social networks. In: Proceedings of the International Conference on Advances in Social Networks Analysis and Mining, pp 379–383
8. Beattie L, Taber D, Cramer H (2022) Challenges in translating research to practice for evaluating fairness and bias in recommendation systems. In: Proceedings of the 16th ACM Conference on Recommender Systems, pp 528–530
9. Centola D (2010) The spread of behavior in an online social network experiment. science 329(5996):1194–1197
10. Chen W, Pacheco D, Yang KC, Menczer F (2020) Neutral bots reveal political bias on social media. arXiv preprint arXiv:200508141
11. Cheng HT, Koc L, Harmsen J, Shaked T, Chandra T, Aradhye H, Anderson G, Corrado G, Chai W, Ispir M, et al. (2016) Wide & deep learning for recommender systems. In: Proceedings of the 1st workshop on deep learning for recommender systems, pp 7–10

12. Donkers T, Ziegler J (2023) De-sounding echo chambers: Simulation-based analysis of polarization dynamics in social networks. Online Social Networks and Media 37:100275
13. El-Kishky A, Markovich T, Park S, Verma C, Kim B, Eskander R, Malkov Y, Portman F, Samaniego S, Xiao Y, et al. (2022) Twhin: Embedding the twitter heterogeneous information network for personalized recommendation. In: Proceedings of the 28th ACM SIGKDD Conference on Knowledge Discovery and Data Mining, pp 2842–2850
14. Galesic M, Olsson H, Rieskamp J (2012) Social sampling explains apparent biases in judgments of social environments. Psychological Science 23(12):1515–1523
15. Galesic M, Bruine de Bruin W, Dumas M, Kapteyn A, Darling J, Meijer E (2018) Asking about social circles improves election predictions. Nature Human Behaviour 2(3):187–193
16. Galesic M, Bruine de Bruin W, Dalege J, Feld SL, Kreuter F, Olsson H, Prelec D, Stein DL, van Der Does T (2021) Human social sensing is an untapped resource for computational social science. Nature 595(7866):214–222
17. González-Bailón S, Lazer D, Barberá P, Zhang M, Allcott H, Brown T, Crespo-Tenorio A, Freelon D, Gentzkow M, Guess AM, et al. (2023) Asymmetric ideological segregation in exposure to political news on facebook. Science 381(6656):392–398
18. Grandi U, Kanesh L, Lisowski G, Ramanujan M, Turrini P (2023) Identifying and eliminating majority illusion in social networks
19. Granovetter MS (1973) The strength of weak ties. American journal of sociology 78(6):1360–1380
20. Guess AM, Malhotra N, Pan J, Barberá P, Allcott H, Brown T, Crespo-Tenorio A, Dimmery D, Freelon D, Gentzkow M, et al. (2023) Reshares on social media amplify political news but do not detectably affect beliefs or opinions. Science 381(6656):404–408
21. Gupta S, Wang H, Lipton Z, Wang Y (2021) Correcting exposure bias for link recommendation. In: International Conference on Machine Learning, PMLR, pp 3953–3963
22. He X, Liao L, Zhang H, Nie L, Hu X, Chua TS (2017) Neural collaborative filtering. In: Proceedings of the 26th international conference on world wide web, pp 173–182
23. Hodas NO, Lerman K (2014) The simple rules of social contagion. Scientific reports 4(1):4343
24. Huszár F, Ktena SI, O'Brien C, Belli L, Schlaikjer A, Hardt M (2022) Algorithmic amplification of politics on twitter. Proceedings of the National Academy of Sciences 119(1):e2025334119
25. Juneja P, Mitra T (2021) Auditing e-commerce platforms for algorithmically curated vaccine misinformation. In: Proceedings of the 2021 chi conference on human factors in computing systems, pp 1–27
26. Kardosh R, Sklar AY, Goldstein A, Pertzov Y, Hassin RR (2022) Minority salience and the overestimation of individuals from minority groups in perception and memory. Proceedings of the National Academy of Sciences 119(12):e2116884119
27. Kumar V, Krackhardt D, Feld S (2018) Network interventions based on inversity: Leveraging the friendship paradox in unknown network structures. Yale University, Tech
28. Lazovich T, Belli L, Gonzales A, Bower A, Tantipongpipat U, Lum K, Huszar F, Chowdhury R (2022) Measuring disparate outcomes of content recommendation algorithms with distributional inequality metrics. Patterns 3(8):100568
29. Lee E, Karimi F, Wagner C, Jo HH, Strohmaier M, Galesic M (2019) Homophily and minority-group size explain perception biases in social networks. Nature human behaviour 3(10):1078–1087
30. Los M, Christoff Z, Grossi D (2023) On the graph theory of majority illusions. arXiv preprint arXiv:230402258
31. Mønsted B, Sapieżyński P, Ferrara E, Lehmann S (2017) Evidence of complex contagion of information in social media: An experiment using twitter bots. PloS one 12(9):e0184148
32. Nikolov D, Flammini A, Menczer F (2021) Right and left, partisanship predicts (asymmetric) vulnerability to misinformation. Harvard Kennedy School (HKS) Misinformation Review
33. Panagiotopoulos P, Barnett J, Bigdeli AZ, Sams S (2016) Social media in emergency management: Twitter as a tool for communicating risks to the public. Technological Forecasting and Social Change 111:86–96

34. Ramaciotti Morales P, Cointet JP (2021) Auditing the effect of social network recommendations on polarization in geometrical ideological spaces. In: Proceedings of the 15th ACM Conference on Recommender Systems, pp 627–632
35. Ribeiro MH, Ottoni R, West R, Almeida VA, Meira Jr W (2020) Auditing radicalization pathways on youtube. In: Proceedings of the 2020 conference on fairness, accountability, and transparency, pp 131–141
36. Rodriguez MG, Gummadi K, Schoelkopf B (2014) Quantifying information overload in social media and its impact on social contagions. In: Proceedings of the international AAAI conference on web and social media, vol 8, pp 170–179
37. Rogers EM (2010) Diffusion of innovations. Simon and Schuster
38. Sandvig C, Hamilton K, Karahalios K, Langbort C (2014) Auditing algorithms: Research methods for detecting discrimination on internet platforms. Data and discrimination: converting critical concerns into productive inquiry 22(2014):4349–4357
39. Sapiezynski P, Zeng W, E Robertson R, Mislove A, Wilson C (2019) Quantifying the impact of user attentionon fair group representation in ranked lists. In: Companion proceedings of the 2019 world wide web conference, pp 553–562
40. Stoica AA, Litvak N, Chaintreau A (2024) Fairness rising from the ranks: Hits and pagerank on homophilic networks. arXiv preprint arXiv:240213787
41. Tomlein M, Pecher B, Simko J, Srba I, Moro R, Stefancova E, Kompan M, Hrckova A, Podrouzek J, Bielikova M (2021) An audit of misinformation filter bubbles on youtube: Bubble bursting and recent behavior changes. In: Proceedings of the 15th ACM Conference on Recommender Systems, pp 1–11
42. Yan S, Altenburger KM, Wang YC, Cheng J (2022) What does perception bias on social networks tell us about friend count satisfaction? In: Proceedings of the ACM Web Conference 2022, pp 2687–2695

The manufacturer's authorised representative in the EU is Springer Nature Customer Service Centre GmbH, Europaplatz 3, 69115 Heidelberg, Germany. If you have any concerns regarding our products, please contact ProductSafety@springernature.com

Printed and bound by CPI Group (UK) Ltd, Croydon, CR0 4YY
01/10/2026
02225910-0013